Biomarkers in Urology

Editor

ADAM S. FELDMAN

UROLOGIC CLINICS
OF NORTH AMERICA

www.urologic.theclinics.com

Consulting Editor
KEVIN R. LOUGHLIN

February 2023 • Volume 50 • Number 1

ELSEVIER

1600 John F. Kennedy Boulevard • Suite 1800 • Philadelphia, Pennsylvania, 19103-2899

http://www.theclinics.com

UROLOGIC CLINICS OF NORTH AMERICA Volume 50, Number 1
February 2023 ISSN 0094-0143, ISBN-13: 978-0-323-94019-1

Editor: Kerry Holland
Developmental Editor: Diana Ang

Urologic Clinics of North America (ISSN 0094-0143) is published quarterly by Elsevier Inc., 360 Park Avenue South, New York, NY 10010-1710. Months of issue are February, May, August, and November. Business and Editorial Offices: 1600 John F. Kennedy Blvd., Suite 1800, Philadelphia, PA 19103-2899. Periodicals postage paid at New York, NY and additional mailing offices. Subscription prices are $415.00 per year (US individuals), $832.00 per year (US institutions), $100.00 per year (US students and residents), $473.00 per year (Canadian individuals), $1040.00 per year (Canadian institutions), $100.00 per year (Canadian students/residents), $546.00 per year (foreign individuals), $1040.00 per year (foreign institutions), and $240.00 per year (foreign students/residents). Foreign air speed delivery is included in all *Clinics* subscription prices. All prices are subject to change without notice. **POSTMASTER:** Send address changes to *Urologic Clinics of North America*, Elsevier Health Sciences Division, Subscription Customer Service, 3251 Riverport Lane, Maryland Heights, MO 63043. **Customer Service: 1-800-654-2452 (US). From outside the United States, call 1-314-447-8871. Fax: 1-314-447-8029. E-mail: JournalsCustomerServiceusa@elsevier.com (for print support)** and **JournalsOnlineSupport-usa@elsevier.com (for online support)**.

Reprints. For copies of 100 or more, of articles in this publication, please contact the Commercial Reprints Department, Elsevier Inc., 360 Park Avenue South, New York, New York 10010-1710. Tel.: 212-633-3874; Fax: 212-633-3820; E-mail: reprints@elsevier.com.

Urologic Clinics of North America is covered in MEDLINE/PubMed (*Index Medicus*), *Excerpta Medica, Current Contents/Clinical Medicine, Science Citation Index,* and *ISI/BIOMED.*

Contributors

CONSULTING EDITOR

KEVIN R. LOUGHLIN, MD, MBA
Emeritus Professor of Surgery (Urology),
Harvard Medical School, Visiting Scientist,
Vascular Biology Research Program at Boston
Children's Hospital, Boston, Massachusetts,
USA

EDITOR

ADAM S. FELDMAN, MD, MPH
Co-Director, The Combined Harvard Medical
School Urologic Oncology Fellowship
Program, Director of Urologic Research,
Urologic Oncology, Massachusetts General
Hospital, Assistant Professor of Surgery,
Harvard Medical School, Boston,
Massachusetts, USA

AUTHORS

BASHIR AL HUSSEIN AL AWAMLH, MD
Department of Urology, Vanderbilt University
Medical Center, Nashville, Tennessee, USA

FADY J. BAKY, MD
Department of Urology, The University of
Texas Southwestern Medical Center, Dallas,
Texas, USA

PETER C. BLACK, MD
Department of Urologic Sciences, University of
British Columbia, Vancouver, Canada

PERIS R. CASTAÑEDA, MD
Division of Urology, Department of Surgery,
Cedars-Sinai Medical Center, Los Angeles,
California, USA

LINA CALDERON, MD
Department of Urology, Weill Cornell Medicine,
New York, New York, USA

JACK G. CAMPBELL, MD
Division of Urology, Lahey Hospital and
Medical Center, Burlington, Massachusetts,
USA

JAD CHAHOUD, MD, MPH
Department of Genitourinary Oncology, H. Lee
Moffitt Cancer Center and Research Institute,
Tampa, Florida, USA

ALBERTO CONTRERAS-SANZ, PhD
Department of Urologic Sciences, University of
British Columbia, Vancouver, Canada

ANNA DORSTE, MLIS
Boston Children's Hospital, Boston,
Massachusetts, USA

JILLIAN EGAN, MD
Department of Urology, Massachusetts
General Hospital, Harvard Medical School,
Boston, Massachusetts, USA

BRIAN H. EISNER, MD
Department of Urology, Massachusetts
General Hospital, Harvard Medical School,
Boston, Massachusetts, USA

ESTHER FINNEY, MD
Boston Children's Hospital, Boston,
Massachusetts, USA

KHURSHID A. GURU, MD
Professor of Oncology, Chairman, Department
of Urology, Roswell Park Comprehensive
Cancer Center, New York, New York, USA

ARVIN HAJ-MIRZAIAN, MD
Department of Radiology, Nuclear Medicine
and Molecular Imaging, Postdoctoral Research
Fellow, Center for Precision Imaging, Athinoula
A. Martinos Center for Biomedical Imaging,
Massachusetts General Hospital, Boston,
Massachusetts, USA

A. ARI HAKIMI, MD
Department of Surgery, Urology Service,
Memorial Sloan Kettering Cancer Center, New
York, New York, USA

JOSHUA P. HAYDEN, MD
Division of Urology, Lahey Hospital and
Medical Center, Burlington, Massachusetts,
USA

PEDRAM HEIDARI, MD
Service Chief, Department of Radiology,
Nuclear Medicine and Molecular Imaging,
Associate Director, Center for Precision
Imaging, Athinoula A. Martinos Center for
Biomedical Imaging, Massachusetts General
Hospital, Assistant Professor of Radiology,
Harvard Medical School, Boston,
Massachusetts, USA

DAVID E. HINOJOSA-GONZALEZ, MD
Department of Urology, Massachusetts
General Hospital, Harvard Medical School,
Boston, Massachusetts, USA

AHMED A. HUSSEIN, MD, PhD
Assistant Professor of Oncology, Department
of Urology, Roswell Park Comprehensive
Cancer Center, New York, New York, USA

ANJALI JHA, MSC
Geisel School of Medicine at Dartmouth,
Hanover, New Hampshire, USA

SARI KHALEEL, MS, MD
Department of Surgery, Urology Service,
Memorial Sloan Kettering Cancer Center, New
York, New York, USA

JAYOUNG KIM, PhD
Division of Urology, Department of Surgery,
Division of Cancer Biology and Therapeutics,
Department of Surgery, Samuel Oschin
Comprehensive Cancer Institute, Cedars-Sinai
Medical Center, Los Angeles, California,
USA

RICHARD J. LEE, MD, PhD
Assistant Professor of Medicine, Harvard
Medical School, Massachusetts General
Hospital Cancer Center, Boston Children's
Hospital Boston, Massachusetts, USA

TED LEE, MD, MSC
Boston Children's Hospital, Boston,
Massachusetts, USA

YAIR LOTAN, MD
Department of Urology, The University of
Texas Southwestern Medical Center, Dallas,
Texas, USA

IKENNA MADUEKE, MD, PhD
Massachusetts General Hospital Cancer
Center, Harvard Medical School, Boston,
Massachusetts, USA

UMAR MAHMOOD, MD, PhD
Chief, Nuclear Medicine and Molecular
Imaging, Department of Radiology, Athinoula
A. Martinos Center for Biomedical Imaging,
Massachusetts General Hospital, Director,
Center for Precision Imaging, Professor of
Radiology, Harvard Medical School, Boston,
Massachusetts, USA

JOHN M. MASTERSON, MD
Division of Urology, Department of Surgery,
Cedars-Sinai Medical Center, Los Angeles,
California, USA

DAVID T. MIYAMOTO, MD, PhD
Assistant Professor of Radiation Oncology,
Harvard Medical School, Investigator, Mass
General Center for Cancer Research,
Associate Member, Broad Institute of Harvard
and MIT, Massachusetts General Hospital
Cancer Center, Boston, Massachusetts, USA

ANDREA NECCHI, MD
Department of Genitourinary Oncology, Vita-Salute San Raffaele University, Milan, Italy

STEPHEN REESE, MD
Department of Surgery, Urology Service, Memorial Sloan Kettering Cancer Center, New York, New York, USA

MORITZ J. REIKE, MD
Department of Urologic Sciences, University of British Columbia, Vancouver, British Columbia, Canada; Department of Urology, Marien Hospital Herne, Ruhr—University Bochum, Herne, Germany

KEYAN SALARI, MD, PhD
Department of Urology, Massachusetts General Hospital, Harvard Medical School, Center for Genitourinary Cancers, Massachusetts General Hospital Cancer Center, Boston, Massachusetts, USA

NATHAN L. SAMORA, MD
Department of Urology, Vanderbilt University Medical Center, Nashville, Tennessee, USA

GARY SMITH, PhD
Professor of Oncology, Department of Urology, Roswell Park Comprehensive Cancer Center, New York, New York, USA

PHILIPPE E. SPIESS, MD, MS, FRCS(C), FACS
Department of Genitourinary Oncology, H. Lee Moffitt Cancer Center and Research Institute, Tampa, Florida, USA

JEFFREY J. TOSOIAN, MD, MPH
Department of Urology, Vanderbilt University Medical Center, Vanderbilt Ingram Cancer Center, Nashville, Tennessee, USA

ALEX J. VANNI, MD
Division of Urology, Lahey Hospital and Medical Center, Burlington, Massachusetts, USA

ALICE YU, MD, MPH
Department of Genitourinary Oncology, H. Lee Moffitt Cancer Center and Research Institute, Tampa, Florida, USA

Contents

> A noninvasive test that can longitudinally assess renal parenchymal status would be incredibly valuable for a wide range of conditions, including neurogenic bladder, renal transplantation, and upper and lower urinary tract anomalies. To address this need, enormous amounts of time, effort, andd resources have been invested to identify biologic molecules that signal the pathologic processes of renal parenchymal defects. In this comprehensive narrative review, the authors summarize biomarkers that have previously been investigated while highlighting the key pitfalls and barriers that have impeded biomarker discovery and translation.

> A variety of biomarkers have been studied in the setting of conditions and scenarios related to kidney stone disease. These biomarkers are commonly serum markers, novel urinary proteins, and inflammatory whose use is aimed at providing clinicians with additional information of underlying processes and improving detection and stratification of patients with kidney stones, acute ureteral obstruction, stone passage, and related infectious complications. Their adoption has been limited, and further evidence is required to determine their role in the care of patients with stone disease.

> Increased understanding of molecular pathophysiology has led to the detection of clinically applicable biomarkers across medicine, which allow for minimally invasive detection, management, and monitoring of disease processes. Although biomarkers have traditionally played a more significant role in malignancy, these goals also pertain to benign disease. Herein, the authors review ongoing research into biomarker investigation and application in urethral stricture disease, benign prostatic hyperplasia, bladder outlet obstruction, and overactive bladder. No biomarkers for these entities are currently in clinical use; however, numerous physiologic pathways provide targets for current and future study.

We performed a narrative review of studies that produced clinically applicable data by examining the combined use of at least one biomarker test and multiparametric MRI to predict GG $\geq$2 prostate cancer on biopsy and by reporting the resultant clinical outcomes (i.e, the proportion of biopsies avoided and GG $\geq$2 cancers missed) following the application of various testing strategies incorporating these diagnostic tests.

Liquid biopsies such as circulating tumor cells (CTCs) and circulating tumor DNA (ctDNA) have great potential to serve as prognostic and predictive biomarkers in urologic cancers. The possibility of using liquid biopsies for real-time noninvasive and dynamic monitoring of response to therapy has been an active area of investigation. In this brief review, we outline the evidence for the potential clinical utility of CTC and ctDNA analyses in prostate, urothelial, and renal cancers.

Urologic malignancies constitute a large portion of annually diagnosed cancers. Timely diagnosis, accurate staging, and assessment of tumor heterogeneity are essential to devising the best treatment strategy for individual patients. The high sensitivity of molecular imaging allows for early and sensitive detection of lesions that were not readily detectable using conventional imaging techniques. Moreover, molecular imaging enables the interrogation of molecular processes used in targeted cancer therapies and predicts cancer response to treatment. Here we review the current advancements in molecular imaging of urologic cancers, including prostatic, vesical, renal testicular, and ureteral cancers.

Biomarkers play a key role in patients with testicular germ cell tumors in a variety of clinical contexts, including initial diagnosis, prognostication, monitoring treatment response, and posttreatment surveillance. Although the classic serum tumor markers for testicular germ cell tumors are essential for clinical management, the low sensitivity (particularly for seminoma and teratoma) and potential for false positives has spurred novel biomarker discovery and validation efforts. Here, we review the current state of serum-based biomarkers for testicular germ cell tumors, with a focus on the classic serum tumor markers and emerging class of microRNA markers.

Penile cancer is relatively rare in North America and Europe (<1% of all malignant neoplasms); however, it remains a significant health concern with a higher propensity of cases in many African, South American, and Asian countries. It occurs primarily in older men with a peak incidence in the 6th decade of life. The etiology of penile cancer is multifactorial and there are many risk factors including lack of neonatal circumcision, chronic inflammation, lichen sclerosis, tobacco use, obesity, poor hygiene, exposure to ultraviolet radiation, history of sexually transmitted diseases, and human papillomavirus (HPV) infection. Pathogenesis of penile squamous cell carcinoma (PSCC) can be broadly dichotomized into HPV related and non–HPV-related pathways which will be discussed in detail in this review.

Stephen Reese, Lina Calderon, Sari Khaleel, and A. Ari Hakimi

Renal cell carcinoma biomarkers include serum, urine, liquid, and tissue biomarkers. There is currently an ongoing search for predictive biomarkers in the detection, recurrence, and treatment of renal cell carcinoma. Emerging signatures in the transcriptomic and translational biomarker space seem promising, although additional work is needed to validate candidates in a larger and more generalizable patient population.

UROLOGIC CLINICS OF NORTH AMERICA

SERIES OF RELATED INTEREST
Surgical Clinics of North America
https://www.surgical.theclinics.com/

Foreword

The Continued Pursuit of Urologic Biomarkers: Beyond Prostate-Specific Antigen

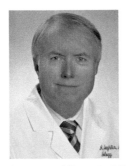

Kevin R. Loughlin, MD, MBA
Consulting Editor

Urologists have utilized biomarkers for almost the past century. Gutman and Gutman[1,2] discovered and reported on the utility of acid phosphatase in the 1930s. Prostate-specific antigen was identified in 1970,[3] and for the next several decades, prostate cancer received most of the attention of biomarker applications in urologic practice.[4]

However, in this century, there has been an explosion in the discovery, application, and interest in urologic biomarkers. In the last issue of the *Urologic Clinics* devoted to Biomarkers, which was published in 2016, we reported that a Medline search for the term "biomarker" revealed a growth of 116 citations in 2000 to 2988 in 2014.[5] That growth has continued unabated up to the present time.

Doctor Feldman has gathered recognized experts to contribute to this latest issue of Biomarkers. What is striking is that urologic biomarkers are no longer confined to prostate disease. This issue not only touches on biomarker applications to several urologic malignancies but also expands the applications to pediatric disease as well as to benign urologic conditions.

Urologic biomarkers have been expanded to aid in the diagnosis, prognosis, selection of therapy, and surveillance in a variety of urologic conditions. Urine, serum, tissue, and radiologic imaging are all current sources for biomarker development.

In addition, the application of molecular markers, some of which are reviewed in this issue, holds particular promise to practice "personalized" biomarkers in selected patients. The next decade holds great promise for even more applications of biomarkers in clinical practice, and this issue of the *Urologic Clinics* provides a state-of-the-art review of this topic.

Kevin R. Loughlin, MD, MBA
Vascular Biology Research Program at
Boston Children's Hospital
300 Longwood Avenue
Boston, MA 02115, USA

E-mail address:
kloughlin@partners.org

REFERENCES

1. Gutman EB, Sproul EE, Gutman AB. Significance of increased phosphatase activity of bone at the site

Urol Clin N Am 50 (2023) xiii–xiv
https://doi.org/10.1016/j.ucl.2022.10.002
0094-0143/23/© 2022 Published by Elsevier Inc.

of osteoblastic metastases secondary to carcinoma of the prostate gland. Am J Cancer 1936;28:485–95.

2. Gutman AB, Gutman EB. An 'acid' phosphatase occurring in the serum of patients with metastasizing carcinoma of the prostate gland. J Clin Invest 1938; 17:473–8.

3. Albin RJ, Soares WA, Bronson P, et al. Precipitating antigens of the normal human prostate. Reprod Fertil 1970;22:573–4.

4. Loughlin KR. PSA velocity: a systematic review of clinical applications. Urol Oncol 2014;32(8):1116–25.

5. Loughlin KR. Preface: biomarkers in urologic cancer. Urol Clin North Am 2016;43:xvii.

Preface
Progress and Promise of Biomarker Discovery and Development in Urologic Disease

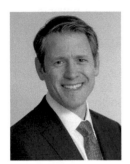

Adam S. Feldman, MD, MPH
Editor

Over the past several years, there has been an enormous amount of research in biomarkers in both benign and malignant urologic conditions. Scientific advances using a multitude of various -omics pathways, including genomics, transcriptomics, proteomics, metabolomics, radiomics, microbiomics, and other methods using olfaction-based research have afforded investigators with multiple new tools to interrogate blood, urine, seminal fluid, and tissue for promising novel biomarkers. Furthermore, the efficiency and cost associated with these analyses have dramatically improved, resulting in an ability to perform larger-scale investigations in a high-throughput manner. Other novel methodologies, including statistical improvements using artificial intelligence, have similarly created new opportunities for the development of clinically meaningful and accurate biomarkers.

Despite an enormous amount of research effort and expenditure, many potential biomarkers have failed to successfully make the leap from bench to bedside, and for those which have become commercially available, understanding their value, cost effectiveness, and how to use them can be challenging for the clinical urologist. This issue of *Urologic Clinics* is dedicated to the practicing urologist to understand what has been the latest research in biomarkers in urology, but also and perhaps more importantly, which biomarkers can be clinically useful at this time.

Our initial article in this issue introduces the various scientific approaches to biomarker discovery and addresses some of the methodologic challenges, using biomarker investigation in pediatric urology as an example. Although the majority of biomarker research in urology has been focused on the genitourinary cancers, there has been significant interest in biomarker development to assist in the management of benign urologic conditions. Biomarkers to determine nephrolithiasis risk, development, and recurrence has become a major area of investigation with significant clinical implications. An understanding of the biologic basis of the pathophysiology of urethral stricture disease can allow us to utilize biologic indicators for improved management of our patients. Similarly, research into the biologic underpinnings of interstitial cystitis may allow us to better characterize and personalize the management of this disease.

Urologic oncology has seen an explosion in biomarker research. Many have investigated biomarkers in both non-muscle-invasive bladder cancer and muscle-invasive disease, improving our understanding of the biology of cancer and attempting to better detect new and recurrent disease, as well as improve patient selection for various treatments options.

Urol Clin N Am 50 (2023) xv–xvi
https://doi.org/10.1016/j.ucl.2022.10.001
0094-0143/23/© 2022 Published by Elsevier Inc.

While prostate-specific antigen (PSA) is one of the best known and investigated biomarkers in all of medicine, an enormous amount of time and money have been spent in an effort to surpass PSA and improve our detection and management of prostate cancer. A PubMed search of "biomarkers AND prostate cancer" results in 43,798 hits for articles, indicating the vast volume and breadth of research in this field. In addition to the classic approach to measurable biomarkers in body fluids and tissues, the use of imaging as a biomarker has exploded in prostate cancer in the form of multiparametric MRI and even more recently targeted molecular imaging using prostate cancer–specific biomarkers.

Testicular cancer, penile cancer, and kidney cancer have had less of a revolution in biomarker discovery than the other urologic malignancies. However, significant improvements in the biologic understanding of these disease processes have led to improvements in biomarker assessment, which, similar to other disease states, have resulted in advances in patient care.

Although it is impossible to cover every aspect and all novel research on biomarkers in all areas of urology, we hope that this issue of *Urologic Clinics* will shed some light on the progress and promise of biomarkers in our field and how we might use them now and in the future to improve the care and management of our patients.

Adam S. Feldman, MD, MPH
Department of Urology
Massachusetts General Hospital
55 Fruit St. GRB 1100
Boston, MA 02114, USA

E-mail address:
afeldman@mgh.harvard.edu

Approaches and Barriers to Biomarker Discovery
The Example of Biomarkers of Renal Scarring in Pediatric Urology

Ted Lee, MD, MSc[a],*, Esther Finney, MD[a], Anjali Jha, MSc[b], Anna Dorste, MLIS[a], Richard Lee, MD[a]

KEYWORDS

- Biomarker • Renal scarring • Renal parenchymal defects

KEY POINTS

- Biomarker for renal scarring and renal parenchymal defects.

Renal preservation is the pillar of pediatric urology. Early detection of renal parenchymal defects or "renal scarring" among children with urinary anomalies allows identification of those who stand to gain the most from early intervention. A noninvasive test that can longitudinally assess renal parenchymal status would be incredibly valuable for a wide range of conditions, including neurogenic bladder, renal transplantation, and upper and lower urinary tract anomalies. To address this need, enormous amounts of time, effort, and resources have been invested to identify biologic molecules that signal the pathologic processes of renal parenchymal defects. In this comprehensive narrative review, the authors summarize biomarkers that have previously been investigated while highlighting the key pitfalls and barriers that have impeded biomarker discovery and translation.

INTRODUCTION

Renal preservation is the pillar of pediatric urology. Early detection of renal parenchymal defects or "renal scarring" among children with urinary anomalies allows identification of those who stand to gain the most from early intervention. Decision making is guided by renal parenchymal status, as opposed to estimated glomerular filtration rates, because the opportunity for maximal renal preservation may have passed by the time decline in renal function is detected. The "ship has sailed," so to speak.

The current gold standard for evaluating renal parenchymal defects is ^{99m}Tc-labeled dimercaptosuccinic acid (DMSA) scintigraphy.[1] However, DMSA studies are not used for longitudinal monitoring due to ionizing radiation exposure. For reference, radiation exposure from a single DMSA is 5- to 10-fold greater than exposure from voiding cystourethrography.[2–4] Furthermore, limited availability of DMSA has resulted in significant problems with access and prohibitive costs within the United States.[5,6]

A noninvasive test that can longitudinally assess renal parenchymal status would be incredibly valuable for a wide range of conditions, including neurogenic bladder, renal transplantation, and upper and lower urinary tract anomalies. To address this need, enormous amounts of time, effort, and resources have been invested to identify biologic molecules that signal the pathologic processes of renal parenchymal defects.

In this comprehensive narrative review, the authors summarize biomarkers that have previously been investigated while highlighting the key pitfalls

[a] Boston Children's Hospital, 300 Longwood Avenue, Hunnewell 350, Boston, MA 02115, USA; [b] Geisel School of Medicine at Dartmouth, Hanover, NH, USA

* Corresponding author.

E-mail address: ted.lee@childrens.harvard.edu

Urol Clin N Am 50 (2023) 1–17
https://doi.org/10.1016/j.ucl.2022.09.005
0094-0143/23/Published by Elsevier Inc.

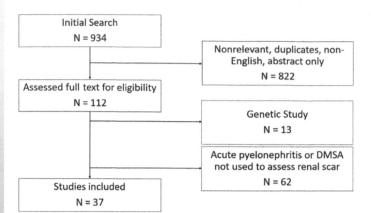

Fig. 1. Flow diagram of study selection.

and barriers that may impede biomarker discovery and translation.

Materials and Methods

Studies for this comprehensive narrative review were extracted from PubMed and Embase using the search run by a medical librarian (A.D.). Strategies were identical except for the translation of syntax between the 2 databases. Controlled vocabulary terms from each database (Medical Subject Headings and Emtree terms, respectively) and associated keywords for each concept were combined logically using Boolean operators. Concepts included terms relating to biomarkers, urinary tract infections, and renal scarring. Biomarker terms consisted not only of plurals and alternate spellings (ie, bio-markers) but also synonyms (ie, "clinical markers," "biochemical markers") and terms that qualify as biomarkers (ie, "serum albumin," "factor IV"). These terms and the associated controlled vocabulary terms were combined using OR; these pieces were layered over the other 2 concepts, which were built similarly, using AND. The results from each database were combined and deduplicated in EndNote using the validated deduplication process described by Bramer and colleagues.[7] Results (934 unique citations) were then sent to the authors T.L. and A.J. for review.

All abstracts were reviewed independently by authors T.L. and A.J. using predetermined criteria. Discrepancies were rereviewed until consensus was reached. After elimination of 822 nonrelevant, duplicate, non-English, or abstract-only articles, 112 abstracts were reviewed. The authors applied stringent criteria to only include studies that assessed outcome of parenchymal defects using delayed DMSA, defined as at least 4 months from time of urinary tract infection, to exclude outcomes capturing parenchymal defects secondary to acute pyelonephritis. Articles pertaining to genetic susceptibility to renal scarring were removed because understanding polymorphisms associated with renal scarring risk is a separate topic for discussion.[8] A narrative review format was used to summarize literature for all biological agents studied for association with renal parenchymal defects.

RESULTS

A total of 37 studies that met the inclusion criteria were identified. Flow diagram of study selection can be referenced in **Fig. 1**. Forty-four different markers were included within the studies. Details regarding sample collection method, timing of sample collection, study design, sample size, and performance characteristics, if available, are included in **Table 1**. A brief description of each biomarker is included in **Table 2**.

DISCUSSION

Despite a myriad of studies testing numerous biomarkers in both plasma and urine over the past 3 decades, the authors' review suggests that stand-alone candidate biomarkers that are worthy of further investigation have not yet surfaced. We are still in the discovery or "qualification" phase of identifying a highly sensitive and highly specific biomarker for renal parenchymal defects.

Challenges in biomarker discovery and translation are universal across all disciplines. Several authorities have published recommendations, short proposals, and information about experimental design requirements and performance characteristics necessary for a biomarker to be successfully translated into practice.[56,57] The following discussion summarizes and highlights key pitfalls and barriers to biomarker discovery and translation, with the hopes of facilitating biomarker research and development within the field of biomarker discovery.

Table 1
Details regarding sample collection method, timing of sample collection, study design, sample size, and biomarker performance characteristics

Biomarker	Study Title	Timing	Urine Collection Method	Adjusted for Concentration	DMSA Obtained Time Period	Significant Difference	Analysis Method	Study Design	Treatment Arm	Control Arm	Threshold Level	Sensitivity	Specificity	PPV	NPV	AUC
IL-6 urine																
	Renata et al,[9] 2013	Acute before antibiotics	Variable (SP aspiration, catheterization, or midstream)	No	6 mo	No	Univariate	Case control	5	26	-	D -	-	-	-	-
	Tramma et al,[10] 2012	6 mo after UTI	Not specified	Yes	6 mo	No	Univariate	Case control	33	17	-	-	-	-	-	-
	Tullus et al,[11] 1994	Within 10 d	Not specified	Yes	10 d (early); 1 y (late)	Yes	Univariate	Case control	27	12	Not specified	-	-	-	-	-
	Sheu et al,[12] 2009	Acute	Not specified	Yes	7 d (early); 6 mo (late)	Yes	Multivariate	Case control	45	15	1000 pg/mg	47%	90%	70%	76%	-
	Gokce et al,[13] 2010	At least 3 wk after UTI	Midstream or bagged	Yes	3–6 mo after UTI, 6 mo before urine specimen	No	Univariate	Case control	60	54	-	-	-	-	-	-
IL-8 urine																
	Renata et al,[9] 2013	Acute before antibiotics	Variable (SP aspiration, catheterization, or midstream)	No	6 mo	Yes	Univariate	Case control	5	26	Not specified	-	-	-	-	-
	Tramma et al,[10] 2012	6 mo following UTI	Not specified	Yes	6 mo	No	Univariate	Case control	33	17	-	-	-	-	-	-
	Tullus et al,[11] 1994	Within 10 d	Not specified	Yes	10 d (early); 1 y (late)	Yes	Univariate	Case control	27	12	Not specified	-	-	-	-	-
	Gokce et al,[13] 2010	At least 3 wk after UTI	Midstream or bagged	Yes	3–6 mo after UTI, 6 mo before urine specimen	Yes	Univariate	Case control	60	54	10.69 pg/mg	85%	44%	-	-	0.67
	Sheu et al,[14] 2009	Acute before antibiotics	Not specified	Yes	7 d (early); 6 mo (late)	Yes	Multivariate	Case control	26	41	4000 pg/mg	77%	90%	83%	86%	0.788,
IL-18 urine																
	Yavuz et al,[15] 2013	At least 3 wk after UTI	Not specified	-	6 mo	No	Univariate	Case control	57	36	-	-	-	-	-	-
Serum CRP																

(continued on next page)

Table 1
(continued)

Biomarker	Study Title	Timing	Urine Collection Method	Adjusted for Concentration	DMSA Obtained Time Period	Significant Difference	Analysis Method	Study Design	Treatment Arm	Control Arm	Threshold Level	Sensitivity	Specificity	PPV	NPV	AUC
	Renata et al,[9] 2013	Acute before antibiotics	-	-	6 mo	No	Univariate	Case control	5	26	-	-	-	-	-	-
	Leroy et al,[16] 2013	Not specified	-	-	7 d (early), 3–24 mo (late)	Yes	Multivariate	Systematic review/meta-analysis	-	-	30 mg/L	0.74	0.54	0.72	0.56	-
	Prat et al,[17] 2003	Acute before antibiotics	-	-	5–6 mo	Yes	Univariate	Case control	77	38	20 mg/_	92%	34%	23%	95%	0.72
	Bellhadj-Tahar et al,[18] 2008	Acute	-	-	7 d (early); 9 mo (late)	No	Univariate	Case control	107	29	-	-	-	-	-	0.624
	Bresse et al,[19] 2009	Acute	-	-	7 d (early) 12 mo (late)	No	Univariate	Case control	-	-	-	-	-	-	-	-
	Sheu et al,[20] 2011	Acute before antibiotics, 3 d after antibiotics	-	-	3 d (early); 6 mo (late)	No	Multivariate	Case control	34	48	-	-	-	-	-	-
	Karavanaki et al,[21] 2019	Acute before antibiotics, 2 d after antibiotics	-	-	6 mo	Yes	Multivariate	Case control	34	114	Not specified	-	-	-	-	-
	Karavanaki et al,[22] 2017	Acute before antibiotics, 2 d after antibiotics	-	-	10 d (early); 6 mo (late)	No	Multivariate	Case control	34	88	-	-	-	-	-	-
	Jakobsson et al,[23] 1994	Acute, not specified	-	-	Acute; 2 mo; 2 y (late)	No	Univariate	Case control	28	31	-	-	-	-	-	-
	Byun et al,[24] 2016	Acute before antibiotics	-	-	6 mo	No	Multivariate	Case control	25	47	-	-	-	-	-	-
	Rodriguez et al,[25] 2013	Acute	-	-	Early; 6–8 mo (late)	Yes	Univariate	Case control	8	10	115 mg/L	62%	88%	62%	88%	0.70
	Stckland et al,[26] 1996	Acute	-	-	Acute; 1 y (late)	Yes	Multivariate	Case control	59	97	20 mg/L	92%	20%	41%	80%	-
	Wang et al,[27] 2005	Acute	-	-	7 d (early); 6 mo (late)	Yes	Univariate	Case control	32	33	70 mg/L	52%	82%	76%	60%	-

Study														
Swerkersson et al,[28] 2006	Acute	-	3 mo (early); 1–2 y (late)	Yes (girls only)	Multivariate	Case control	80	223	Not specified	-	-	-	-	-
Kotoula et al,[29] 2008	Acute before antibiotics	-	7 d (early); 6 mo (late)	Yes	Univariate	Case control	27	30	66 mg/L	74%	100%	100%	81%	0.957
Yilmaz et al,[30] 2018	Acute	-	6 mo	Yes	Univariate	Case control	19	57	Not specified	-	-	-	-	-
Serum WBC														
Renata et al,[9] 2013	Acute before antibiotics	-	6 mo	No	Univariate	Case control	5	26	-	-	-	-	-	-
Leroy et al,[16] 2013	Not specified	-	7 d (early), 3–24 mo (late)	Yes	Multivariate	Systematic review/meta-analysis	-	-	15,000	0.68	0.51	0.33	0.82	-
Prat et al,[17] 2003	Acute before antibiotics	-	5–6 mo	No	Univariate	Case control	77	38						0.622
Bresse et al,[19] 2009	Acute	-	7 d (early); 12 mo (late)	No	Univariate	Case control	-	-						-
Sheu et al,[20] 2011	Acute before antibiotics, 3 d after antibiotics	-	3 d (early); 6 mo (late)	No	Multivariate	Case control	34	48						-
Jakobsson et al,[23] 1994	Acute, not specified	-	Acute; 2 mo; 2 y (late)	No	Univariate	Case control	28	31						-
Byun et al,[24] 2016	Acute before antibiotics	-	6 mo	No	Multivariate	Case control	25	47	-	-	-	-	-	-
Serum PCT														
Leroy et al,[16] 2013	Not specified	-	7 d (early), 3–24 mo (late)	Yes	Multivariate	Systematic review/meta-analysis	-	-	0.05 ng/mL	0.88	0.5	0.51	0.87	0.87
Prat et al,[17] 2003	Acute before antibiotics	-	5–6 mo	Yes	Univariate	Case control	77	38	1 ng/mL	92%	62%	32%	97%	0.83
Bellhadj-Tahar et al,[18] 2008	Acute	-	7 d (early); 9 mo (late)	Yes (early)	Univariate	Case control	107	29	Not specified	-	-	-	-	0.624
Bressan et al,[19] 2009	Acute	-	7 d (early); 12 mo (late)	Yes (late)	Univariate	Case control	52	20	1.0 ng/mL	79%	64%	-	-	0.74
Sheu et al,[20] 2011	Acute before antibiotics,	-	3 d (early); 6 mo (late)	Yes	Multivariate	Case control	34	48	3.5 ng/mL (acute)	94% (acute)	95% (acute)	95% (acute)	94% (acute); 66% (3 d)	0.942 (acute); 0.963 (3 d)

(continued on next page)

Table 1
(continued)

Biomarker	Study Title	Timing	Urine Collection Method	Adjusted for Concentration	DMSA Obtained Time Period	Significant Difference	Analysis Method	Study Design	Treatment Arm	Control Arm	Threshold Level	Sensitivity	Specificity	PPV	NPV	AUC
		3 d after antibiotics									1.0 ng/mL (3 c)	68% (3 d)	95% (3 d)	94% (3 d)	-	-
	Karavanaki et al,[22] 2017	Acute before antibiotics, 2 d after antibiotics	-	-	10 d (early); 6 mo (late)	No	Multivariate	Case control	34	88	-	-	-	-	-	-
	Liao et al,[31] 2014	Acute before antibiotics	-	-	3 d (early); 6 mo (late)	Yes	Multivariate	Case control	75	203	1.0 ng/mL	100%	57%	46%	100%	-
	Kotoula et al,[29] 2008	Acute before antibiotics	-	-	7 d (early); 6 mo (late)	Yes	Univariate	Case control	27	30	0.85 ng/mL	89%	97%	96%	91%	0.988
Serum ANC																
	Bresse et al,[19] 2009	Acute	-	-	7 d (early) 12 mo (late)	No	Univariate	Case control	-	-	-	-	-	-	-	-
	Karavanaki et al,[22] 2017	Acute before antibiotics, 2 d after antibiotics	-	-	10 d (early); 6 mo (late)	No	Multivariate	Case control	34	88	-	-	-	-	-	-
Serum ESR																
	Byun et al,[24] 2016	Acute before antibiotics	-	-	6 mo	No	Multivariate	Case control	25	47	-	-	-	-	-	-
	Kotoula et al,[29] 2008	Acute before antibiotics	-	-	7 d (early); 6 mo (late)	Yes	Univariate	Case control	27	30	25 mm/h	100%	75%	75%	100%	0.883
Serum vitamin A																
	Kavukcu et al,[32] 1998	Acute	-	-	6 mo	No	Univariate	Case control	23	91	-	-	-	-	-	-
Serum β-carotene																
	Kavukcu et al,[32] 1998	Acute	-	-	6 mo	No	Univariate	Case control	23	91	-	-	-	-	-	-
Serum ST2																
	Onta et al,[33] 2019	Acute	-	-	4 mo	Yes	Univariate	Case control	28	13	38.7 ng/mL	0.929	0.643	-	-	0.79
Serum IFN-γ																

Biomarker	Study														
	Ohta et al,[33] 2019	Acute	-	4 mo	No	Univariate	Case control	28	13	-	-	-	-	-	-
IL-2 serum	Ohta et al,[33] 2019	Acute	-	4 mo	No	Univariate	Case control	28	13	-	-	-	-	-	-
IL-4 serum	Ohta et al,[33] 2019	Acute	-	4 mo	No	Univariate	Case control	28	13	-	-	-	-	-	-
IL-6 serum	Ohta et al,[33] 2019	Acute	-	4 mo	No	Univariate	Case control	28	13	-	-	-	-	-	-
	Sheu et al,[12] 2009	Acute	Not specified	7 d (early); 6 mo (late)	Yes	Multivariate	Case control	45	15	120 pg/mL	33%	93%	71%	73%	-
	Rodriguez et al,[25] 2013	Acute	-	Early; 6–8 mo (late)	Yes	Univariate	Case control	8	10	20 pg/mL	50%	92%	67%	85%	0.75
IL-8 serum	Sheu et al,[14] 2009	Acute before antibiotics	Not specified	7 d (early); 6 mo (late)	Yes	Multivariate	Case control	26	41	55 pg/mL	65%	93%	85%	81%	0.785
IL-10 serum	Ohta et al,[33] 2019	Acute	-	4 mo	No	Univariate	Case control	28	13	-	-	-	-	-	-
IL-18 serum	Yavuz et al,[15] 2013	At least 3 wk after UTI	-	6 mo	No	Univariate	Case control	57	36	-	-	-	-	-	-
Serum TNF-α	Ohta et al,[33] 2019	Acute	-	4 mo	No	Univariate	Case control	28	13	-	-	-	-	-	-
sTNFR1	Ohta et al,[33] 2019	Acute	-	4 mo	No	Univariate	Case control	28	13	-	-	-	-	-	-
Serum TGF-β	Ohta et al,[33] 2019	Acute	-	4 mo	No	Univariate	Case control	28	13	-	-	-	-	-	-
Urine AGT															

(continued on next page)

Table 1
(continued)

Biomarker	Study Title	Timing	Urine Collection Method	Adjusted for Concentration	DMSA Obtained Time Period	Significant Difference	Analysis Method	Study Design	Treatment Arm	Control Arm	Threshold Level	Sensitivity	Specificity	PPV	NPV	AUC
	Kitao et al,[34] 2015	4 mo	Catheterization	Yes	4 mo	Yes	Multivariate	Case control	32	17	7.27 mg/g Cr	81%	76%	-	-	-
Urine NGAL																
	Kitao et al,[34] 2015	4 mo	Catheterization	Yes	4 mo	No	Multivariate	Case control	32	17	-	-	-	-	-	-
	Rafiei et al,[35] 2C15	72 h after initiating antibiotics	Variable (SP aspiration, catheterization, or midstream)	Yes	Early (not specified); 4–6 mo (late)	Yes	Univariate	Case control	16	38	7.32 ng/mL	81%	66%	-	-	0.73
R	Lee et al,[36] 2015	Acute before antibiotics	Variable (catheterization or bagged)	Yes	Early (not specified); 6 mo (late)	No	Univariate	Case control	18	15	-	-	-	-	-	-
	Yamanouchi et al,[37] 2018	4 mo	Not specified	Yes	4 mo	No	Multivariate	Case control	23	14	-	-	-	-	-	0.64
Urine L-FABP																
	Kitao et al,[34] 2015	4 mo	Catheterization	Yes	4 mo	No	Multivariate	Case control	32	17	-	-	-	-	-	-
	Yamanouchi et al,[37] 2018	4 mo	Not specified	Yes	4 mo	No	Multivariate	Case control	23	14	-	-	-	-	-	0.61
Urine NAG																
	Kitao et al,[34] 2015	4 mo	Catheterization	Yes	4 mo	No	Multivariate	Case control	32	17	-	-	-	-	-	-
	Yamanouchi et al,[37] 2018	4 mo	Not specified	Yes	4 mo	No	Multivariate	Case control	23	14	-	-	-	-	-	0.43
	Islekel et al,[38] 2007	6 mo	24-h urine collection	No	6 mo	No	Univariate	Case control	19	9	-	-	-	-	-	-
Urine BMG																
	Kitao et al,[34] 2015	4 mo	Catheterization	Yes	4 mo	No	Multivariate	Case control	32	17	-	-	-	-	-	-
	Yamanouchi et al,[37] 2018	4 mo	Not specified	Yes	4 mo	No	Multivariate	Case control	23	14	-	-	-	-	-	0.42
Urine C-megalin																

Biomarker	Study															
Serum AGT	Yamanouchi et al,[37] 2018	4 mo	Not specified	Yes	4 mo	Yes	Multivariate	Case control	23	14	6.5 pmol/nmol	74%	93%	94%	68%	0.85
sTNF-RI	Kitao et al,[34] 2015	4 mo	Catheterization	Yes	4 mo	No	Multivariate	Case control	32	17	-	-	-	-	-	-
sTNF-RII	Tullus et al,[39] 1997	Acute; 6 wk	Not specified	Yes	Within 10 d; 1 y	No	Univariate	Case control	43	31	-	-	-	-	-	-
sIL-6R	Tullus et al,[39] 1997	Acute; 6 wk	Not specified	Yes	Within 10 d; 1 y	No	Univariate	Case control	43	31	-	-	-	-	-	-
	Tullus et al,[39] 1997	Acute; 6 wk	Not specified	Yes	Within 10 d; 1 y	No	Univariate	Case control	43	31	-	-	-	-	-	-
Urine IL-1α	Tullus et al,[40] 1996	Acute; 6 wk	Not specified	Yes	Within 10 d; 1 y	Yes	Univariate	Case control	40	34	Not specified	-	-	-	-	-
Urine 1L-Ira	Tullus et al,[40] 1996	Acute; 6 wk	Not specified	Yes	Within 10 d; 1 y	No	Univariate	Case control	40	34	-	-	-	-	-	-
MMP9	Abedi et al,[41] 2017	72 h after initiating antibiotics	Variable (SP aspiration, catheterization, or midstream)	No	4–5 mo	Yes	Univariate	Case control	16	31	75.5 ng/mL	62%	71%	48%	82%	0.681
TIMP1	Abedi et al,[41] 2017	72 h after initiating antibiotics	Variable (SP aspiration, catheterization, or midstream)	No	4–5 mo	Yes	Univariate	Case control	16	31	16.1 ng/mL	75%	55%	41%	84%	0.699
Urine PTX3	Becerir et al,[42] 2019	3 wk	Variable (clean catch, bagged)	Yes	6 mo	Yes	Univariate	Case control	52	36	Not specified	-	-	-	-	0.67
Serum PTX3	Becerir et al,[42] 2019	3 wk	Variable (clean catch, bagged)	Yes	6 mo	No	Univariate	Case control	52	36	-	-	-	-	-	-
Urine KIM-1																

(continued on next page)

Table 1
(continued)

Biomarker	Study Title	Timing	Urine Collection Method	Adjusted for Concentration	DMSA Obtained Time Period	Significant Difference	Analysis Method	Study Design	Treatment Arm	Control Arm	Threshold Level	Sensitivity	Specificity	PPV	NPV	AUC
Serum cystatin-C	Lee et al,[36] 2015	Acute before antibiotics	Variable (catheterization or bagged)	Yes	Early (not specified); 6 mo (late)	Yes	Univariate	Case control	18	15	Not specified	-	-	-	-	0.71
	Islekel et al[38] 2007	6 mo	24-h urine collection	No	6 mo	No	Univariate	Case control	19	9	-	-	-	-	-	-
Urine cystatin-C	Islekel et al[38] 2007	6 mo	24-h urine collection	Yes	6 mo	No	Univariate	Case control	19	9	-	-	-	-	-	-
Urine endothelin-1	Yilmaz et al,[43] 2012	No active UTI	Variable (midstream or bagged)	Yes	6 mo	Yes	Univariate	Case control	44	32	1.67 fmol/mg	95%	84%	86%	95%	0.945
IL-1b urine	Sheu et al,[44] 2007	Acute before antibiotics; 2 wk after	Not specified	Yes	7 d (early); 6-12 mo (late)	Yes	Multivariate	Case control	12	29	Not specified	-	-	-	-	-
IL-32 urine	Rafiei et al,[45] 2017	Acute	Not specified	Yes	Early (not specified); 6 mo (late)	Yes	Univariate	Case control	19	23	1.4 pg/g	67%	73%	63%	76%	0.682
Serum IL-3yi2	Rafiei et al,[45] 2017	Acute	-	-	Early (not specified); 6 mo (late)	No	Univariate	Case control	19	23	-	-	-	-	-	-

Abbreviations: ANC; AGT; AUC, area under the curve; BMG, beta-2-microglobulin; Cr; CRP; ESR; IFN-γ, interferon γ; IL, interleukin; L-FABP, liver-type fatty acid binding protein; MMP, matrix metalloproteinase 9; NAG, N-acetyl-β-ᴅ-glucosaminidase; NGAL, neutrophil gelatinase-associated lipocalin; NPV, negative predictive value; PCT, procalcitonin; PPV, positive predictive value; sIL-6R; SP; sTNF-RI; TGF-β, tissue growth factor β; TIMP1, tissue inhibitor of metalloproteinases a; TNF-α; UTI, urinary tract infection; WBC, white blood cell.

Table 2
Brief description of each biomarker

Biomarker	Description
C-megalin	Multiligand receptor expressed in proximal tubular cells that reabsorbs filtered albumin[46]
CRP	Acute-phase reactant, a protein made by the liver and released into the blood within a few hours after tissue injury[47]
Cystatin-C	A cysteine proteinase inhibitor that is freely filtered by the glomeruli, reabsorbed, and catabolized in the proximal tubular cells; used as indicator of GFR[38]
Endothelin-1	Released by renal mesangial cells in response to glomerular injury, contributes to fibrosis by increasing collagen synthesis, decreasing ECM degradation, and stimulating mesangial contraction[43]
IFN-γ	Important activator of macrophages and inducer of major histocompatibility complex class II molecule expression[48]
IL-1	Acts as a leukocytic pyrogen and inducer of several components of the acute-phase response and lymphocyte-activating factor[49]
IL-1ra	Interleukin-1 receptor antagonist
IL-2	Secreted by activated T cells and represents a key player in the cell-mediated immune response[33]
IL-4	Regulator of immunity secreted primarily by mast cells, Th2 cells, eosinophils, and basophils. IL-4 increases type I collagen production by fibroblasts[50]
IL-6	Acts as an endogenous pyrogen, activating hepatocyte C-reactive protein production and stimulates mucosal B cells to produce IgA antibodies[9]

(continued on next page)

Table 2
(*continued*)

Biomarker	Description
IL-6R	Soluble IL-6 receptor thought to downregulate proinflammatory cascade by binding free cytokines in biological fluids[39]
IL-8	Chemotactic for neutrophils, forming a gradient across the mucosa and allowing neutrophils to cross the mucosal barrier into the urine[9]
IL-10	Potent inhibitor of antigen presentation; it inhibits major histocompatibility complex class II expression as well as the upregulation of costimulatory molecules[51]
IL-18	Proinflammatory cytokine role in renal ischemia-reperfusion injury[15]
IL-1β	Endogenous pyrogen that appears early during the inflammatory cascade and is found free in biological fluids[44]
IL-32	Pluripotent, proinflammatory cytokine that induces several other proinflammatory cytokines, including TNF, IL-1β, IL-6 and IL-8[45]
KIM1	Transmembrane protein upregulated in dedifferentiated proximal tubule cells after ischemic injury[52]
L-FABP	Localizes in renal proximal tubules, is excreted into the urine in response to oxidative stress-induced tubular injury[53]
MMP9	Zinc-dependent endopeptidase, degrades extracellular matrix components with specific activity for type IV collagen[41]
NAG	Lysosomal enzyme present dominantly in proximal tubules[54]

(continued on next page)

Table 2 (continued)	
Biomarker	Description
NGAL	Mediates inflammation by covalently binding to matrix metalloproteinase 9[35]
Pentraxin 3	Mediator of inflammation synthesized in peripheral tissues and stimulated by proinflammatory cytokines[42]
PCT	Produced by thyroid C-cells and found at a high concentration in critically ill patients, although role is unclear[18]
ST2	Membrane-bound IL-33 receptor, which activates immune cells and induces inflammation[33]
TGF-β	Proofibrotic and immunomodulatory cytokine[55]
TIMP1	Prevents degradation of extracellular matrix components by inhibiting matrix metalloproteinases[41]
TNF	Following hypoxia or ischemic injury to kidney, apoptotic pathway can be triggered by binding of ligands to TNF[33]
TNF-R and TNF-RII	Soluble TNF receptors thought to downregulate proinflammatory cascade by binding free cytokines in biological fluids[39]

Abbreviations: CRP; ECM; GFR; IFN- γ, interferon γ; IL-1, interleukin 1; IL-1ra, interleukin 1 receptor antagonist; IL-6R, interleukin 6 receptor; KIM1, kidney injury molecule-1; L-FABP, liver-type fatty acid binding protein; MMP9, matrix metalloproteinase 9; NAG, N-acetyl- β-D-glucosaminidase; NGAL, neutrophil gelatinase-associated lipocalin; PCT, procalcitonin; TGF- β, tissue growth factor β; TIMP1, tissue inhibitor of metalloproteinases 1; TNF, tissue necrosis factor; TNF-R and TNF-RII, tissue necrosis factor receptors.

Batch Effects

Inconsistencies in experiment times, handlers, reagent lots, or instruments can introduce unwanted confounding, commonly referred to as "batch effects," which can result in invalid study results.[58] Stringent criteria are needed to standardize the way specimens are collected, handled, stored, and processed. This issue is heightened in studies in which specimens are collected from multiple institutions. Whether it be serum, plasma, urine, saliva, or tissue, samples need to be snap frozen shortly after collection and stored in consistent temperatures (−20°C if less than 1–2 weeks, and −70°C if more than 2 weeks).[59] Similarly, specimens should be stored and processed in a consistent manner, blind to case-control status.[60]

One possible method to overcome variations secondary to sample processing is creating replicates of samples. Drucker and Krapfenbauer[56] recommend that samples be analyzed in triplicates to overcome variations in which specimens are processed and analyzed. Furthermore, there are statistical methods to adjust for batch effects. However, batch effect correction through computational methods often incompletely mitigates confounding effects and can unintentionally remove true biological differences.[61]

Last, studies assessing biomarkers within the urine should always control for dilutional effects using specific gravity or creatinine, which are known to impact urinary levels of biologic molecules.[62]

Selection of Cases and Controls

At the study design level, it is important to attempt to balance the cases and control groups with respect to as many characteristics as possible. Sampling based on convenience often results in major differences between the cases and controls with respect to factors such as age, sex, and medical comorbidities. Sampling methods to consider include matching or randomization. Although statistical methods can be applied to adjust for differences in baseline characteristics between cases and controls, this requires larger sample sizes to prevent overfit models that can produce invalid results.[63]

Sample Size

Careful attention must be paid to the number of samples needed to achieve reasonable statistical power to detect biomarkers, especially given the finite resources and time allotted for sample accrual. Too often, insufficient sample sizes result in lack of sample sizes necessary to document meaningful differences between the diseased and controls. Even if there was a true difference between cases and controls, incomplete sample size may lead to "false-negative" results (eg, type 2 error). Power calculations must be performed at the study design stage, not after data accrual. This critical shortcoming in study design has plagued the field of biomarker discovery. Several authorities have outlined ways to address some of these barriers.[64–66]

Heterogeneous Outcome

Study outcomes have to be clearly defined and correctly measured. Using renal parenchymal defects as an example, both baseline congenital dysplasia and acquired renal scarring can appear as renal parenchymal defects on DMSA studies. Distinguishing between the congenital dysplasia and acquired renal scarring may not be critical for making management decisions because both reflect diminished renal health. However, it would be critical to distinguish between the 2 because they likely differ in metabolites or proteins that are excreted in the urine or detected within the serum. Furthermore, there are varying degrees of renal parenchymal defects, ranging from one of a few small cortical defects to significant global atrophy. It may be useful to create subcategories among those with renal parenchymal defects or treat the outcome of renal scarring as a continuous variable (eg, percentage split function), to properly assess variations in biomarker expression across the full spectrum of disease.

Statistical Analyses and Performance Characteristics

Many biomarker discovery studies use t-statistics and their P values as a method to identify candidate biomarkers. Unfortunately, these measures do not quantify biomarker performance in a clinically relevant way. The t-statistic is based on the difference in mean biomarker values between the case and controls but does not quantify the usefulness of the biomarker for clinical application. Instead, performance methods related to the research question at hand, including sensitivity and specificity at different diagnostic thresholds as well as negative predictive and positive predictive values that take into consideration prevalence of disease, should be reported to assess whether the biomarker of interest can help test for renal parenchymal defects.[67] It is also critical that analyses account for multiplicity to avoid inflated type 1 errors, resulting in false-positive findings.[68]

The "Bottleneck" Effect

Traditional approaches of assessing the candidacy of biomarkers involved testing a handful of preselected biomolecules selected based on small sample animal physiology models or other similarly designed clinical studies. This type of study design creates a "bottleneck" to discovery. Considering the sheer number of protein-coding genes ($\sim$20,000) and variations of this code

through polymorphisms and posttranscriptional and posttranslational modifications, important proteins may be missed without casting a wide net for differential expression between diseased versus controls.[69] Similarly, dynamic anabolic and catabolic processes within the cell and organ can result in a wide range of metabolites present in a biological system.[70,71]

Integration of modern bioinformatics techniques has helped other fields circumvent this problem. Methods that rely on chromatographic methods for biomolecule separation and mass spectrometry methods for identification of those biomolecules in tissue or fluid samples have led to a recent explosion of candidate biomarker discovery within cancer, nephrology, and cardiology.[72–75] Proteins, and more recently, metabolites, have been the main subjects of biomarker discovery and clinical translation due to their enormous abundance and variation of products produced as response to physiologic stimuli. Mass spectrometry-based techniques allow scientists to simultaneously study thousands of molecules within tissue samples. This comprehensive assessment of a set of molecules is referred to as an "-omics" approach.[71,76]

Another important benefit of mass spectrometry-based approaches to biomarker discovery is the streamlined process of combining or "multiplexing" various proteins; this contrasts from traditional approaches that relied on single-protein immunoassays (eg, enzyme-linked immunosorbent assay) for discovery. Although immunoassays can be multiplexed to include multiple candidate proteins to create a diagnostic test following discovery, immunoassays are typically not multiplexed at the discovery stage.[77,78]

Following Discovery: Verification, Validation, and Clinical Translation

Advancing through the biomarker pipeline following biomarker discovery is an enormously complex process that consumes significant time and resources.[79,80] For this reason, the yield rate of clinically useful biomarkers has remained low despite an explosion of candidate biomarkers identified following the emergence of "-omics" technology.[71] In order for clinical translation, however, biomarkers need to be properly verified and validated.

Following identification of candidate biomarkers that are differentially expressed in the discovery stage, verification through replicated analyses is needed to confirm differential expression. Animal models should be made to replicate findings, which may aid in understanding the mechanism of action of the disease process.[76] At this stage, it is important to develop high-throughput, precise, and affordable assays that can be used during clinical validation.

Following the verification stage, biomarkers must be clinically validated; this involves clinical studies with clear outcomes that are well controlled and rigorously analyzed. Clinical validation requires significant resource utilization, and the bar for validation at the clinical level is extremely high.[80]

What is the Level of Biomarker Performance Needed for Clinical Utility?

The following excerpt provides an example of how challenging it is to find a biomarker with high-enough performance characteristics to provide clinical utility.

Although the area under the curve measure from receiver operator curves is frequently used to assess biomarker performance, a much more practical way to conceptualize whether a test is ready to be used clinically is through Bayes' theorem, which takes into account the prevalence of disease.[81]

Say we were to use a hypothetical biomarker for diagnosis of renal parenchymal defects in children with vesicoureteral reflux suffering from a first-time febrile urinary tract infection. The sensitivity and specificity of this biomarker is 0.80 and 0.80, respectively, for the designated diagnostic threshold. The hypothetical prevalence of renal parenchymal defects within this population is approximately 15%. From a population of 10,000 patients with vesicoureteral reflux and urinary tract infection, we would expect our population to have 1500 patients with parenchymal defects and 8500 without it (15% disease prevalence). Of the 1500 children with parenchymal defects, we would expect about 1200 to test positive for the biomarker (based on 80% sensitivity). Of the 8500 without the disease, we would then expect 1700 to test positive based upon a 20% false-positive test rate for the biomarker.

The logical following question is: what is the probability of renal parenchymal defects given the positive result? Calculated by using Bayes' theorem, only 41.4% of patients with a positive test result will actually have the disease.[82] If the sensitivity and specificity of the biomarker were to be raised to 0.90 and 0.90, respectively, 61.4% of patients with a positive test result will have the disease. In other words, the performance of a biomarker is slightly better than a coin flip despite a significantly higher sensitivity and specificity than any of the biomarkers studied to date.

SUMMARY

A noninvasive test that can longitudinally assess renal parenchymal status would be incredibly valuable for a wide range of conditions. Yet, stand-alone candidate biomarkers for renal parenchymal defects that are worthy of further investigation have not yet surfaced. With recent developments in high-throughput technology and bioinformatics techniques, biomarker research is progressing at an unprecedented rate. It is crucial that researchers continue to implement rigorous experimental and study design methods while understanding the challenges that lie ahead for biomarker discovery and translation.

CLINICS CARE POINTS

- Biomarker research is progressing at an unprecedented rate with recent developments in high-throughput technology and bioinformatics techniques.

- It is crucial that researchers continue to implement rigorous experimental and study design methods while understanding the challenges that lie ahead for biomarker discovery and translation.

DISCLOSURE

None of the authors have commercial or financial conflicts of interest. No funding sources related to this study.

REFERENCES

1. Shanon A, et al. Evaluation of renal scars by technetium-labeled dimercaptosuccinic acid scan, intravenous urography, and ultrasonography: a comparative study. J Pediatr 1992;120(3):399–403.

2. Abdelhalim A, Khoury AE. Critical appraisal of the top-down approach for vesicoureteral reflux. Investig Clin Urol 2017;58(Suppl 1):S14–22.

3. Herz D, et al. 5-year prospective results of dimercapto-succinic acid imaging in children with febrile urinary tract infection: proof that the top-down approach works. J Urol 2010;184(4 Suppl): 1703–9.

4. Ward VL, et al. Pediatric radiation exposure and effective dose reduction during voiding cystourethrography. Radiology 2008;249(3):1002–9.

5. Paolino J, Treves ST. Availability of (99m)Tc-DMSA. J Nucl Med 2017;58(11):16N.

6. Lim R, Bar-Sever Z, Treves ST. Is Availability of (99m) Tc-DMSA insufficient to meet clinical needs in the United States? A Survey. J Nucl Med 2019;60(8): 14N–6N.

7. Bramer WM, et al. De-duplication of database search results for systematic reviews in EndNote. J Med Libr Assoc 2016;104(3):240–3.

8. Zaffanello M, et al. Genetic susceptibility to renal scar formation after urinary tract infection: a systematic review and meta-analysis of candidate gene polymorphisms. Pediatr Nephrol 2011;26(7): 1017–29.

9. Renata Y, et al. Urinary concentration of cytokines in children with acute pyelonephritis. Eur J Pediatr 2013;172(6):769–74.

10. Tramma D, et al. Interleukin-6 and interleukin-8 levels in the urine of children with renal scarring. Pediatr Nephrol 2012;27(9):1525–30.

11. Tullus K, et al. Urine interleukin-6 and interleukin-8 in children with acute pyelonephritis, in relation to DMSA scintigraphy in the acute phase and at 1-year follow-up. Pediatr Radiol 1994;24(7):513–5.

12. Sheu JN, et al. Relationship between serum and urine interleukin-6 elevations and renal scarring in children with acute pyelonephritis. Scand J Urol Nephrol 2009;43(2):133–7.

13. Gokce I, et al. Urinary levels of interleukin-6 and interleukin-8 in patients with vesicoureteral reflux and renal parenchymal scar. Pediatr Nephrol 2010; 25(5):905–12.

14. Sheu JN, et al. The role of serum and urine interleukin-8 on acute pyelonephritis and subsequent renal scarring in children. Pediatr Infect Dis J 2009;28(10):885–90.

15. Yavuz S, Anarat A, Bayazit AK. Interleukin-18, CRP and procalcitonin levels in vesicoureteral reflux and reflux nephropathy. Ren Fail 2013;35(10):1319–22.

16. Leroy S, et al. Association of procalcitonin with acute pyelonephritis and renal scars in pediatric UTI. Pediatrics 2013;131(5):870–9.

17. Prat C, et al. Elevated serum procalcitonin values correlate with renal scarring in children with urinary tract infection. Pediatr Infect Dis J 2003;22(5): 438–42.

18. Belhadj-Tahar H, et al. Procalcitonin implication in renal cell apoptosis induced by acute pyelonephritis in children. Infect Drug Resist 2008;1:17–20.

19. Bressan S, et al. Procalcitonin as a predictor of renal scarring in infants and young children. Pediatr Nephrol 2009;24(6):1199–204.

20. Sheu JN, et al. The role of procalcitonin for acute pyelonephritis and subsequent renal scarring in infants and young children. J Urol 2011;186(5):2002–8.

21. Karavanaki K, et al. Fever duration during treated urinary tract infections and development of permanent renal lesions. Arch Dis Child 2019;104(5): 466–70.

22. Karavanaki KA, et al. Delayed treatment of the first febrile urinary tract infection in early childhood increased the risk of renal scarring. Acta Paediatr 2017;106(1):149–54.

23. Jakobsson B, Berg U, Svensson L. Renal scarring after acute pyelonephritis. Arch Dis Child 1994; 70(2):111–5.

24. Byun HJ, et al. The impact of obesity on febrile urinary tract infection and renal scarring in children with vesicoureteral reflux. J Pediatr Urol 2017; 13(1):67 e1–6.

25. Rodriguez LM, et al. Do serum C-reactive protein and interleukin-6 predict kidney scarring after urinary tract infection? Indian J Pediatr 2013;80(12): 1002–6.

26. Stokland E, et al. Renal damage one year after first urinary tract infection: role of dimercaptosuccinic acid scintigraphy. J Pediatr 1996;129(6):815–20.

27. Wang YT, et al. Correlation of renal ultrasonographic findings with inflammatory volume from dimercaptosuccinic acid renal scans in children with acute pyelonephritis. J Urol 2005;173(1):190–4 [discussion: 194].

28. Swerkersson S, et al. Relationship among vesicoureteral reflux, urinary tract infection and renal damage in children. J Urol 2007;178(2):647–51 [discussion: 650-1].

29. Kotoula A, et al. Comparative efficacies of procalcitonin and conventional inflammatory markers for prediction of renal parenchymal inflammation in pediatric first urinary tract infection. Urology 2009; 73(4):782–6.

30. Yilmaz I, et al. Association of vesicoureteral reflux and renal scarring in urinary tract infections. Arch Argent Pediatr 2018;116(4):e542–7.

31. Liao PF, et al. Comparison of procalcitonin and different guidelines for first febrile urinary tract infection in children by imaging. Pediatr Nephrol 2014; 29(9):1567–74.

32. Kavukcu S, et al. Serum vitamin A and beta-carotene concentrations and renal scarring in urinary tract infections. Arch Dis Child 1998;78(3): 271–2.

33. Ohta N, et al. Serum soluble ST2 as a marker of renal scar in pediatric upper urinary tract infection. Cytokine 2019;120:258–63.

34. Kitao T, et al. Urinary Biomarkers for Screening for Renal Scarring in Children with Febrile Urinary Tract Infection: Pilot Study. J Urol 2015;194(3):766–71.

35. Rafiei A, et al. Urinary neutrophil gelatinase-associated lipocalin (NGAL) might be an independent marker for anticipating scar formation in children with acute pyelonephritis. J Ren Inj Prev 2015;4(2):39–44.

36. Lee HE, et al. The diagnosis of febrile urinary tract infection in children may be facilitated by urinary biomarkers. Pediatr Nephrol 2015;30(1):123–30.

37. Yamanouchi S, et al. Urinary C-megalin for screening of renal scarring in children after febrile urinary tract infection. Pediatr Res 2018;83(3):662–8.

38. Islekel H, et al. Serum and urine cystatin C levels in children with post-pyelonephritic renal scarring: a pilot study. Int Urol Nephrol 2007;39(4):1241–50.

39. Tullus K, et al. Soluble receptors to tumour necrosis factor and interleukin-6 in urine during acute pyelonephritis. Acta Paediatr 1997;86(11):1198–202.

40. Tullus K, et al. Interleukin-1 alpha and interleukin-1 receptor antagonist in the urine of children with acute pyelonephritis and relation to renal scarring. Acta Paediatr 1996;85(2):158–62.

41. Abedi SM, et al. Urinary matrix metalloproteinase 9 and tissue inhibitor of metalloproteinase 1 biomarkers for predicting renal scar in children with urinary tract infection. Turk J Urol 2017;43(4):536–42.

42. Becerir T, et al. Urinary excretion of pentraxin-3 correlates with the presence of renal scar following acute pyelonephritis in children. Int Urol Nephrol 2019;51(4):571–7.

43. Yilmaz A, et al. Urine endothelin-1 levels as a predictor of renal scarring in children with urinary tract infections. Clin Nephrol 2012;77(3):219–24.

44. Sheu JN, et al. Urine interleukin-1beta in children with acute pyelonephritis and renal scarring. Nephrology (Carlton) 2007;12(5):487–93.

45. Rafiei A, et al. The urinary and serum levels of IL-32 in children with febrile urinary tract infections. Future Sci OA 2017;3(4):FSO242.

46. Nishiwaki H, et al. Urinary C-megalin as a novel biomarker of progression to microalbuminuria: a cohort study based on the diabetes Distress and Care Registry at Tenri (DDCRT 22). Diabetes Res Clin Pract 2022;186:109810.

47. Yildiz B, et al. High sensitive C-reactive protein: a new marker for urinary tract infection, VUR and renal scar. Eur Rev Med Pharmacol Sci 2013;17(19):2598–604.

48. Schoenborn JR, Wilson CB. Regulation of interferon-gamma during innate and adaptive immune responses. Adv Immunol 2007;96:41–101.

49. Kaneko N, et al. The role of interleukin-1 in general pathology. Inflamm Regen 2019;39:12.

50. Gadani SP, et al. IL-4 in the brain: a cytokine to remember. J Immunol 2012;189(9):4213–9.

51. Mosser DM, Zhang X. Interleukin-10: new perspectives on an old cytokine. Immunol Rev 2008;226:205–18.

52. Chevalier RL. The proximal tubule is the primary target of injury and progression of kidney disease: role of the glomerulotubular junction. Am J Physiol Renal Physiol 2016;311(1):F145–61.

53. Kamijo A, et al. Urinary excretion of fatty acid-binding protein reflects stress overload on the proximal tubules. Am J Pathol 2004;165(4):1243–55.

54. Yoo JJ, et al. The role of urinary N-Acetyl-beta-d-glucosaminidase in cirrhotic patients with acute kidney injury: multicenter, prospective cohort study. J Clin Med 2021;10(19):4328.

55. Gilbert RE, et al. Urinary transforming growth factor-beta in patients with diabetic nephropathy: implications for the pathogenesis of tubulointerstitial pathology. Nephrol Dial Transpl 2001;16(12):2442–3.

56. Drucker E, Krapfenbauer K. Pitfalls and limitations in translation from biomarker discovery to clinical utility in predictive and personalised medicine. EPMA J 2013;4(1):7.

57. Waerner T, Thurnher D, Krapfenbauer K. The role of laboratory medicine in healthcare: quality requirements of immunoassays, standardisation and data management in prospective medicine. EPMA J 2010;1(4):619–26.

58. Goh WWB, Wang W, Wong L. Why batch effects matter in omics data, and how to avoid them. Trends Biotechnol 2017;35(6):498–507.

59. Issaq HJ, Waybright TJ, Veenstra TD. Cancer biomarker discovery: opportunities and pitfalls in analytical methods. Electrophoresis 2011;32(9):967–75.

60. Simon RM, Paik S, Hayes DF. Use of archived specimens in evaluation of prognostic and predictive biomarkers. J Natl Cancer Inst 2009;101(21):1446–52.

61. Nygaard V, Rodland EA, Hovig E. Methods that remove batch effects while retaining group differences may lead to exaggerated confidence in downstream analyses. Biostatistics 2016;17(1):29–39.

62. Weaver VM, et al. Challenges for environmental epidemiology research: are biomarker concentrations altered by kidney function or urine concentration adjustment? J Expo Sci Environ Epidemiol 2016;26(1):1–8.

63. Pepe MS, Li CI, Feng Z. Improving the quality of biomarker discovery research: the right samples and enough of them. Cancer Epidemiol Biomarkers Prev 2015;24(6):944–50.

64. Rodriguez H, et al. Analytical validation of protein-based multiplex assays: a workshop report by the NCI-FDA interagency oncology task force on molecular diagnostics. Clin Chem 2010;56(2):237–43.

65. Regnier FE, et al. Protein-based multiplex assays: mock presubmissions to the US Food and Drug Administration. Clin Chem 2010;56(2):165–71.

66. Skates SJ, et al. Statistical design for biospecimen cohort size in proteomics-based biomarker discovery and verification studies. J Proteome Res 2013;12(12):5383–94.

67. Soreide K. Receiver-operating characteristic curve analysis in diagnostic, prognostic and predictive biomarker research. J Clin Pathol 2009;62(1):1–5.

68. Ioannidis JP. Biomarker failures. Clin Chem 2013;59(1):202–4.

69. International Human Genome Sequencing, C. Finishing the euchromatic sequence of the human genome. Nature 2004;431(7011):931–45.

70. Wishart DS. Metabolomics for investigating physiological and pathophysiological processes. Physiol Rev 2019;99(4):1819–75.

71. Srivastava A, Creek DJ. Discovery and validation of clinical biomarkers of cancer: a review combining metabolomics and proteomics. Proteomics 2019;19(10):e1700448.

72. Crutchfield CA, et al. Advances in mass spectrometry-based clinical biomarker discovery. Clin Proteomics 2016;13:1.

73. Hawkridge AM, Muddiman DC. Mass spectrometry-based biomarker discovery: toward a global proteome index of individuality. Annu Rev Anal Chem (Palo Alto Calif) 2009;2:265–77.

74. Zou W, She J, Tolstikov VV. A comprehensive workflow of mass spectrometry-based untargeted metabolomics in cancer metabolic biomarker discovery using human plasma and urine. Metabolites 2013;3(3):787–819.

75. Seger C, Salzmann L. After another decade: LC-MS/MS became routine in clinical diagnostics. Clin Biochem 2020;82:2–11.

76. Hasin Y, Seldin M, Lusis A. Multi-omics approaches to disease. Genome Biol 2017;18(1):83.

77. Tighe PJ, et al. ELISA in the multiplex era: potentials and pitfalls. Proteomics Clin Appl 2015;9(3–4):406–22.

78. Pappireddi N, Martin L, Wuhr M. A review on quantitative multiplexed proteomics. Chembiochem 2019;20(10):1210–24.

79. Rifai N, Gillette MA, Carr SA. Protein biomarker discovery and validation: the long and uncertain path to clinical utility. Nat Biotechnol 2006;24(8):971–83.

80. Boja E, et al. Restructuring proteomics through verification. Biomark Med 2010;4(6):799–803.

81. Lopez Puga J, Krzywinski M, Altman N. Points of significance: Bayes' theorem. Nat Methods 2015;12(4):277–8.

82. Python for the life sciences : a gentle introduction to Python for life scientistsz. Lancaster, Alexander ; Webster, Gordon. Berkeley, CA: Apress; 2019.

Biomarkers in Urolithiasis

David E. Hinojosa-Gonzalez, MD, Brian H. Eisner, MD*

KEYWORDS

- Urolithiasis • Biomarkers • Kidney stones • Nephrolithiasis

KEY POINTS

- Biomarker use in endourology and stone disease has seen limited use without widespread adoption to date.
- There are many potential applications of biomarkers for the study of patients with urolithiasis, both for clinical and research purposes.
- Further studies are needed to define the role of novel biomarkers in the evaluation and treatment of patients with kidney stone disease.

INTRODUCTION

Urolithiasis is one of the most common urologic diseases. It is estimated that the lifetime prevalence in the United States is approximately 1 in 11. Trend analysis has determined that stone disease is on the increase, with prevalence numbers nearly doubling over the prior 2 decades.[1] Stones that form in the kidney may detach from the renal papilla and obstruct the ureter, leading to acute obstructive episodes that require emergency care and/or intervention; this has resulted in emergency department visits and health care cost utilization estimated at more than $5 billion spending per year.[2]

Urolithiasis is the result of alterations in the renal tubular and renal pelvic pH and solute concentration. Renal handling of calcium, oxalate, phosphate, and citrate among others may be disrupted by underlying metabolic, lifestyle, and genetic factors as well as local and systemic processes. Disturbances to the regulation of excretion and secretion of these substances leads to solute crystallization and aggregation, which in turn grow into kidney stones. Given the variety of substrates handled by the renal filtration system in the convergence of multiple pathways, it is clear that different alterations may lead to different compositions of stones. Urolithiasis most commonly involves calcium oxalate stones with a degree of phosphate components. Other common types of stones are composed of struvite, uric acid, and cystine, which are estimated to represent 10%, 9%, and 1%, respectively.[3]

"Biomarker" is a broad term whose actual definition has undergone various revisions by organizations such as the World Health Organization and the National Institutes of Health, among others. Current definitions are wide encompassing, denominating a biomarker any consistent measurement that reflects underlying processes.[4] This review focuses on measurements of serum, urinary and genetic structures, substances, proteins, and bacteria. As previously mentioned, urolithiasis is the result of underlying alterations in metabolic and/or genetic processes. Therefore, biomarkers can be surrogates, reflecting underlying biological aberrations. These markers, including inflammasomes, serum and urinary proteins, RNA/DNA, and bacteria, may provide detailed insight into stone formation risk, as well as track complications such as kidney injury and sepsis.

MARKERS OF URETERAL OBSTRUCTION AND KIDNEY INJURY

Kidney stones, regardless of composition, may dislodge and cause obstruction during passage down the ureter or grow enough to partially or

Department of Urology, Massachusetts General Hospital, Harvard Medical School, 55 Fruit Street, GRB 1102, Boston, MA 02114, USA
* Corresponding author.
E-mail address: beisner@mgh.harvard.edu

Urol Clin N Am 50 (2023) 19–29
https://doi.org/10.1016/j.ucl.2022.09.004
0094-0143/23/© 2022 Published by Elsevier Inc.

completely obstruct renal outflow. In both cases, renal damage may ensue both acutely and chronically. Creatinine has been classically used as a surrogate of kidney function; however, it is nonspecific and lacks sensitivity to identify early renal damage, as serum levels may lag and not accurately depict undergoing renal injury. Various biomarkers have been proposed and studied as more accurate identifiers of ongoing renal injury with mixed success.

Kidney Injury Molecule 1

Kidney injury molecule 1 (KIM-1), a type 1 transmembrane protein in the proximal tubule, was identified to be upregulated in rat kidneys undergoing ischemic injury by Ichimura and colleagues in 1998.[5] These findings were then verified in human kidneys biopsies in 2002 by Han and colleagues.[6] They also proposed that urine levels of KIM-1 were higher in patients with ischemic acute tubular necrosis than in patients with other forms of renal injury, such as contrast nephropathy, systemic lupus erythematosus, diabetes mellitus, postrenal obstruction, chronic kidney disease, and healthy controls.[6] These findings gathered worldwide interest, resulting in more than a thousand studies that have been published on this protein in various settings. Among these studies, some have been dedicated to ureteral obstruction and urolithiasis, which found increased urinary levels of KIM-1 in obstructive nephropathy.[7–9] However, further studies attempting to determine the role and utility of KIM-1 in urolithiasis have been inconclusive.

Fahmy and colleagues[10] analyzed KIM-1 urinary expression levels in patients undergoing retrograde intrarenal surgery (RIRS) and shockwave lithotripsy (SWL) and compared them with healthy controls. Among their findings, patients with stone disease had increased KIM-1 urinary levels compared with controls. Patients who underwent SWL had increased KIM-1 levels after treatment, whereas those who underwent RIRS did not. These findings contrast to those of Urbschat and colleagues[11] who compared urinary levels of KIM-1 in patients with acute obstructive uropathy with that of healthy controls and found no significant differences. Olvera-Posada and colleagues[7] also analyzed urinary levels of KIM-1 in patients with hydronephrosis. They found the presence of KIM-1 successfully identified hydronephrosis and decreased after treatment; however, it was not found to be a specific marker for urolithiasis, as various obstructing pathologies were included.

Bansal and colleagues[12] analyzed the ratio of KIM-1 to creatinine in urine in patients undergoing various endourological interventions for urolithiasis. They found significant correlation between KIM-1/creatinine and stone size. In addition, they found that their interventions with low stone-free rates had persistently high KIM-1/creatinine ratios after intervention, whereas RIRS and percutaneous nephrolithotomy (PCNL) had significant decreased urinary concentrations of KIM-1/creatinine in urine. These investigators concluded these combinations of KIM-1 and creatinine could be an effective indicator of underlying stone disease. KIM-1 is currently approved by the Food and Drug Administration as a marker, currently in use in various clinical trials for monitoring renal damage related to drugs.[13]

Neutrophil Gelatinase–Associated Lipocalin

Neutrophil gelatinase–associated lipocalin (NGAL) is a protein bound to gelatinase from neutrophils that mediates cellular proliferation and differentiation and exerts a bacteriostatic effect. NGAL's expression is upregulated during inflammatory events.[14] Its utility in renal damage and various other renal injuries remains contested by mixed evidence.[14–16]

Bolgeri and colleagues[15] studied NGAL as a potential renal injury marker in acute obstructive uropathy. They found both urinary and serum as well as the ratio of urinary NGAL to creatinine elevated in patients with both urolithiasis and acute obstructive uropathy compared with healthy controls. There were no differences in these values between both study groups. However, patients who experienced spontaneous stone expulsion and those who underwent surgical management also had significant reductions of these values. Hughes and colleagues[16] compared baseline and post-shockwave levels of NGAL, finding increased levels at 30 and 120 minutes post-shockwave, with levels trending toward normalization at 240 minutes. Hughes and colleagues[17] also performed a similar study by analyzing patients undergoing flexible ureteroscopy (URS) testing various biomarkers. In the setting of URS, they concluded similar findings of increased NGAL post-URS. These findings are consistent with those of Dede and colleagues.[18] Although increased markers in the setting of SWL are explained by trauma from soundwave shock, in the setting of URS increases may be explained by renal manipulation, stone movement, and/or laser heat and damage.

Olvera-Posada and colleagues[7] as well as Urbschat and colleagues[11] presented similar findings when they studied NGAL. Both studies found that although NGAL was increased in obstruction, it was more intimately correlated to pyuria and other inflammatory processes. These results are further supported by the findings presented by Zhu and colleagues[19] in which they found the NGAL was significantly higher in patients with urinary tract infections and was a sensitive and specific predictor of systemic inflammatory response syndrome.

Carbohydrate Antigen 19-9

Carbohydrate antigen 19-9 (CA19-9) has been most widely studied as a biomarker for pancreatic and other gastrointestinal tract cancers. Prior investigators have established that serum and urinary levels of CA19-9 may have potential as biomarkers of renal injury related to obstruction.[20] Amini and colleagues'[20] analysis of patients with urolithiasis and healthy controls determined CA19-9 levels to be increased in patients with urolithiasis and hydronephrosis; however, further studies found a closer association with hydronephrosis and no relation with urolithiasis, urinary tract infections, and proteinuria. CA19-9 may also be elevated in other systemic conditions, limiting its use.[21]

N-acetyl-B-D-glucosaminidase

N-acetyl-B-D-glucosaminidase (NAG) is upregulated and found in increased concentration in tubular damage.[22] Fahmy and colleagues[10] found nonincreased levels of NAG in patients with kidney stone disease; however, they determined NAG increased shortly after SWL, suggesting that NAG may be a marker for renal damage associated to SWL.

Cystatin-C

Cystatin-C is a freely filtered protein that has been previously used as a biomarker for renal damage following surgery.[23] Hughes and colleagues[17] compared pre-URS with post-URS cystatin C levels, finding no significant differences; however, their study may be limited by a small sample size.

Myeloperoxidase

Myeloperoxidase (MPO) is an enzyme involved in the generation of oxygen radicals by neutrophils allowing for host defense. It has previously been used as a marker for inflammatory states and cardiovascular disease.[23-25] Hughes and colleagues[17] compared pre-URS with post-URS MPO levels, finding no significant differences; however, their study may be limited by a small sample size.

Urinary Genes, Proteins, and Cytokines

Various biomarkers may provide insight into renal pathophysiology when quantified. Underlying cellular changes occurring as response or in relation to stone formation and related complications may be tracked through expression and excretion of proteins and genetic material. Inflammation may be tracked through the measurement of mediators such as cytokines, of which various have been studied in the context of urological biomarkers; these have been previously used to detect acute and chronic kidney injuries, as there is often an ongoing underlying inflammatory reaction related to endothelial and tissue injury.[26,27]

Among studied cytokines are the following: interleukin-6 (IL-6) is a multifunctional cytokine that is involved in various processes, ranging from hematopoiesis, inflammation, and regulation. Increased urinary levels of IL-6 have been identified in patients with sepsis and acute kidney injury.[26,27] IL-8 targets neutrophils avidly and is also currently used as a marker of inflammation. It has previously been measured in urine of patients with pyelonephritis, hemolytic uremic syndrome, as well as graft rejection.[28] IL-10 has also been shown in the past to be elevated in infections as well as neoplasia.[29,30] IL-18 is upregulated during inflammatory responses. Although it is typically released by macrophages, it has also been determined to be present in the renal tubular epithelium. Thus, urinary concentrations of IL-18 have been confirmed to be significantly increased in patients with AKI and is able to discern between AKI and other urological pathologies such as urinary tract infections and renal syndromes.[31,32] Tumor necrosis factor alpha (TNF-α) is a multifunctional cytokine that is heavily involved in priming and sustaining inflammatory responses.[33] Hughes and colleagues[16] performed a comparative analysis in patients undergoing SWL in which they compared baseline levels of the aforementioned cytokines with various post-SWL levels and various timepoints. Among their findings, they determined IL-6 and TNF-α to increase significantly within 30 to 120 minutes post-shockwave. These findings could suggest these specific cytokines could be used to assess early renal damage.

Long noncoding RNA (lncRNA) accurately reflects intranuclear processes and is thought to provide specific insight in ongoing cellular processes. Tawfick and colleagues[34] analyzed urinary levels of RNA in patients undergoing SWL against healthy controls and also tracked changes in urinary concentrations after the intervention. They found that lncRNAs SBF2-AS1 and FENDRR-19 and messenger RNAs (mRNA) GBP1 and NLRP3 were increased in patients after undergoing SWL. They concluded that urinary markers may be potential markers for renal damage. In addition, they identified these RNA markers to be significantly increased in urolithiasis patients as compared with healthy controls. They found absence of these 4 measured urinary RNA markers in healthy controls, whereas 40% to 80% of patients with urolithiasis had increased urinary levels. These biomarkers are reflections of established inflammasome pathways and thus may suggest underlying renal inflammation in patients with urolithiasis. An overall summary of identified biomarkers is displayed in **Table 1**.

Spontaneous stone passage

As previously mentioned, stones may dislodge from the kidney and migrate into the ureter where they may either spontaneously pass or become affected. Current guidelines endorse medical expulsive therapy (MFT) for ureteral stones less than 10 mm in selected patients with varying degrees of success.[35] The role of biomarkers in this setting as possible indicators of passage has also been thoroughly studied.

Table 1 Summary of identified biomarkers related to kidney injury and acute obstruction	
Biomarker	**Function**
Kidney injury molecule 1 (KIM-1)	Increased in renal damage and obstruction Unclear if elevated by nonobstructing stones
Neutrophil gelatinase–associated lipocalin (NGAL)	Increased in renal damage and infectious/inflammatory processes
Carbohydrate antigen 19-9/CA19-9	Increased in renal obstruction
N-acetyl-B-D-glucosaminidase (NAG)	Possibly increased in renal damage
Cystatin-C	Marker of renal function
Myeloperoxidase (MPO)	Marker of inflammation, unclear role in urolithiasis
Cytokines	Interleukins: possible markers of renal damage and infection/inflammation
Gene-related products	LncRNA/mRNA: possible markers of renal damage

Cilesiz and colleagues[36] analyzed serum procalcitonin levels in patients undergoing MET. They found patients who failed MET had higher procalcitonin levels than those who achieved spontaneous passage. A cutoff of 160pg/mL was proposed with an 86.7% sensitivity and 70.8% specificity. The investigators hypothesized that increased procalcitonin reflects underlying inflammation from stone impaction. Similar to procalcitonin, C-reactive protein (CRP) has been studied and demonstrated similar effects. Özcan and colleagues[37] performed a similar analysis with CRP, suggesting a cutoff of 0.506 mg/L to have significant predictive value in stone passage. These findings are supported by Aldaqadossi and colleagues[38] who proposed a cutoff of 21.9 mg/L for CRP and Jain and colleagues[39] who proposed a cutoff of 4.1 mg/L. Given the wide range of reported values, further research is needed to clarify optimal cutoff points.

It is hypothesized that inflammatory reactions are proportional to stone impaction based on the aforementioned evidence, and thus multiple other markers such as neutrophil percentage, neutrophil-to-lymphocyte ratio, and platelet-to-lymphocyte ratio (PLR) have been proposed as potential adjunct biomarkers.[40,41]

Stones and stone types

Metabolic disorders and endothelial dysfunction have long been linked to urolithiasis. Prior meta-analyses have established a significant association between diseases linked to endothelial dysfunction such as coronary artery disease, stroke and myocardial infarction, and urolithiasis.[42–44] Some have identified that patients with these disorders have lower urinary excretion of citrate and magnesium and have signaled these findings as possible related factors.[45] Certain markers such as CRP have been long used as surrogates of ongoing underlying inflammation in cardiovascular disease and other inflammatory conditions. Shoag and colleagues[46] determined increased risk of urolithiasis in young patients with elevated CRP. This database analysis of 11,033 patients found that increasing quintiles of CRP values in this population had increased odds of prevalent urolithiasis.

The triglyceride-glucose index incorporates fasting triglyceride and glucose levels and has been previously used as an accurate indicator of insulin resistance. Qin and colleagues[47] performed a large database analysis of 20,970 patients, in which they determined the triglyceride-glucose index and the prevalence as well as recurrence of urolithiasis. The mean triglyceride-glucose index was 8.71, and the investigators concluded that there was an increase of urolithiasis incidence with an odds ratio (OR) 1.12 and an increased recurrence with an OR of 1.26 per unit increase in the index. These findings remained significant when models were adjusted for gender, age, body mass index, hypertension, and diabetes.

Urinary Proteins

Osteopontin was originally isolated from bone matrix and was later identified through many systems within the human body, as it serves various functions. In the renal epithelium it has been proposed to act as a potent inhibitor of adhesion of mineral crystals.[48] This protein is influenced by nutrition and anthropometric conformation.[49,50] Icer and colleagues[51] compared urinary levels of osteopontin in patients with urolithiasis with that in matched cohorts. Interestingly, this study found that patients in the urolithiasis cohort had significantly lower levels of urinary osteopontin when compared with the control group. The role of osteopontin in stone prevention, especially among calcium oxalate stone formers, is supported by in vitro and animal studies where it has been shown to inhibit nucleation, crystallization, and growth as well as attachment to the renal epithelium. Experiments in mice have also shown that knockout mice were more likely to form stones.[52]

Matrix Gla protein (MGP), similar to osteopontin, was first identified in the bone matrix and was later found in other tissues.[53] Because of its expression in vascular tissue, it has been proposed as an inhibitor of calcification.[54] Although in vitro and animal models have found alterations in levels of MGP, these have not been identified to be significantly altered in stone formers.[55]

Tamm-Horsfall protein (THP), also known as uromodulin, is a protein found mainly within the renal epithelium. It lines the thick ascending limb of Henle loop and serves multiple functions.[56,57] THP is normally found in urine, and although its presence has been suggested to inhibit crystallization, this finding has been contested by studies that suggest the opposite. THP's behavior has been theorized by various studies to depend on its concentration as well as that of other solutes. A recent study determined THP has concentration-dependent crystallization inhibitory effects by avidly binding calcium,[58] whereas prior studies have suggested that in settings with increased calcium concentrations, THP increases crystal aggregation.[59]

Urinary prothrombin fragment-1 (UPTF-1) is a component of the thrombin protein. In vitro findings of its inhibitory effects on crystallization have been further sustained by results from epidemiological studies that associated increased incidences of urolithiasis in populations with lower UPTF-1.[60,61]

Some investigators have hypothesized that urolithiasis generates a constant inflammatory environment in the kidney and thus may elevate some of the damage markers previously mentioned. In children, Kovacevic and colleagues[62] compared the levels of NGAL, cystatin C, and lysozyme C in patients with urolithiasis against healthy controls. Out of these 3 markers, cystatin C and NGAL were found to be significantly increased in patients with urolithiasis. Further proteomic analysis revealed that these markers were elevated within patients with urolithiasis regardless of urinary levels of calcium and citrate. Lastly, both cystatin C and NGAL were elevated in patients with a history of stones regardless of stone status at the time of urine collection. Fan and colleagues[63] analyzed the urinary protein components' differences between patients with unilateral and bilateral urolithiasis. They found patients with higher urinary NAG-to-creatinine ratios had increased odds of bilateral stones.[63]

Cadieux and colleagues[64] analyzed various urinary proteins through a surface-enhanced laser desorption/ionization–time-of-flight mass spectrometry in patients with urolithiasis and compared them with healthy controls. They found patients with urolithiasis had increased levels of proteinuria, oxalate, p67:p24, and albumin while having similar levels of osteopontin. Zhu and colleagues[65] performed a similar proteomics analysis, in which they found that in patients with calcium oxalate urolithiasis, fibrinogen alpha chain precursor and apolipoprotein A-1 were accurate markers.[65] Wang, and colleagues[66] identified altered metabolism of involved caffeine, phenylalanine, galactose, and tyrosine metabolism.

Metabolomics

Duan and colleagues[67] performed a nuclear magnetic resonance–based metabolomic analysis to create a metabolomic profile for stone formers. They found various pathways, notably glyoxylate and dicarboxylate metabolism, as well as the metabolism of glycine, serine, threonine, phenylalanine, and the Krebs cycle to be associated with urolithiasis. Primiano and colleagues[68] further analyzed the urinary amino acid signatures of patients with urolithiasis and compared them with healthy controls by quantifying the amount of certain amino acids in the urine. This analysis involved 15 stone formers and 12 controls who were tested using a panel of 25 amino acids and derivatives. Resulting urinary amino acid profiles revealed stone formers had lower urinary levels of α-aminobutyric acid, asparagine, ethanolamine, isoleucine, methionine, phenylalanine, serine, tryptophan, and valine. These findings are consistent with prior studies analyzing altered metabolic pathways in urolithiasis and its traces in urine that have found low urinary levels of ethanolamine, serine, tryptophan, oxalate, calcium, citrate, and cystine.[64,66,67] It is theorized that alterations in the glycine metabolism may result in increased oxalate production and thus increased risk of urolithiasis.[67] Other amino acids such as alanine, tryptophan, and threonine are proposed to have inhibitory effects on crystallization.[68,69] Similarly, Wen and colleagues[70–73] performed a metabolomic analysis on children with urolithiasis and compared it with a control group. They identified 40 metabolites related to retinol metabolism, steroid hormone biosynthesis, porphyrin, and chlorophyll metabolism, and these translated to lower levels of serum bilirubin, with increased levels of retinal, all-trans retinoic acid, progesterone, and prostaglandin E2.[70] Overall findings are summarized in **Table 2**.

SEPSIS

Sepsis is an immune phenomenon resulting from dysregulated inflammatory response to infectious insults. It is termed urosepsis when the original infectious insult originates from within the urinary tract. Urolithiasis may result in sepsis when stones become infected, and obstruction occurs with concomitant infection or as a postoperative complication of a urologic procedure. Procedures such as PCNL may carry up to 5% rates of postoperative sepsis.[74] Prior literature is abundant in modeling attempts to determine risk factors in order to better predict and prevent sepsis.

Although leukocytosis is common in infections and other inflammatory processes, attention has been paid to the degree in which various specific cell counts increase or decrease in relation to another. Although in the past, specific cell counts have been used as biomarkers in the evaluation of oncology patients, it has only recently been explored in urolithiasis.[75] Kriplani and colleagues[76] analyzed a cohort of patients undergoing PCNL and determined that patients who developed sepsis had significantly higher leukocyte count, higher neutrophil-to-lymphocyte ratio (NLR), higher PLR, and lower lymphocyte-to-monocyte ratio (LMR). They established various cutoffs for these findings. At a cutoff of 2.45, NLR was found to have an 87% sensitivity and on receiver operating characteristic curve analysis, an area under the curve (AUC) of 0.639. PLR had a sensitivity of 80.2% at a cutoff of 110, with an AUC of 0.663.

Table 2 Summary of identified biomarkers and proposed applications for kidney stone detection	
Marker	**Function**
CRP	Possibly increased in younger patients with urolithiasis. Possibly related to underlying metabolic disorders
Triglyceride-glucose index	Possibly increased in patients with urolithiasis in relation to underlying metabolic disorders
Osteopontin	Thought to be decreased in stone formers
Matrix Gla protein (MGP)	In vitro evidence of possible mineralization inhibitor
Tamm-Horsfall protein (THP)	Concentration-dependent function. Possibly decreased in stone formers. In high-calcium scenarios increases mineralization
Urinary prothrombin fragment 1	Possible inhibitor of crystallization, decreased in stone formers
Amino acid and other metabolic pathways	Various metabolic pathways altered identified in patients with urolithiasis including • Glyoxylate and dicarboxylate metabolism • Glycine, ethanolamine, serine, and others

Lastly LMR had a sensitivity of 87.5 with a cutoff of 3.23 and an AUC of 0.649.

Some of the previously mentioned biomarkers such as NGAL, cystatin-C, MPO, and others were analyzed in the context of infectious complications due to a urologic source. Hughes and colleagues,[17] although limited by a small sample size, found that there may be a role for these biomarkers in monitoring infections. Patients with urinary tract infections had increased levels compared with the rest of the cohort of cystatin-C; however, the patient who developed sepsis had average levels of cystatin C. NGAL was average in 2 patients with urinary tract infections and normal in the patient with sepsis and was elevated only in 1 of the 3 patients with a urinary tract infection. On the other hand, MPO was increased in the patient with sepsis and elevated in 1 of the 3 patients with urinary tract infections. The investigators encouraged future experiments involving these biomarkers in larger cohorts. Qi and colleagues [77] performed similar measurements in patients undergoing PCNL and found that serum IL-6 drawn within 2 hours of the operation was found to have an AUC of 1 at identifying postoperative urosepsis. Procalcitonin was also found to be accurate with an AUC of 0.954 when drawn on the third postoperative day. Thus, the investigators suggest that IL-6 may be a very accurate early marker of sepsis in patients undergoing PCNL.[77,78] In a similar analysis, Liu and colleagues[79] analyzed sepsis rates after endourological surgery and found that procalcitonin levels of greater than 0.1 ng/mL had significantly increased odds of postoperative gram-negative sepsis. Studies have also found ratios of procalcitonin to albumin to be accurate identifiers of patients with urosepsis after endourological stone procedures.[80]

GENETICS

Genetic analysis may provide insight into the multiple pathways that may be altered and ultimately increase the risk of urolithiasis. CD44 is a cell adhesion molecule that is known to play a role in various biologic processes and has been associated with cancer pathogenesis. Among its notable functions, it has been established as an important receptor for osteopontin. Qiao and colleagues[81] studied the possible role of CD44 rs13347 locus polymorphisms in Chinese patients with urolithiasis. The investigators identified 4 genotypes for this gene, cytosine cytosine (CC), cytosine thymine (CT), thymine thymine (TT), and cytosine thymine + thymine thymine(CT + TT). In their analysis, CT, TT, and CT + TT had increased odds of urolithiasis compared with CC (OR 1.98, OR 2.69, and OR 2.21, respectively). Further stratified analysis revealed CT and TT to demonstrate an increased risk of stone recurrence. They also concluded markedly increased risk of urolithiasis in male populations. Jabalameli and colleagues[82] analyzed SLC25A25 variants in European, theorizing that mutations in this transporter altered mitochondrial ATP production and renal solute transport.

Liu and colleagues[83] analyzed subsets of patients with urolithiasis to determine if their genetics played a role as a predisposition to renal damage from stone disease. They analyzed various genes in patients relative to the quantification of several markers, such as NAG. Their analysis concluded that rs4880 and rs5746135 of manganese superoxide dismutase could increase susceptibility to renal damage in patients with urolithiasis. Similarly, Mehdi and colleagues[84] analyzed polymorphisms

in human transcription factor 7-like 2, β-defensin, and CD14 as possible links between these genes and urolithiasis. Further studies by Liang and colleagues[85] support the possible polygenic causes of urolithiasis, as they found alterations in the expression of 9 microRNAs, 883 mRNAs, and 1002 lncRNAs in patients with calcium oxalate urolithiasis.

Current evidence suggests there are a variety of involved genes and pathways in urolithiasis; however, a study by Halbritter and colleagues[86] determined that 14 monogenic genes were responsible for 15% of diagnosed patients with nephrolithiasis. Although germline genetic analysis is not truly a biomarker, per se, and is beyond the scope of this review, current evidence suggests a possible future role in the identification and screening of stone formers.[86]

Gastrointestinal and Urinary Microbiota

The human intestinal and urinary tracts are the hosts of complex, dynamic symbiosis with microbial organisms. In particular, gut microbiota have been extensively linked to metabolic diseases, autoimmune diseases, and urolithiasis. Some of these organisms, such as Oxalobacter formigenes play an important role in the downstream prevention of stones by regulating intestinal absorption of oxalate through degradation.[87] Although deficiency of this bacterial population was thought to increase the risk of stones, further studies found normal populations in stone formers.[88–91] However, clinical studies have suggested that O formigenes colonization can significantly reduce the risk of calcium oxalate stone recurrence[88]; this is probably due to the complex interplay of various pathways related to stone formation.

As the human intestinal tract hosts more than thousands of species of bacteria, scientists have studied the balance and proportions of these bacteria and their possible impact on measured outcomes. Decreased microbial diversity and alterations of specific bacterial populations have been identified in patients with urolithiasis by various investigators.[92–95] Among them, Lachnospiraceae, Ruminiclostridium, Dorea, Christensenellaceae, and Enterobacter have been found to be reduced, whereas Bacteroides, Bifidobacterium, and Faecalibacterium were found to be increased.[95] Studies attempting to determine the accuracy of gut bacteria in identifying patients with nephrolithiasis have returned mixed results.[92] However, Tang and colleagues[95] concluded Escherichia coli and Pseudomonas aeruginosa could identify patients with urolithiasis correctly with statistical significance.

Chen and colleagues[96] performed a similar study by analyzing the gut flora of patients with calcium oxalate urolithiasis and compared them with healthy controls. The investigators determined that the urolithiasis groups had decreased populations of *Firmicutes*, *Verrucomicrobia*, *Akkermansia* spp, *Faecalibacterium* spp, and *Lactobacillus* spp while having higher populations of *Bacteroidetes* and *Phascolarctobacterium*. Through Spearman correlation analysis, they determined that renal calculi had a negative correlation with *Akkermansia* spp, *Faecalibacterium* spp, *Streptococcus* spp, and *Lactobacillus* spp, whereas *Phascolarctobacterium* spp, *Blautia* spp, *Lachnospiraceae*, and *Bacteroides* spp were positively correlated with urolithiasis. Ultimately, the investigators concluded that *Lactobacillus* spp contributed the most (76%) to reducing the risk of kidney stone disease. These 5 bacteria had an AUC of 0.871 and 95% confidence interval (CI) (0.785–0.957) for predicting patients with calcium oxalate kidney stone disease.

Additional analysis of short-chain fatty acid contents determined that urolithiasis was correlated with valeric acid positively and with propionic acid, acetic acid, and butyric acid negatively. These short-chain amino acids were associated with various bacteria such as the aforementioned *Roseburia* and *Megamonas*. Lastly, the investigators concluded that these variations in microbiota can be related to tea consumption and thus may represent an opportunity for effective intervention at normalizing gut microbiota.[96]

Cao and colleagues[97] analyzed the gut microbiomes of uric acid stone formers with and without gout and compared them with normal controls. They identified increased colonization of *Bacteroides* and *Fusobacterium* in patients with uric acid stones, identifying a correlation between the population of this bacteria and serum uric acid levels. These bacteria have been found to be proinflammatory.

SUMMARY

Biomarker research in urolithiasis represents an array of potential applications ranging from diagnosis and detection, assessment of risk of stone development, kidney injury, ureteral obstruction, postsurgical alterations, infection, and stone passage. Even with such potential utilities, biomarkers currently face limited adoption and use stemming from an incomplete understanding of their application in these settings and require further studies to better define their role in the evaluation and treatment of patients with kidney stone disease.

CLINICS CARE POINTS

- Biomarkers are underutialized in the evaluation of stone patients.-Some biomarkers which may be useful are included in the standard evaluation of stone patients while others are not.
- The future utilization of biomarkers may help in understanding various aspects of stone disease including risk of stone formation and recurrence, risk of infection related to stones, and risks of surgical procedures.

REFERENCES

1. Litwin MS, Saigal CS, Yano EM, et al. Urologic diseases in America Project: analytical methods and principal findings. J Urol 2005;173(3):933–7.
2. Fwu CW, Eggers PW, Kimmel PL, et al. Emergency department visits, use of imaging, and drugs for urolithiasis have increased in the United States. Kidney Int 2013;83(3):479–86.
3. Evan AP. Physiopathology and etiology of stone formation in the kidney and the urinary tract. Pediatr Nephrol 2010;25(5):831–41.
4. WHO International Programme on Chemical Safety. Biomarkers and risk assessment: concepts and principles. 1993. Available at: http://www.inchem.org/documents/ehc/ehc/ehc155.htm.
5. Ichimura T, Bonventre JV, Bailly V, et al. Kidney injury molecule-1 (KIM-1), a putative epithelial cell adhesion molecule containing a novel immunoglobulin domain, is up-regulated in renal cells after injury. J Biol Chem 1998;273(7):4135–42.
6. Han WK, Bailly V, Abichandani R, et al. Kidney Injury Molecule-1 (KIM-1): a novel biomarker for human renal proximal tubule injury. Kidney Int 2002;62(1):237–44.
7. Olvera-Posada D, Dayarathna T, Dion M, et al. KIM-1 is a potential urinary biomarker of obstruction: results from a prospective cohort study. J Endourol 2017;31(2):111–8.
8. Xie Y, Xue W, Shao X, et al. Analysis of a urinary biomarker panel for obstructive nephropathy and clinical outcomes. PLoS One 2014;9(11):e112865.
9. Xue W, Xie Y, Wang Q, et al. Diagnostic markers for acute kidney injury. Nephrology 2014;19:186–94.
10. Fahmy N, Sener A, Sabbisetti V, et al. Urinary expression of novel tissue markers of kidney injury after ureteroscopy, shockwave lithotripsy, and in normal healthy controls. J Endourol 2013;27(12):1455–62.
11. Urbschat A, Gauer S, Paulus P, et al. Serum and urinary NGAL but not KIM-1 raises in human postrenal AKI. Eur J Clin Invest 2014;44(7):652–9.

12. Balasar M, Pişkin MM, Topcu C, et al. Urinary kidney injury molecule-1 levels in renal stone patients. World J Urol 2016;34(9):1311–6.

13. Dieterle F, Sistare F, Goodsaid F, et al. Renal biomarker qualification submission: a dialog between the FDA-EMEA and Predictive Safety Testing Consortium. Nat Biotechnol 2010;28(5):455–62.

14. Devarajan P. Neutrophil gelatinase-associated lipocalin–an emerging troponin for kidney injury. Nephrol Dial Transpl 2008;23(12):3737–43.

15. Bolgeri M, Whiting D, Reche A, et al. Neutrophil gelatinase-associated lipocalin (NGAL) as a biomarker of renal injury in patients with ureteric stones: a pilot study. J Clin Urol 2021;14(1):21–8.

16. Hughes SF, Jones N, Thomas-Wright SJ, et al. Shock wave lithotripsy, for the treatment of kidney stones, results in changes to routine blood tests and novel biomarkers: a prospective clinical pilot-study. Eur J Med Res 2020;25(1):18.

17. Hughes SF, Moyes AJ, Lamb RM, et al. The role of specific biomarkers, as predictors of postoperative complications following flexible ureterorenoscopy (FURS), for the treatment of kidney stones: a single-centre observational clinical pilot-study in 37 patients. BMC Urol 2020;20(1):122.

18. Dede O, Dağguli M, Utanğaç M, et al. Urinary expression of acute kidney injury biomarkers in patients after RIRS: it is a prospective, controlled study. Int J Clin Exp Med 2015;8(5):8147–52.

19. Zhu W, Liu M, Wang GC, et al. Urinary neutrophil gelatinase-associated lipocalin, a biomarker for systemic inflammatory response syndrome in patients with nephrolithiasis. J Surg Res 2014;187(1):237–43.

20. Amini E, Pishgar F, Hojjat A, et al. The role of serum and urinary carbohydrate antigen 19-9 in predicting renal injury associated with ureteral stone. Ren Fail 2016;38(10):1626–32.

21. Aybek H, Aybek Z, Sinik Z, et al. Elevation of serum and urinary carbohydrate antigen 19-9 in benign hydronephrosis. Int J Urol 2006;13(11):1380–4.

22. Wellwood JM, Ellis BG, Price RG, et al. Urinary N-acetyl- beta-D-glucosaminidase activities in patients with renal disease. Br Med J 1975;3(5980):408–11.

23. Tenstad O, Roald AB, Grubb A, et al. Renal handling of radiolabelled human cystatin C in the rat. Scand J Clin Lab Invest 1996;56(5):409–14.

24. Hughes SF, Cotter MJ, Evans SA, et al. Role of leucocytes in damage to the vascular endothelium during ischaemia-reperfusion injury. Br J Biomed Sci 2006;63(4):166–70.

25. van der Veen BS, de Winther MP, Heeringa P. Myeloperoxidase: molecular mechanisms of action and their relevance to human health and disease. Antioxid Redox Signal 2009;11(11):2899–937.

26. Chawla LS, Seneff MG, Nelson DR, et al. Elevated plasma concentrations of IL-6 and elevated APACHE II score predict acute kidney injury in patients with severe sepsis. Clin J Am Soc Nephrol 2007;2(1):22–30.

27. Kwon O, Molitoris BA, Pescovitz M, et al. Urinary actin, interleukin-6, and interleukin-8 may predict sustained ARF after ischemic injury in renal allografts. Am J Kidney Dis 2003;41(5):1074–87.

28. Rao WH, Evans GS, Finn A. The significance of interleukin 8 in urine. Arch Dis Child 2001;85(3):256–62.

29. Sabat R, Grütz G, Warszawska K, et al. Biology of interleukin-10. Cytokine Growth Factor Rev 2010;21(5):331–44.

30. Rabinovich A, Medina L, Piura B, et al. Expression of IL-10 in human normal and cancerous ovarian tissues and cells. Eur Cytokine Netw 2010;21(2):122–8.

31. Faust J, Menke J, Kriegsmann J, et al. Correlation of renal tubular epithelial cell-derived interleukin-18 upregulation with disease activity in MRL-Faslpr mice with autoimmune lupus nephritis. Arthritis Rheum 2002;46(11):3083–95.

32. Parikh CR, Mishra J, Thiessen-Philbrook H, et al. Urinary IL-18 is an early predictive biomarker of acute kidney injury after cardiac surgery. Kidney Int 2006;70(1):199–203.

33. Chandrasekharan UM, Siemionow M, Unsal M, et al. Tumor necrosis factor alpha (TNF-alpha) receptor-II is required for TNF-alpha-induced leukocyte-endothelial interaction in vivo. Blood 2007;109(5):1938–44.

34. Tawfick A, Matboli M, Shamloul S, et al. Predictive urinary RNA biomarkers of kidney injury after extracorporeal shock wave lithotripsy. World J Urol 2022;40(6):1561–7.

35. Pearle MS, Goldfarb DS, Assimos DG, et al. Medical management of kidney stones: AUA guideline. J Urol 2014;192(2):316–24.

36. Cilesiz NC, Ozkan A, Kalkanli A, et al. Can serum procalcitonin levels be useful in predicting spontaneous ureteral stone passage? BMC Urol 2020;20(1):42.

37. Özcan C, Aydoğdu O, Senocak C, et al. Predictive factors for spontaneous stone passage and the potential role of serum c-reactive protein in patients with 4 to 10 mm distal ureteral stones: a prospective clinical study. J Urol 2015;194(4):1009–13.

38. Jain A, Sreenivasan SK, Manikandan R, et al. Association of spontaneous expulsion with C-reactive protein and other clinico-demographic factors in patients with lower ureteric stone. Urolithiasis 2020;48(2):117–22.

39. Aldaqadossi HA. Stone expulsion rate of small distal ureteric calculi could be predicted with plasma C-reactive protein. Urolithiasis 2013;41(3):235–9.

40. Ramasamy V, Aarthy P, Sharma V, et al. Role of inflammatory markers and their trends in predicting the outcome of medical expulsive therapy for distal ureteric calculus. Urol Ann 2022;14(1):8–14.

41. Abou Heidar N, Labban M, Bustros G, et al. Inflammatory serum markers predicting spontaneous

ureteral stone passage. Clin Exp Nephrol 2020; 24(3):277–83.

42. Peng JP, Zheng H. Kidney stones may increase the risk of coronary heart disease and stroke: A PRISMA-Compliant meta-analysis. Medicine (Baltimore) 2017;96(34):e7898.

43. Liu Y, Li S, Zeng Z, et al. Kidney stones and cardiovascular risk: a meta-analysis of cohort studies. Am J Kidney Dis 2014;64(3):402–10.

44. Cheungpasitporn W, Thongprayoon C, Mao MA, et al. The risk of coronary heart disease in patients with kidney stones: a systematic review and meta-analysis. N Am J Med Sci 2014;6(11):580–5.

45. Bargagli M, Moochhala S, Robertson WG, et al. Urinary metabolic profile and stone composition in kidney stone formers with and without heart disease. J Nephrol 2022;35(3):851–7.

46. Shoag J, Eisner BH. Relationship between C-reactive protein and kidney stone prevalence. J Urol 2014;191(2):372–5.

47. Qin Z, Zhao J, Geng J, et al. Higher Triglyceride-Glucose Index Is Associated With Increased Likelihood of Kidney Stones. Front Endocrinol (Lausanne) 2021;12:774567.

48. Okada A, Nomura S, Saeki Y, et al. Morphological conversion of calcium oxalate crystals into stones is regulated by osteopontin in mouse kidney. J Bone Miner Res 2008;23(10):1629–37.

49. Siener R, Glatz S, Nicolay C, et al. The role of overweight and obesity in calcium oxalate stone formation. Obes Res 2004;12(1):106–13.

50. Mansour A, Aboeerad M, Qorbani M, et al. Association between low bone mass and the serum RANKL and OPG in patients with nephrolithiasis. BMC Nephrol 2018;19(1):172.

51. Icer MA, Gezmen-Karadag M, Sozen S. Can urine osteopontin levels, which may be correlated with nutrition intake and body composition, be used as a new biomarker in the diagnosis of nephrolithiasis? Clin Biochem 2018;60:38–43.

52. Khan A. Prevalence, pathophysiological mechanisms and factors affecting urolithiasis. Int Urol Nephrol 2018;50(5):799–806.

53. Price PA, Urist MR, Otawara Y. Matrix Gla protein, a new gamma-carboxyglutamic acid-containing protein which is associated with the organic matrix of bone. Biochem Biophys Res Commun 1983;117(3): 765–71.

54. Luo G, Ducy P, McKee MD, et al. Spontaneous calcification of arteries and cartilage in mice lacking matrix GLA protein. Nature 1997;386(6620):78–81.

55. Castiglione V, Pottel H, Lieske JC, et al. Evaluation of inactive Matrix-Gla-Protein (MGP) as a biomarker for incident and recurrent kidney stones. J Nephrol 2020;33(1):101–7.

56. Goldberg H, Grass L, Vogl R, et al. Urine citrate and renal stone disease. CMAJ 1989;141(3):217–21.

57. Rose GA, Sulaiman S. Tamm-Horsfall mucoproteins promote calcium oxalate crystal formation in urine: quantitative studies. J Urol 1982;127(1):177–9.

58. Noonin C, Peerapen P, Yoodee S, et al. Systematic analysis of modulating activities of native human urinary Tamm-Horsfall protein on calcium oxalate crystallization, growth, aggregation, crystal-cell adhesion and invasion through extracellular matrix. Chem Biol Interact 2022;357:109879.

59. Hess B. Tamm-Horsfall glycoprotein–inhibitor or promoter of calcium oxalate monohydrate crystallization processes? Urol Res 1992;20(1):83–6.

60. Doyle IR, Ryall RL, Marshall VR. Inclusion of proteins into calcium oxalate crystals precipitated from human urine: a highly selective phenomenon. Clin Chem 1991;37(9):1589–94.

61. Webber D, Rodgers A, Sturrock E. Synergism between Urinary Prothrombin Fragment 1 and Urine: a comparison of inhibitory activities in stone-prone and stone-free population groups. Clin Chem Lab Med 2002;40(9):930–6.

62. Kovacevic L, Lu H, Kovacevic N, et al. Cystatin C, Neutrophil gelatinase-associated lipocalin, and lysozyme C: urinary biomarkers for detection of early kidney dysfunction in children with urolithiasis. Urology 2020;143:221–6.

63. Fan X, Ye W, Ma J, et al. Metabolic differences between unilateral and bilateral renal stones and their association with markers of kidney injury. J Urol 2022;207(1):144–51.

64. Cadieux PA, Beiko DT, Watterson JD, et al. Surface-enhanced laser desorption/ionization-time of flight-mass spectrometry (SELDI-TOF-MS): a new proteomic urinary test for patients with urolithiasis. J Clin Lab Anal 2004;18(3):170–5.

65. Zhu W, Liu M, Wang GC, et al. Fibrinogen alpha chain precursor and apolipoprotein A-I in urine as biomarkers for noninvasive diagnosis of calcium oxalate nephrolithiasis: a proteomics study. Biomed Res Int 2014;2014:415651.

66. Wang X, Wang M, Ruan J, et al. Identification of urine biomarkers for calcium-oxalate urolithiasis in adults based on UPLC-Q-TOF/MS. J Chromatogr B Analyt Technol Biomed Life Sci 2019;1124: 290–7.

67. Duan X, Zhang T, Ou L, et al. 1H NMR-based metabolomic study of metabolic profiling for the urine of kidney stone patients. Urolithiasis 2020;48:27–35.

68. Primiano A, Persichilli S, Ferraro PM, et al. A specific urinary amino acid profile characterizes people with kidney stones. Dis Markers 2020;2020:1–7.

69. Khan SR, Pearle MS, Robertson WG, et al. Kidney stones. Nat Rev Dis Primers 2016;2:16008.

70. Taranets YV. Institute for Single Crystals, STC "Institute for Single Crystals", National Academy of Sciences of Ukraine, 60 Nauky Ave., 61001 Kharkiv, Ukraine. Crystallization kinetics of calcium oxalate

monohydrate in he presence of amino acids. FunctMater 2018;25(2):381–5.

71. Taranets YV, Bezkrovnaya ON, Pritula IM, et al. L-threonine amino acid as a promoter of the growth of pathogenic calcium oxalate monohydrate crystals. J Nanomater Mol Nanotechnol 2017;6(5). https://doi.org/10.4172/2324-8777.1000229.

72. Gao S, Yang R, Peng Z, et al. Metabolomics analysis for hydroxy-L-proline-induced calcium oxalate nephrolithiasis in rats based on ultra-high performance liquid chromatography quadrupole time-of-flight mass spectrometry. Sci Rep 2016;6:30142.

73. Wen J, Cao Y, Li Y, et al. Metabolomics analysis of the serum from children with urolithiasis using UPLC-MS. Clin Transl Sci 2021;14(4):1327–37.

74. Michel MS, Trojan L, Rassweiler JJ. Complications in percutaneous nephrolithotomy. Eur Urol 2007;51(4):899–906.

75. de Martino M, Pantuck AJ, Hofbauer S, et al. Prognostic impact of preoperative neutrophil-to-lymphocyte ratio in localized nonclear cell renal cell carcinoma. J Urol 2013;190(6):1999–2004.

76. Kriplani A, Pandit S, Chawla A, et al. Neutrophil-lymphocyte ratio (NLR), platelet-lymphocyte ratio (PLR) and lymphocyte-monocyte ratio (LMR) in predicting systemic inflammatory response syndrome (SIRS) and sepsis after percutaneous nephrolithotomy (PNL). Urolithiasis 2022;50(3):341–8.

77. Qi T, Lai C, Li Y, et al. The predictive and diagnostic ability of IL-6 for postoperative urosepsis in patients undergoing percutaneous nephrolithotomy. Urolithiasis 2021;49(4):367–75.

78. Zheng J, Li Q, Fu W, et al. Procalcitonin as an early diagnostic and monitoring tool in urosepsis following percutaneous nephrolithotomy. Urolithiasis 2015;43(1):41–7.

79. Liu M, Zhu Z, Cui Y, et al. The value of procalcitonin for predicting urosepsis after mini-percutaneous nephrolithotomy or flexible ureteroscopy based on different organisms. World J Urol 2022;40(2):529–35.

80. Luo X, Yang X, Li J, et al. The procalcitonin/albumin ratio as an early diagnostic predictor in discriminating urosepsis from patients with febrile urinary tract infection. Medicine (Baltimore) 2018;97(28):e11078.

81. Qiao Y, Liu G, Zhou W, et al. The rs13347 Polymorphism of the CD44 Gene Is Associated with the Risk of Kidney Stones Disease in the Chinese Han Population of Northeast Sichuan, China. Comput Math Methods Med 2022;2022(Article ID 6481260):6.

82. Jabalameli MR, Fitzpatrick FM, Colombo R, et al. Exome sequencing identifies a disease variant of the mitochondrial ATP-Mg/Pi carrier SLC25A25 in two families with kidney stones. Mol Genet Genomic Med 2021;9(12):e1749.

83. Liu CC, Wu CF, Lee YC, et al. Genetic Polymorphisms of MnSOD Modify the Impacts of Environmental Melamine on Oxidative Stress and Early Kidney Injury in Calcium Urolithiasis Patients. Antioxidants (Basel) 2022;11(1):152.

84. Mehdi WA, Mehde AA, Raus RA, et al. Genetic polymorphisms of human transcription factor-7 like 2 (TCF7L2), β-defensin (DEFB1) and CD14 genes in nephrolithiasis patients. Int J Biol Macromol 2018;118(Pt A):610–6.

85. Liang X, Lai Y, Wu W, et al. LncRNA-miRNA-mRNA expression variation profile in the urine of calcium oxalate stone patients. BMC Med Genomics 2019;12(1):57.

86. Halbritter J, Baum M, Hynes AM, et al. Fourteen monogenic genes account for 15% of nephrolithiasis/nephrocalcinosis. J Am Soc Nephrol 2015;26(3):543–51.

87. Siva S, Barrack ER, Reddy GP, et al. A critical analysis of the role of gut Oxalobacter formigenes in oxalate stone disease. BJU Int 2009;103(1):18–21.

88. Kaufman DW, Kelly JP, Curhan GC, et al. Oxalobacter formigenes may reduce the risk of calcium oxalate kidney stones. J Am Soc Nephrol 2008;19(6):1197–203.

89. Kumar R, Mukherjee M, Bhandari M, et al. Role of Oxalobacter formigenes in calcium oxalate stone disease: a study from North India. Eur Urol 2002;41(3):318–22.

90. Abratt VR, Reid SJ. Oxalate-degrading bacteria of the human gut as probiotics in the management of kidney stone disease. Adv Appl Microbiol 2010;72:63–87.

91. Miller AW, Dearing D. The metabolic and ecological interactions of oxalate-degrading bacteria in the Mammalian gut. Pathogens 2013;2(4):636–52.

92. Tavasoli S, Alebouyeh M, Naji M, et al. Association of intestinal oxalate-degrading bacteria with recurrent calcium kidney stone formation and hyperoxaluria: a case-control study. BJU Int 2020;125(1):133–43.

93. Ticinesi A, Milani C, Guerra A, et al. Understanding the gut-kidney axis in nephrolithiasis: an analysis of the gut microbiota composition and functionality of stone formers. Gut 2018;67(12):2097–106.

94. Jiang S, Xie S, Lv D, et al. Alteration of the gut microbiota in Chinese population with chronic kidney disease. Sci Rep 2017;7(1):2870.

95. Tang R, Jiang Y, Tan A, et al. 16S rRNA gene sequencing reveals altered composition of gut microbiota in individuals with kidney stones. Urolithiasis 2018;46(6):503–14.

96. Chen F, Bao X, Liu S, et al. Gut microbiota affect the formation of calcium oxalate renal calculi caused by high daily tea consumption. Appl Microbiol Biotechnol 2021;105:789–802.

97. Cao C, Fan B, Zhu J, et al. Association of gut microbiota and biochemical features in a chinese population with renal uric acid stone. Front Pharmacol 2022;13:888883.

Biomarkers in Urethral Stricture Disease and Benign Lower Urinary Tract Disease

Jack G. Campbell, MD, Joshua P. Hayden, MD, Alex J. Vanni, MD*

KEYWORDS

- Biomarkers • Urethral stricture • Lichen sclerosus • Benign prostatic hyperplasia
- Bladder outlet obstruction • Overactive bladder

KEY POINTS

- Hypogonadism plays a significant role in urethral hypervascularity and therefore hold promise for future biomarker discovery in urethral stricture disease.
- Lichen sclerosus (LS) and non-LS related urethral stricture disease (USD) appear to have significantly different biomarker expression.
- Numerous inflammatory biomarkers are elevated in Benign Prostatic Hyperplasia (BPH), however a lack of specificity limits their clinical use.

INTRODUCTION

Increased understanding of molecular pathophysiology has led to the detection of clinically applicable biomarkers across medicine, which allow for minimally invasive detection, management, and monitoring of disease processes. Although biomarkers have traditionally played a more significant role in malignancy, these goals also pertain to benign disease. Herein, we review the ongoing research of biomarker application in urethral stricture disease (USD), benign prostatic hyperplasia (BPH), bladder outlet obstruction (BOO), and overactive bladder (OAB).

Urethral Stricture Disease

The incidence of USD in men is approximately 0.6% in the United States.[1] USD cause is variable including idiopathic, iatrogenic, infectious, lichen sclerosus (LS), radiation, and previous hypospadias, with idiopathic strictures accounting for approximately 63% of all USD.[2] The heterogeneous nature of USD has been a barrier to

understanding the underlying pathophysiology; however, recent investigation into the roles of hypogonadism and inflammation has identified pathways, which could be targets for biomarker identification. There is also promising research into LS USD In both tissue studies and the urinary microbiome, which have implications for biomarker discovery in the future.

Hypogonadism

Hypogonadism is not a specific marker for USD; however, recent studies demonstrate a key role for testosterone and the androgen receptor in urethral vascularity and overall health. In 2016,[3] identified hypogonadism in 18/20 (90%) of men with artificial urinary sphincter (AUS) cuff erosion.[3] In this study, hypogonadism was an independent risk factor for cuff erosion even when accounting for prior AUS, radiation, androgen deprivation therapy, and concomitant penile implant. Subsequent studies confirm hypogonadism in nearly half (45%) of all men undergoing AUS placement[4] and an odds ratio of 2.519 (P = .021) for AUS cuff

Division of Urology, Lahey Hospital and Medical Center, 41 Mall Road, Burlington, MA 01805, USA
* Corresponding author
E-mail address: alex.j.vanni@lahey.org

Urol Clin N Am 50 (2023) 31–38
https://doi.org/10.1016/j.ucl.2022.09.001
0094-0143/23/© 2022 Published by Elsevier Inc.

erosion in hypogonadal versus eugonadal men.[5] Additionally, hypogonadism has been identified in 45% to 57% of men with history of USD.[6,7] In fact,[7] detected increased severity of USD in hypogonadal men, with a mean stricture length of 7.2 versus 4.8 cm for eugonadal men.

Considered together, studies on hypogonadism in AUS cuff erosion and USD highlight the importance of testosterone in urethral vascularity. Androgen-induced angiogenesis occurs via vascular endothelial growth factor (VEGF), angiopoietin, and a downstream androgen receptor TIE-2,[8] and this mechanism has recently been highlighted in USD.[6] Hofer et al evaluated 5 hypogonadal men and 6 eugonadal men with history of urethroplasty, and compared the immunohistochemical expression of AR, TIE-2, and blood vessel counts. Hypogonadal men were found to have a significantly lower expression of AR, TIE-2, and overall vessel counts, and the expression levels of AR and TIE-2 were directly correlated with serum testosterone levels.[6] These findings suggest that hypogonadism leads to decreased periurethral vascularity through the AR–TIE-2 pathway. Testosterone supplementation has been shown to improve periurethral vascularity in rats at autopsy and in rats undergoing urethroplasty[9,10]; however further study is necessary in human subjects to determine if this would be a beneficial treatment modality.

Systemic Inflammation

Systemic inflammation is also thought to play a role in USD pathophysiology. Recently, neutrophil to lymphocyte ratio (NLR) and platelet to lymphocyte ratio (PLR) have emerged as biomarkers of systemic inflammation associated with poor prognosis in both malignant and benign disease.[11,12] Studies have evaluated the prognostic value of NLR and PLR in USD but with mixed results.[13] Urkmez and colleagues evaluated 512 patients who underwent direct vision internal urethrotomy for USD from 2010 to 2018 and identified a significantly higher median NLR in patients with recurrent USD compared with those without recurrence.[13] The authors concluded that patients with a higher NLR value may be better served by urethroplasty rather than repeat endoscopic treatments. Interestingly, these authors did not observe a difference in NLR for patients with or without stricture recurrence following urethroplasty.[14]

Inflammation is also implicated in the development of iatrogenic USD. This accounts for 13% of bulbar USD and 23% of penile USD according to a recent multi-institutional study.[2] The incidence of USD after transurethral resection of the prostate (TURP) is 1% to 6%,[15,16] representing a significant disease burden given the prevalence of BPH. Although inflammation after TURP may be significant, multiple studies suggest preoperative inflammation is also higher in patients who ultimately go on to develop USD after TURP.[17–19] Histopathology of resected TURP specimens show increased inflammatory cells in periurethral, stromal, and periglandular areas in patients who develop USD compared with controls.[17] Additionally, higher preoperative white blood cell count and PLR have both been associated with a higher risk of USD after TURP.[18,19] Although future study is necessary to find sensitive and specific biomarkers for this process, reduction of inflammation after TURP with postoperative Cox-2 inhibitor administration has been shown to decrease the risk of subsequent USD (0% vs 17%, $P = .0039$).[20]

Lichen Sclerosus Urethral Stricture Disease

The prevalence of genital LS is approximately 70 per 100,000[21] and up to 30% will develop USD.[22] Surgical management carries a higher rate of failure than other causes of USD,[23] and the most severe cases may require urinary diversion.[24] The pathophysiology of LS is believed to be multifactorial, including genetic predisposition,[25] autoimmunity,[26] and systemic inflammation.[23] Erickson and colleagues identified an association with higher body mass index, hypertension, and active tobacco use, and proposed a 2-hit mechanism for the development of LS, which emphasizes the importance of both local and systemic factors.[23] Recently, tissue microarray studies and investigation into the urinary microbiome have revealed differences between LS and non-LS USD, which is promising for future biomarker identification.

Levy and colleagues evaluated protein expression in LS USD versus non-LS USD and identified a higher proportion of T lymphocytes and expression of the inflammatory Chemokine C-C Motif Ligand 4 (CCL-4) in LS USD.[27] Epstein-Barr Virus (EBV) RNA, p16, and identified a higher proportion of T lymphocytes and expression of the inflammatory chemokine CCL-4 in LS USD.[27] EBV RNA, p16, and varicella zoster virus were also found in significantly more LS USD, suggesting a possible infectious cause. Subsequently, authors at the same institution evaluated microRNA expression profiles and found 15 total microRNAs differentially expressed in LS USD, which offer the potential to serve as tissue biomarkers for LS USD.[28] MiR-155-5p is a microRNA involved in fibroblast proliferation,[29] which was upregulated 11-fold in

LS USD. Overall, most differentially expressed miRNAs are involved with angiogenesis, fibrosis, and immune responses. There also seems to be heterogeneity within LS USD, which affects the likelihood of successful urethroplasty.[30] Levy and colleagues evaluated stricture tissue from patients with LS who had undergone urethroplasty and found decreased Ki-67 mitotic index, decreased expression of inflammatory markers C-Reactive Protein (CRP), Interleukin 1β (IL-1β), and Tumor Necrosis Factor α (TNF-α), and increased VEGF expression in LS USD, which recurred after urethroplasty.[30]

The urinary microbiome is another area of promise for finding future biomarkers in USD and specifically LS USD.[31] Cohen and colleagues recently identified a unique urinary microbiome profile for men with LS USD.[31] The urine of men with LS-USD revealed significantly more Bacillales, Bacteroidales, and Pasteurellales. The significance of these specific orders of bacteria is currently unknown; however, a urinary profile for LS USD would be useful because it could avoid the necessity for tissue biopsy for diagnosis and potentially serve as a biomarker for the risk of future cancer development.[32]

Because many causes of USD are understood at a deeper molecular level, opportunities to identify biomarkers in blood and urine will undoubtedly expand.

Benign Prostatic Hyperplasia and Bladder Outlet Obstruction

BPH affects approximately 70% of men aged 60 to 69 years and 80% of men aged 70 years or older.[33] Progression of BPH results in BOO and lower urinary tract symptoms (LUTSs), and the prevalence of male LUTS increases approximately 10% per decade from 40 years to 79 years of age.[34] Given this widespread prevalence, it is advantageous to identify minimally invasive means of BPH diagnosis and monitoring. Although specific biomarkers are not yet in clinical use, numerous molecules have been investigated in BPH/BOO as potential biomarkers in both blood and urine. Herein, we separate the discussion into biomarkers based on inflammation and noninflammatory pathways.

Inflammation

There is no consensus on the exact mechanism of BPH development and progression; however, it has been widely demonstrated that BPH nodules frequently involve chronic inflammatory infiltrates of activated T lymphocytes.[35,36] Activated T lymphocytes produce inflammatory cytokines that promote the proliferation of prostatic epithelial cell lines.[37] These cytokines also damage surrounding cells, leaving space to be filled by fibromuscular nodules.[38] Inflammatory infiltrates have been associated with larger prostate volume and LUTS progression in both the Medical Therapies of Prostate Symptoms trial[39] and the Reduction by Dutasteride of Prostate Cancer Events trial.[40]

The multiple inflammatory pathways involved in the inflammatory model of BPH provide numerous potential biomarkers. C-C motif chemokine ligand 1 (CCL1) is one potential biomarker and can be easily measured in human serum. CCL1 is produced by activated T-cells in the prostatic microenvironment[41,42] and serves as a ligand for G-protein coupled receptor CCR8.[43] Elevated CCL1 levels have been observed in the serum of men with BPH[44] and in the seminal plasma from patients with BPH,[45] so it may represent a serum marker for T lymphocele expansion, proliferation of prostatic epithelial cells, and ultimately symptomatic BPH.

From a more general inflammatory framework, IL-6, IL-8, and TNF-α serve as widely studied markers of systemic inflammation and are known to be secreted by T lymphocytes in the prostatic stroma.[37] Milasheuski et al[46] detected a statistically significant difference in serum levels of IL-6, IL-8, and TNF-α in men with BPH compared with controls without BPH ($P = .02$). Additionally, IL-8 and TNF-α were also found to be higher in patients who experienced progression of BPH. An association between higher IL-6 levels and LUTS severity was detected in the Prostate Cancer Prevention Trial[47]; however, [48] it did not identify any association between prostate size or LUTS severity with IL-6, IL-8, TNF-α, and IL-1β.[48] In fact, in this study, the authors actually observed a trend toward higher IL-6 and IL-1β levels with lower LUTS severity.

Markers of systemic inflammation such as TNF-α, TGF-β, and most interleukins are also easily detected in urine,[49] and therefore, they have also been studied as urinary biomarkers. TGF-β represents the most promising molecule, although human data is minimal to date.[50] Kim and colleagues identified increased mRNA expression of TGF-β in the urine of rats with a model of severe BOO ($P < .05$),[50] and there is evidence that urinary TGF-β levels increase with the duration of BOO.[51] Shi and colleagues observed a negative correlation between detrusor contractility in rats and levels of urinary TGF-β, suggesting that higher levels of TGF-β may signal new bladder fibrosis resulting from BOO.[51] There is only one study on urinary TGF-β in human subjects.[52] The authors evaluated 23 men with LUTS using noninvasive uroflowmetry, cystometrogram, and voiding pressure flow studies, and observed a strong correlation between urinary TGF-β levels and BOO defined by the Abrams-Griffith nomogram ($P = .025$).[52]

Noninflammation

Biomarkers for BPH/BOO independent of inflammation include markers of oxidative stress, prostate specific antigen (PSA), adenosine triphosphate, and neurotrophins. Markers of oxidative stress also play a role in the pathophysiology of BPH/BOO. BPH/BOO causes oxidative stress that leads to free radial production and direct bladder injury.[53,54] Oxidative damage can be detected in the plasma and urine of obstructed rabbits as 8-OhdG and plasma malondialdehyde,[55] and these authors have demonstrated that levels of these markers will return to normal after surgical unobstruction.[56] Another marker of oxidative stress is F2-isoprostane (F2iP), which measures in vivo lipid peroxidation, and elevated levels of F2iP have been detected in bladder tissue samples of mice with BOO,[57] although not specifically in urine. Finally, PGE2/PGE-M is a marker of oxidative stress via cyclo-oxygenase (COX) activity, which has been detected as increased levels in the urine of men with BPH.[48]

PSA is likely the most-studied biomarker in all of urology given the role in prostate cancer screening. Despite this primary use, it is clear that PSA functions as a biomarker for BPH and specifically for prostate size.[58–60] In fact,[58] authors identified good predictive value for PSA for assessing prostate size (Receiver operating curve analyses 0.76–0.78) in an analysis of previous trial data including 4627 total men.[58] Similarly, the Baltimore Longitudinal Study of Aging observed that for men aged 60 to 69 years, the 10-year probability of freedom from prostate enlargement was 83% with PSA less than 1.7 ng/mL but decreased to 27% with PSA greater than 1.7 ng/mL.[59] Therefore, although the decision to obtain a PSA level will likely remain one primarily relating to prostate cancer screening,[61] it is also important to recognize the relationship between PSA and BPH.

Another potential noninflammatory biomarker for BPH/BOO is adenosine triphosphate (ATP). ATP is released by urothelium in response to stretch and other stimuli.[62] It is preferentially released in higher amounts on the luminal side of urothelial cells leading to its accumulation within the urine[63,64] The authors demonstrated that urothelial strips from patients with BPH release more ATP into the urine than non-BPH controls[64]; however, the role as a biomarker for BPH/BOO may be limited as it seems to be relatively nonspecific and

is often elevated in cases of urinary tract infection.[65]

The final noninflammatory biomarker for BPH/BOO is nerve growth factor (NGF). NGF is a neurotrophin, which is a class of tissue-derived NGFs secreted by both smooth muscle and urothelium in the bladder thought to be important for neuronal survival.[66] NGF is involved in the micturition pathway,[67] and higher levels of bladder tissue NGF have been observed in BOO-associated detrusor overactivity (DO), neurogenic DO, mixed stress and urge incontinence, diabetic cystopathy, and bladder inflammation/cystitis.[68,69] Studies focusing on urinary detection of NGF in regards to BPH and BOO are more limited.[70] The authors have demonstrated higher urinary NGF levels in male patients with BOO and also observed that urinary NGF levels return to normal after successful medical treatment of overactivity symptoms in patients with both BOO and DO.[70] Similarly,[71] observed decreased urinary NGF levels after treatment of BPH/BOO with dutasteride.[71] In this study, the decrease in urinary NGF correlated with change in prostatic volume.

In summary, although there is a lack of specificity in potential biomarkers for BPH/BOO, there are numerous targets for future study. Opportunities will only increase as the understanding of the underlying pathophysiology deepens.

Overactive Bladder

OAB is a clinical diagnosis characterized by LUTS such as urinary urgency, urge urinary incontinence, urinary frequency, and nocturia. The prevalence of patients with OAB ranges from 27% to 43%, and it is estimated to affect around 29.8 million adults aged older than 40 years.[72] The pathophysiology of OAB likely involves a complex interplay of multiple processes including urothelium signaling, aberrant signaling from the urethra, metabolic syndrome, sex hormone deficiency, and autonomic nervous system dysfunction.[73] There is significant overlap with biomarker study in BPH/BOO, specifically with ATP and NGF.

ATP mediates pathologic detrusor contractions in OVBs.[74] Higher urinary ATP has been observed in women with OAB compared with healthy controls,[74] and there also seems to be a correlation between urinary ATP levels and OAB severity.[75] Additionally, higher levels of urinary ATP may predict an enhanced response to antimuscarinic agents when used to treat OAB.[76]

The potential utility of NGF as a biomarker for OAB is highlighted by a recent systematic review and meta-analysis, which identified 12 total studies comparing women with OAB and controls.[77] The authors concluded that urinary NGF and NGF to creatinine ratio could both be potentially useful as diagnostic and management tools in women with OAB based on a standard mean difference of 1.45 and 1.23, respectively. Data is mixed regarding what effect OAB treatment has on levels of urinary NGF. Normalization of urinary NGF levels has been observed after treating patients with OAB with antimuscarinic agents and botulinum toxin.[78] In contrast, the authors failed to identify any predictive value for NGF or brain-derived neurotrophic factor regarding which of 90 total patients with OAB would respond to 1 month of solifenacin treatment.[79] Although no biomarkers for OAB are in clinical use, further investigation is warranted as future biomarkers could potentially fill the role of more invasive urodynamic testing.

SUMMARY

In spite of a significant amount of research, there are currently no clinically used biomarkers for benign lower urinary tract disease. However, as our understanding of the underlying pathophysiology progresses, there will be increasingly numerous opportunities for biomarker identification, which will help reduce the morbidity of diagnosis, management, and monitoring of benign lower urinary tract disease.

CLINICS CARE POINTS

- There is evidence that preoperative inflammation independent of transurethral resection of the prostate (TURP) increases the risk of urethral stricture disease (USD) after transurethral resection of the prostate (TURP).
- It is important to remember that while PSA is used for prostate cancer screening, it is a relatively accurate marker of prostate size and BPH.
- ATP and Nerve Growth Factor (NGF) are linked to both BPH and Overactive Bladder (OAB), and there is promise that NGF levels may assist in monitoring successful OAB Therapy.
- No biomarkers are currently in clinical use for benign lower urinary tract disease.

DISCLOSURE

The authors have no commercial or financial conflicts of interest to disclose.

REFERENCES

1. Santucci R, Joyce G, Wise M, et al. Male urethral stricture disease. J Urol 2007;177(5):1667–74.
2. Cotter K, Hahn A, Voelzke B, et al. Trends in urethral stricture disease etiology and urethroplasty technique from a multi-institutional surgical outcomes research group. Urology 2019;130:167–74.
3. Hofer M, Morey A, Sheth K, et al. Low serum testosterone level predisposes to artificial urinary sphincter cuff erosion. Urology 2016;97:245–9.
4. McKibben M, Fuentes J, Shakir N, et al. Low serum testosterone is present in nearly half of men undergoing artificial urinary sphincter placement. Urology 2018;118:208–12.
5. Wolfe A, Ortiz N, Baumgarten A, et al. Most men with artificial urinary sphincter cuff erosion have low serum testosterone levels. Neurourol Urodyn 2021; 40(4):1035–41.
6. Hofer M, Kapur P, Cordon B, et al. Low testosterone levels result in decreased periurethral vascularity via an androgen receptor-mediated process: pilot study in urethral stricture tissue. Urology 2017;105:175–80.
7. Spencer J, Mahon J, Daugherty M, et al. Hypoandrogenism is prevalent in males with urethral stricture disease and is associated with longer strictures. Urology 2018;114:218–23.
8. Johansson A, Rudolfsson S, Wikström P, et al. Altered levels of angiopoietin 1 and tie 2 are associated with androgen-regulated vascular regression and growth in the ventral prostate in adult mice and rats. Endocrinology 2005;146(8):3463–70.
9. Yura E, Bury M, Chan Y, et al. Reversing urethral hypovascularity through testosterone and estrogen supplementation. Urology 2020;146:242–7.
10. Gerbie E, Bury M, Chan Y, et al. Testosterone and Estrogen Repletion in a Hypogonadal Environment Improves Post-operative Angiogenesis. Urology 2021;152:9–e11.
11. Luo H, He L, Zhang G, et al. Normal reference intervals of neutrophil-to-lymphocyte ratio, platelet-to-lymphocyte ratio, lymphocyte-to-monocyte ratio, and systemic immune inflammation index in healthy adults: a large multi-center study from Western China. Clin Lab 2019;65(3):255–65.
12. Gasparyan A, Ayvazyan L, Mukanova U, et al. The platelet-to-lymphocyte ratio as an inflammatory marker in rheumatic diseases. Ann Lab Med 2019; 39(4):345–57.
13. Urkmez A, Topaktas R, Ozsoy E, et al. Is neutrophil to lymphocyte ratio a predictive factor for recurrence of urethral stricture? Rev Assoc Med Bras 2020;65: 1448–53.
14. Topaktaş R, Ürkmez A, Tokuç E, et al. Hematologic parameters and neutrophil/lymphocyte ratio in the prediction of urethroplasty success. Int Braz J Urol 2019;45:369–75.

15. Autorino R, Damiano R, Di Lorenzo G, et al. Four-year outcome of a prospective randomised trial comparing bipolar plasmakinetic and monopolar transurethral resection of the prostate. Eur Urol 2009;55(4):922–31.

16. Michielsen D, Coomans D. Urethral strictures and bipolar transurethral resection in saline of the prostate: fact or fiction? J Endourol 2010;24(8):1333–7.

17. Aydın A, Oltulu P, Balasar M, et al. The role of prostate inflammation in the pathogenesis of urethral strictures occurring after transurethral resections. Rev Int Androl 2022;20(2):86–95.

18. Afandiyev F, Ugurlu O. Factors predicting the development of urethral stricture after bipolar transurethral resection of the prostate. Rev Assoc Med Bras 2022;68:50–5.

19. Gül M, Altıntaş E, Kaynar M, et al. The predictive value of platelet to lymphocyte and neutrophil to lymphocyte ratio in determining urethral stricture after transurethral resection of prostate. Turk J Urol 2017;43(3):325.

20. Sciarra A, Salciccia S, Albanesi L, et al. Use of cyclooxygenase-2 inhibitor for prevention of urethral strictures secondary to transurethral resection of the prostate. Urology 2005;66(6):1218–22.

21. Nelson D, Peterson A. Lichen sclerosus: epidemiological distribution in an equal access health care system. J Urol 2011;185(2):522–5.

22. Kulkarni S, Barbagli G, Kirpekar D. Lichen sclerosus of the male genitalia and urethra: surgical options and results in a multicenter international experience with 215 patients. Eur Urol 2009; 55(4):945–56.

23. Erickson B, Elliott S, Myers J, et al. Understanding the relationship between chronic systemic disease and lichen sclerosus urethral strictures. J Urol 2016;195(2):363–8.

24. Peterson A, Palminteri E, Lazzeri M, et al. Heroic measures may not always be justified in extensive urethral stricture due to lichen sclerosus (balanitis xerotica obliterans). Urology 2004;64(3):565–8.

25. Sherman V, McPherson T, Baldo M, et al. The high rate of familial lichen sclerosus suggests a genetic contribution: an observational cohort study. J Eur Acad Dermatol Venereol 2010;24(9):1031–4.

26. Oyama N, Chan I, Neill S, et al. Autoantibodies to extracellular matrix protein 1 in lichen sclerosus. Lancet 2003;362(9378):118–23.

27. Levy A, Browne B, Fredrick A, et al. Insights into the pathophysiology of urethral stricture disease due to lichen sclerosus: comparison of pathological markers in lichen sclerosus induced strictures vs nonlichen sclerosus induced strictures. J Urol 2019;201(6):1158–63.

28. Kohli H, Childs B, Sullivan TB, et al. Differential expression of miRNAs involved in biological processes responsible for inflammation and immune response in lichen sclerosus urethral stricture disease. PLoS One 2021;16(12):e0261505. https://doi.org/10.1371/journal.pone.0261505.

29. Ren L, Zhao Y, Huo X, et al. MiR-155-5p promotes fibroblast cell proliferation and inhibits FOXO signaling pathway in vulvar lichen sclerosis by targeting FOXO3 and CDKN1B. Gene 2018;653: 43–50.

30. Levy A, Moynihan M, Bennett J, et al. Protein Expression Profiles among Lichen Sclerosus Urethral Strictures—Can Urethroplasty Success be Predicted? J Urol 2020;203(4):773–8.

31. Cohen A, Gaither T, Srirangapatanam S, et al. Synchronous genitourinary lichen sclerosus signals a distinct urinary microbiome profile in men with urethral stricture disease. World J Urol 2021;39(2): 605–11.

32. Sfanos K, Yegnasubramanian S, Nelson W, et al. The inflammatory microenvironment and microbiome in prostate cancer development. Nat Rev Urol 2018; 15(1):11–24. BPH and BOO.

33. Wei J, Calhoun E, Jacobsen S. Urologic diseases in America project: benign prostatic hyperplasia. J Urol 2005;173(4):1256–61.

34. Boyle P, Robertson C, Mazzetta C, et al. The prevalence of lower urinary tract symptoms in men and women in four centres. The UrEpik study. BJU Int 2003;92(4):409–14.

35. Kramer G, Marberger M. Could inflammation be a key component in the progression of benign prostatic hyperplasia? Cur Opin Urol 2006;16(1):25–9.

36. Kramer G, Mitteregger D, Marberger M. Is benign prostatic hyperplasia (BPH) an immune inflammatory disease? Eur Urol 2007;51(5):1202–16.

37. McDowell K, Begley L, Mor-Vaknin N, et al. Leukocytic promotion of prostate cellular proliferation. Prostate 2010;70(4):377–89.

38. Steiner G, Stix U, Handisurya A, et al. Cytokine expression pattern in benign prostatic hyperplasia infiltrating T cells and impact of lymphocytic infiltration on cytokine mRNA profile in prostatic tissue. Lab Invest 2003;83(8):1131–46.

39. Delongchamps N, de la Roza G, Chandan V, et al. Evaluation of prostatitis in autopsied prostates—is chronic inflammation more associated with benign prostatic hyperplasia or cancer? J Urol 2008; 179(5):1736–40.

40. Nickel J, Roehrborn C, O'Leary M, et al. The relationship between prostate inflammation and lower urinary tract symptoms: examination of baseline data from the REDUCE trial. Eur Urol 2008;54(6): 1379–84.

41. Miller M, Krangel M. The human cytokine I-309 is a monocyte chemoattractant. Proc Natl Acad Sci 1992;89(7):2950–4.

42. Zingoni A, Soto H, Hedrick J, et al. Cutting edge: the chemokine receptor CCR8 is preferentially

expressed in Th2 but not Th1 cells. J Immunol 1998; 161(2):547–51.

43. Roos R, Loetscher M, Legler D, et al. Identification of CCR8, the receptor for the human CC chemokine I-309. J Biol Chem 1997;272(28):17251–4.

44. Agarwal M, He C, Siddiqui J, et al. CCL11 (eotaxin-1): A new diagnostic serum marker for prostate cancer. Prostate 2013;73(6):573–81.

45. Penna G, Mondaini N, Amuchastegui S, et al. Seminal plasma cytokines and chemokines in prostate inflammation: interleukin 8 as a predictive biomarker in chronic prostatitis/chronic pelvic pain syndrome and benign prostatic hyperplasia. Eur Urol 2007; 51(2):524–33.

46. Milasheuski P, Nitkin D, Gres A, et al. Immunological status biomarkers as the risk factors of BPH progression. Eur Urol Supp 2019;18(3):e2494–5.

47. Schenk J, Kristal A, Neuhouser M, et al. Biomarkers of systemic inflammation and risk of incident, symptomatic benign prostatic hyperplasia: results from the prostate cancer prevention trial. Am J Epidemiol 2010;171(5):571–82.

48. Fowke J, Koyama T, Fadare O, et al. Does inflammation mediate the obesity and BPH relationship? An epidemiologic analysis of body composition and inflammatory markers in blood, urine, and prostate tissue, and the relationship with prostate enlargement and lower urinary tract symptoms. PloS one 2016; 11(6):e0156918.

49. Anukam K, Hayes K, Summers K, et al. Probiotic Lactobacillus rhamnosus GR-1 and Lactobacillus reuteri RC-14 may help downregulate TNF-Alpha, IL-6, IL-8, IL-10 and IL-12 (p70) in the neurogenic bladder of spinal cord injured patient with urinary tract infections: a two-case study. Adv Urol 2009; 2009:680363.

50. Kim J, Seo S, Park Y, et al. Changes in detrusor and urinary growth factors according to detrusor function after partial bladder outlet obstruction in the rat. Urology 2001;57(2):371–5.

51. Shi B, Zhu Y, Laudon V, et al. Alterations of urine tgf-β1 and bFGF following bladder outlet obstruction: a predictor for detrusor contractibility? Urol Int 2009; 82(1):43–7.

52. Monga M, Gabal-Shehab L, Stein P. Urinary transforming growth factor-β1 levels correlate with bladder outlet obstruction. Int J Urol 2001;8(9): 487–9.

53. Mitterberger M, Pallwein L, Gradl J, et al. Persistent detrusor overactivity after transurethral resection of the prostate is associated with reduced perfusion of the urinary bladder. BJU Int 2007;99(4):831–5.

54. de Jongh R, Dambros M, Haenen G, et al. Partial bladder outlet obstruction reduces the tissue antioxidant capacity and muscle nerve density of the guinea pig bladder. Neurourol Urodyn 2009;28(5): 461–7.

55. Lin W, Chen C, Wu S, et al. Oxidative stress biomarkers in urine and plasma of rabbits with partial bladder outlet obstruction. BJU Int 2011;107(11): 1839–43.

56. Lin W, Wu S, Lin Y, et al. Reversing bladder outlet obstruction attenuates systemic and tissue oxidative stress. BJU Int 2012;110(8):1208–13.

57. Clayton D, Stephany H, Ching C, et al. F2-isoprostanes as a biomarker of oxidative stress in the mouse bladder. J Urol 2014;191(5):1597–601.

58. Roehrborn C, Boyle P, Gould A, et al. Serum prostate-specific antigen as a predictor of prostate volume in men with benign prostatic hyperplasia. Urology 1999;53(3):581–9.

59. Wright E, Fang J, Metter E, et al. Prostate specific antigen predicts the long-term risk of prostate enlargement: results from the Baltimore Longitudinal Study of Aging. J Urol 2002;167(6):2484–7.

60. Pinsky P, Kramer B, Crawford E, et al. Prostate volume and prostate-specific antigen levels in men enrolled in a large screening trial. Urology 2006; 68(2):352–6.

61. Lilja H, Ulmert D, Vickers A. Prostate-specific antigen and prostate cancer: prediction, detection and monitoring. Nat Rev Cancer 2008;8(4):268–728.

62. Birder L. Urinary bladder urothelium: molecular sensors of chemical/thermal/mechanical stimuli. Vasc Pharm 2006;45(4):221–6.

63. Wang E, Lee J, Ruiz W, et al. ATP and purinergic receptor–dependent membrane traffic in bladder umbrella cells. J Clin Invest 2005;115(9):2412–22.

64. Silva-Ramos M, Silva I, Oliveira J, et al. Increased urinary adenosine triphosphate in patients with bladder outlet obstruction due to benign prostate hyperplasia. Prostate 2016;76(15):1353–63.

65. Gill K, Horsley H, Kupelian A, et al. Urinary ATP as an indicator of infection and inflammation of the urinary tract in patients with lower urinary tract symptoms. BMC Urol 2015;15(1):1–9.

66. Cruz C. Neurotrophins in bladder function: what do we know and where do we go from here? Neurourol Urodyn 2014;33(1):39–45.

67. Steers WD, Tuttle JB. Mechanisms of disease: the role of nerve growth factor in the pathophysiology of bladder disorders. Nat Clin Pract Urol 2006;3(2): 101–10.

68. Cruz F. Mechanisms involved in new therapies for overactive bladder. Urology 2004;63(3):65–73.

69. Ochodnický P, Cruz C, Yoshimura N, et al. Nerve growth factor in bladder dysfunction: contributing factor, biomarker, and therapeutic target. Neurourol Urodyn 2011;30(7):1227–41.

70. Liu H, Kuo H. Urinary nerve growth factor levels are increased in patients with bladder outlet obstruction with overactive bladder symptoms and reduced after successful medical treatment. Urology 2008; 72(1):104–8.

71. Wada N, Matsumoto S, Kita M, et al. Decreased urinary nerve growth factor reflects prostatic volume reduction and relief of outlet obstruction in patients with benign prostatic enlargement treated with dutasteride. Int J Urol 2014;21(12):1258–62.

72. Coyne K, Sexton C, Vats V, et al. National community prevalence of overactive bladder in the United States stratified by sex and age. Urology 2011; 77(5):1081–7.

73. Peyronnet B, Mironska E, Chapple C, et al. A comprehensive review of overactive bladder pathophysiology: on the way to tailored treatment. Eur Urol 2019 Jun;75(6):988–1000.

74. Silva-Ramos M, Silva I, Oliveira O, et al. Urinary ATP may be a dynamic biomarker of detrusor overactivity in women with overactive bladder syndrome. PloS one 2013;8(5):e64696.

75. Firouzmand S, Young J. A pilot study to investigate the associations of urinary concentrations of NO, ATP and derivatives with overactive bladder symptom severity. Exp Physiol 2020;105(6):932–9.

76. Sugaya K, Nishijima S, Kadekawa K, et al. Relationship between lower urinary tract symptoms and urinary ATP in patients with benign prostatic hyperplasia or overactive bladder. Biomed Res J 2009;30(5):287–94.

77. Tsiapakidou S, Apostolidis A, Pantazis K, et al. The use of urinary biomarkers in the diagnosis of overactive bladder in female patients. A systematic review and meta-analysis. Int Urogyn J 2021;7:1–3.

78. Kuo H, Hsin-Tzu L, Chancellor M. Can urinary nerve growth factor be a biomarker for overactive bladder? Rev Urol 2010;12:e69.

79. Alkis O, Zumrutbas A, Toktas C, et al. The use of biomarkers in the diagnosis and treatment of overactive bladder: Can we predict the patients who will be resistant to treatment? Neurourol Urodyn 2017; 36(2):390–3.

Pathophysiology and Clinical Biomarkers in Interstitial Cystitis

John M. Masterson, MD[a], Peris R. Castañeda, MD[a], Jayoung Kim, PhD[a,b],*

KEYWORDS

• Interstitial cystitis • Bladder pain syndrome • Biomarkers • Autoimmune • Inflammation

KEY POINTS

- IC/BPS is a heterogeneous disease both in presentation and pathophysiology, making characterization and reliable biomarker identification challenging.
- The emergence of omics research and collaboration by the MAPP Network has allowed for rapid expansion of our understanding of IC/BPS pathophysiology and introduced numerous candidate biomarkers of disease.
- There still exists no perfect biomarker for the diagnosis of IC/BPS or response to treatment.

Interstitial cystitis/bladder pain syndrome (IC/BPS) is a poorly understood chronic pain condition that affects 2.5% to 6.7% of American women and accounts for roughly 2.5% of urology office visits. Patients present with pain, pressure, or discomfort of the urinary bladder with associated lower urinary tract symptoms (LUTS) for more than 6 weeks without an identifiable cause. IC/BPS is highly comorbid with other chronic pain conditions suggesting a common pathophysiology. Owing to the heterogeneous nature of disease, identification of a reliable biomarker in IC/BPS has been a challenging and an active area of research. Candidate biomarkers include abnormally expressed bladder epithelial proteins, mast cells, neurotransmitters, and inflammatory proteins, among others. As our understanding of IC/BPS pathophysiology continues to expand, so does the search for the ideal biomarker.

INTRODUCTION

IC/BPS is a poorly understood yet prevalent disease that urologists face in daily practice. Prevalence estimates range from 2.5% to 6.7% of American women, with lower estimates among men.[1,2] Approximately 2.5% of urologist visits are related to IC/BPS, and its detrimental impact on patient quality of life leading to missed work, depression, and impaired sexual function is well studied in the literature.[3–7] IC/BPS symptoms are wide ranging and often overlap with those of other conditions; symptoms include bladder/pelvic pain and associated urinary frequency, urgency, nocturia, and dyspareunia, in the setting of sterile urine.[8–10] Patients can experience chronic symptoms every day for years, intermittent symptoms with periods of acquiescence, or a combination of acute-on-chronic symptom flares.[9,10]

Given the heterogeneous presentation and manifestations of disease, identifying the true IC/BPS population has been a challenge, placing increased importance on ruling out other symptom causes.[10] Common conditions that can often masquerade as IC/BPS include endometriosis, noninfectious cystitis, vulvodynia, pudendal nerve entrapment, pelvic floor dysfunction, and prostatitis in men.[10] Perhaps the most important and

[a] Division of Urology, Department of Surgery, Cedars-Sinai Medical Center, Los Angeles, CA, USA; [b] Division of Cancer Biology and Therapeutics, Department of Surgery, Samuel Oschin Comprehensive Cancer Institute, Cedars-Sinai Medical Center, 8635 W 3rd St #930E, Los Angeles, CA 90048, USA
* Corresponding author. Department of Biomedical Sciences, Samuel Oschin Comprehensive Cancer Institute, Cedars-Sinai Medical Center, 8635 W 3rd St #930E, Los Angeles, CA 90048.
E-mail address: Jayoung.Kim@cshs.org

Urol Clin N Am 50 (2023) 39–52
https://doi.org/10.1016/j.ucl.2022.09.006
0094-0143/23/© 2022 Elsevier Inc. All rights reserved.

difficult condition to distinguish from IC/BPS is overactive bladder (OAB), because nearly all patients with IC/BPS present with urinary urgency and frequency.[11] As knowledge of IC/BPS has evolved and become more nuanced, it is now understood that patients with IC/BPS void frequently to avoid pain from overdistention, whereas patients with OAB tend to void frequently to avoid incontinence.[11] IC/BPS was once considered to be a disease of the bladder alone—on the spectrum of OAB—but is now considered to be a chronic pain syndrome with pelvic manifestations.[8–10]

The Society for Urodynamics and Female Urology officially defines IC/BPS as an unpleasant sensation (pain, pressure, and discomfort) perceived to be related to the urinary bladder, associated with LUTS for more than 6 weeks duration, in the absence of infection or other identifiable causes.[12] This definition is the product of much refinement because the understanding of IC/BPS has expanded through research and more accurately captures the true IC/BPS population.[1,12,13] The definition also acknowledges that IC/BPS may not be a primary bladder or urinary tract disorder, despite presenting symptoms being urologic in nature.

There is high concordance with IC/BPS and other idiopathic medical conditions such as fibromyalgia, irritable bowel syndrome, chronic fatigue syndrome, and chronic headaches,[9,14,15] which suggests that there may be a unified underlying abnormality in certain patient groups. Thus, unsurprisingly, the pathophysiology of IC/BPS is poorly understood and remains an active area of research.[8–10] Several etiologic mechanisms have been proposed including intrinsic dysfunction of the protective glycosaminoglycan (GAG) layer of the urothelial surface, mast cell infiltration of the urothelium, infection, neural changes causing hypersensitivity, and chronic inflammation due to autoimmune processes.[16–20]

Identification of useful biomarkers for IC/BPS has been a challenging area of research given the heterogeneous and likely multifactorial nature of the disease. However, as our understanding of IC/BPS continues to expand and as gene sequencing technology has improved leading to the emergence of omics research, candidate biomarkers are being frequently identified.[21] As with all disease processes, the ideal biomarker in IC/BPS not only would identify patients with IC/BPS with suitable sensitivity and specificity but also would reflect response to treatment or disease progression.[9] In addition, IC/BPS biomarkers would ideally be obtained via urine or blood specimen rather than tissue biopsy.[9] With these parameters in mind, herein the current literature pertaining to IC/BPS biomarker discovery is reviewed with emphasis on recent, novel findings.

METHODS

A search of original articles available on PubMed was performed using the search terms "IC/BPS" and "biomarker." To capture the most current trends in biomarker research and application, the authors limited the search to articles published within the past 10 years. Only articles originally published in English were included in the initial screening. Review articles and editorial comments were excluded. Finally, animal model studies and cadaver studies were excluded (**Fig. 1**).

RESULTS

Before 2008, much of the research and understanding of IC/BPS pathophysiology was focused on bladder-centric processes.[22] Leading theories included "leaky epithelium," mast cell activation, neurogenic inflammation, or some combination of these, among others.[22] The urothelium of patients with IC/BPS has been shown to produce lower concentrations of GAGs, which serve as a protective, impermeable barrier to noxious stimuli in urine—compared with controls.[23] This GAG deficiency causes a "leaky epithelium" and increases bladder susceptibility to infection and inflammatory proteins.[24–26] Mast cells are proinflammatory cells that excrete primarily histamine among other compounds when activated.[27] Mast cells are primarily involved in allergic and acute inflammatory responses but have also been shown to infiltrate the urothelium of patients with IC/BPS.[27,28] Although unlikely the root cause of IC/BPS, mast cells are thought to serve as the final common pathway through which IC/BPS symptoms are mediated.[27–29] Increased sympathetic nervous system activity has been demonstrated in IC/BPS along with increased sensory nerve fiber density in the suburothelium.[30,31] This increased sympathetic tone within the bladder is thought to create a hypersensitive bladder mucosa and contribute to mast cell degranulation.[30,31] Each of these theories helped elucidate features of IC/BPS that were previously unrecognized; however, none provide a satisfactory explanation for the cause of IC/BPS. In addition, features of these mechanisms are implicated in other chronic pain syndromes such as irritable bowel syndrome and fibromyalgia, which commonly co-occur with IC/BPS, suggesting that there may be a shared, systemic mechanism of disease.[32]

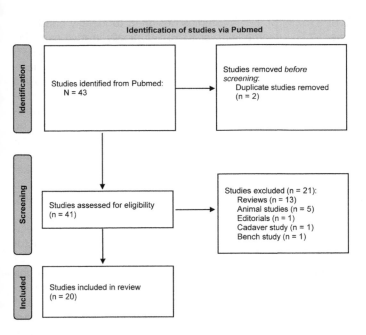

Fig. 1. Flow diagram for literature review and study inclusion.

These insights have shifted the focus of IC/BPS research beyond the bladder alone. In 2008 the National Institute of Diabetes and Digestive and Kidney Diseases established the Multidisciplinary Approach to the Study of Chronic Pelvic Pain (MAPP) Research Network. The network consists of 6 different research centers across the United States and a single Data Coordinating Center, which manages and stores clinical data, and a Tissue and Technology Center to centrally process, store, and disburse clinical samples.[33] MAPP investigators represent a wide array of medical disciplines working together with the shared goal of improving our understanding of IC/BPS and its relationship to other pain conditions.[33] In this shared resource model, large-scale basic science and clinical research studies can be conducted in an efficient manner allowing for rapid advancement of our IC/BPS knowledge.

The MAPP Network has made significant strides in advancing our understanding of IC/BPS symptoms and pain. Studies have shown that approximately three-quarters of patients with IC/BPS experience pain at other sites beyond the pelvis, one-third experience pain at more than 3 nonpelvic sites, and only one-quarter of patients with IC/BPS experience pain only in the pelvis.[33–35] Patients with widespread extrapelvic pain are reported to have more severe pelvic pain symptoms and more psychosocial difficulties and depression.[34] MAPP investigators have also established the importance of differentiating IC/BPS symptoms and pelvic pain from urinary

symptoms. IC/BPS symptoms, but not urinary symptoms, are associated with depression suggesting that urologic pain versus urinary symptoms differ in their overall impact on patient quality of life.[33,36] These findings encourage practitioners to assess IC/BPS symptoms and urinary symptoms with separate measurement tools and measure response to therapy separately.[36–38] The significant impact of nonpelvic and nonurinary symptoms on the lives of patients with IC/BPS further supports the hypothesis that the pathophysiology of IC/BPS is likely more far-reaching than the bladder itself.[33,39] Some of the leading theories to explain the high prevalence of extravesical pain in IC/BPS include central sensitization and pelvic visceral organ cross-sensitization.[33] The central sensitization theory is based on evidence that nociceptive pathways in the brain and spinal cord have been shown to be tonically upregulated in patients with IC/BPS.[33,40] Pelvic visceral organ cross-sensitization describes stimuli from one organ inducing physiologic changes in other organs with shared sensory pathways; these changes can persist even after withdrawal of painful stimuli.[33,41]

Also important in understanding IC/BPS symptoms is the role of flare symptoms—the acute worsening or intensifying of symptoms on top of a patient's chronic or steady-state symptom profile. Some of the early MAPP Network efforts sought to systematically study symptom flares and the influence of flares on patients as investigators performed studies on both multicenter and single-site focus groups of patients with IC/BPS to better elucidate the role of flare symptoms.[42–44] These studies revealed a heterogeneous mix of IC/BPS flare symptoms in terms of frequency, character, physical location, and intensity but did reveal a consistent negative impact on patient quality of life. Investigators found that anticipation and avoidance of flare symptoms are a significant source of stress for patients with IC/BPS and even leads to social anxiety. Given the significant impact of flare symptoms on patient quality of life, identification of flare symptom triggers has naturally garnered the attention of IC/BPS investigators.

One of the more significant triggers of IC/BPS symptom flares identified in the literature is diet.[33,45] Diet modification is often among the earliest and simplest interventions recommended to patients with IC/BPS with bothersome symptoms. Acidic foods are commonly reported to cause IC/BPS symptom exacerbation among survey studies despite evidence that acidic urinary pH alone does not seem to cause symptom flares.[46,47] Caffeine and alcohol are also frequently reported to exacerbate IC/BPS symptoms. Several prospective studies on healthy subjects have identified caffeine as a bladder irritant, causing de novo urinary frequency and in one study, urinary incontinence; however, these effects are generally mild and wash out as patients develop caffeine tolerance.[45,48,49] In a survey of 535 patients with IC/BPS, 94% reported exacerbation of bladder symptoms when consuming alcohol.[45] In other large survey studies directed toward patients with IC/BPS, citrus fruits, tomatoes, vitamin C, coffee, tea, and alcoholic beverages continue to be common culprits for IC/BPS symptom exacerbation.[50,51] Based on findings such as these, practitioners frequently recommend that patients with IC/BPS perform an elimination diet, in which patients carefully record their dietary intake and bladder symptoms, and iteratively remove then reintroduce triggering foods.[45] Dietary modification serves as simple, inexpensive, and potentially efficacious method of limiting IC/BPS symptom flare and quality of life.

Diet has also been implicated in the cause of IC/BPS and explored as a potential therapy.

MAPP Network studies have contributed to the identification of several candidate biomarkers for IC/BPS including matrix metalloproteinase 2 (MMP2), MMP9, neutrophil gelatinase-associated lipocalin (NGAL), the MMP9-NGAL complex, vascular endothelial growth factor (VEGF) and VEGF receptor 1, toll-like receptor 2 (TLR2), TLR4, and etiocholan-3α-ol-17-one sulfate (Etio-S).[33,52–54] Studies designed to identify candidate biomarkers for IC/BPS typically involve sampling bladder tissue or urine from patients with IC/BPS and comparing its features with those of unaffected control patients. This paradigm has evolved over time from comparing urothelial histology under a light microscope and culturing urine specimens to performing genome sequencing on bladder biopsy, urine, serum, and saliva samples.[33,55,56] Both as part of the MAPP Network and within individual research centers, biomarker investigation has moved beyond the bladder to the realms of genomics, epigenomics, proteomics, and metabolomics.[33,53,57,58]

One example of this paradigm shift is the evolution of our understanding of antiproliferative factor (APF). Although not quite pathognomonic for IC/BPS, urinary APF is generally considered the most promising biomarker for disease with reported sensitivity and specificity of 94% and 95%, respectively, for IC/BPS urine versus control urine.[9,59] First described in 1996 via urine culture, APF is present in the urine of patients with IC/BPS and is associated with inhibition of urothelial cell proliferation, thereby contributing to the "leaky epithelium" mechanism of IC/BPS.[60] Further study has precisely characterized the structure of APF as a Frizzled-8 protein-related sialoglycopeptide and is secreted by bladder epithelial cells from patients with IC.[60–62] Taking a step further, proteomic analysis of urothelial cells exposed to APF compared with APF-naive controls found approximately 100 differentially regulated proteins that formed a protein network involved in cell adhesion substantially altered by APF.[63,64] These findings help elucidate the mechanism of APF-induced urothelial damage on the cellular level.

In addition to bioinformatics techniques, given the neurologic implications of IC/BPS, functional MRI (fMRI) has also gained popularity as a methodology of interest in IC/BPS research and introduces the possibility of fMRI findings as biomarkers of disease.[65,66] MAPP Network investigators have identified fMRI alterations in patients with IC/BPS compared with controls.[65,66] One study identified altered resting functional connectivity within centers related to pain; sensory, motor, and emotion regulation processes; reward; and higher executive functioning.[65] The investigators also described decoupling of 2 brain regions from the brain's resting network, which regulates undisturbed, task-free, introspective thought.[65] These findings suggest that while experiencing symptoms, patients with IC/BPS are unable to focus on anything other than their symptoms and have diminished ability to regulate their neurologic resting state.[65]

The authors report examples of many of these techniques that have proposed candidate biomarkers. Results of their literature search yielded 43 articles, 20 of which were excluded based on their criteria: there were 2 duplicate study results, 13 review articles, 5 animal studies, 1 editorial, 1 cadaver study, and 1 bench study of human bladder cells. The 20 studies included in their analysis reported on original clinical data proposing candidate biomarkers for IC/BPS (**Table 1**). The authors also report the sensitivity and specificity of biomarkers for which these data were either reported or calculable (**Table 2**).

DISCUSSION
Clinical Biomarkers: Anesthetic Bladder Capacity

One of the cardinal symptoms thought to be specific for IC/BPS, especially when differentiating between IC/BPS and OAB, is pain associated with bladder filling or bladder distention.[67] Urinary urgency and frequency associated with IC/BPS is believed to be the result of fear of a full bladder rather than intrinsic detrusor overactivity.[11] Along these lines, patients with IC/BPS are thought to have a lower bladder capacity than patients

Table 1
Studies included from literature review with description of biomarkers

	Biomarker	Mechanism	Sample	Change	Reference
1	Anesthetic bladder capacity	Clinical	Bladder capacity	Decreased	Plair et al,[69] 2021
2	Histology/bladder capacity	Clinical	Bladder tissue	Different	Schachar JS, et al,[70] 2019
3	Gene expression/ bladder capacity	Clinical	Bladder tissue	Increased	Colaco et al,[68] 2014
4	WNT11	Genomic	Bladder tissue	Decreased	Choi et al,[71] 2018
5	MCP-1, CXCL10, eotaxin-1, RANTES	Inflammatory	Urine	Increased	Jiang YH, et al,[82] 2020
6	MIP-1β, eotaxin, CXCL10, and RANTES	Inflammatory	Bladder tissue/urine	Increased	Jiang YH, et al,[83] 2021
7	MIF	Inflammatory	Urine	Elevated	Vera et al,[85] 2018
8	Apoptotic cells	Inflammatory	Bladder tissue	Increased	Liu et al,[78] 2015
9	NGF, MMP-13, VEGF	Inflammatory	Urine	Decreased s/p PRP	Jiang et al,[102] 2020
10	Uroplakin	Urothelial barrier	Urine	Elevated	Cho et al,[72] 2020
11	Prefrontal cortex changes	Neurogenic	Brain	Different	Pang and Liao,[86] 2021
12	NGF	Neurogenic	Urine	Increased	Tonyali et al,[81] 2018
13	Etio-S	Metabolomic	Urine	Increased	Parker et al,[53] 2016
14	CD38, ITGAL, KLRB1, and IL-7	Inflammatory	Bladder tissue/urine	Differently expressed	Saha et al,[94] 2020
15	CXCL8, CXCL1, IL-6	Inflammatory	Bladder tissue/urine	Differently expressed	Wu et al,[97] 2021
16	IL-4, TNF-α, MIP-1β, AAA, Tie2	Inflammatory	Urine	Increased	Ma et al,[84] 2016
17	MAPK pathway	Genomic	Urine	Differentially methylated	Bradley et al,[57] 2018
18	IL-4, VEGF, IL-9	Inflammatory	Urine	Decreased s/p LI-ESWT	Shen et al,[104] 2021
19	VEGF	Inflammatory	Bladder tissue	Decreased s/p botox	Peng et al,[103] 2013
20	MCP-1	Inflammatory	Urine	Decreased s/p interstim	Peters et al,[105] 2015

Abbreviations: IL, interleukin; MAPK, mitogen-activated protein kinase; MIF, macrophage migration inhibitory factor; MIP-1β, macrophage inflammatory protein 1β; NGF, nerve growth factor; TNF, tumor necrosis factor.

Table 2
Reported areas under the curve, sensitivity, and specificity of inflammatory biomarkers

Biomarker	AUC	Sensitivity	Specificity
IL-7[94]	0.756	71.1	67.9
MCP-1[82]	0.753	60.3	72.4
Eotaxin-1[82]	0.720	52.2	85.7
MIF[85]	0.718	74.4	61.8
IL-4[84]	0.703	54.4	86.2
CXCL 10[82]	0.685	66.2	65.5
MIP-1β[83]	0.674	92.2	44.8
RANTES[83]	0.666	53.8	75.9
IL-6[97]	0.631	50.0	79.3
Eotaxin[83]	0.604	40.3	80.0
TNF-α[84]	0.527	41.1	71.4

Abbreviations: AUC, area under curve; IL, interleukin; MIF, macrophage migration inhibitory factor; MIP-1β, macrophage inflammatory protein 1β; TNF, tumor necrosis factor.

without IC/BPS. Several studies have explored this hypothesis by comparing anesthetic bladder capacity between patients with IC/BPS and controls.[68–70] Plair and colleagues[69] reported their findings from a retrospective case series of 257 women with a diagnosis of IC/BPS who underwent bladder hydrodistension at their center. The investigators found on multiple regression analysis that patients with normal bladder capacities were more likely to carry a concomitant diagnosis of pelvic pain syndrome, endometriosis, or one of several neurologic, autoimmune, system pain diagnoses.[69] Meanwhile, patients with low bladder capacity were more likely to have bladder-specific and voiding symptoms, suggesting that decreased bladder capacity provides specificity for the diagnosis of bladder-centric IC/BPS rather than diagnosing pain syndromes with associated pelvic symptoms.[69]

Schachar and colleagues[70] built upon this hypothesis and sought to provide histologic supporting evidence for low bladder capacity as a biomarker for bladder-centric IC/BPS. The investigators performed a retrospective review of bladder biopsy pathology slides from 41 patients with IC/BPS and anesthetic bladder capacity below 400 mL compared with 41 patients with IC/BPS with anesthetic bladder capacity greater than 400 mL. Pathology review was performed by a single, blinded pathologist using a standardized, predefined grading scale. The investigators found that the low bladder capacity group demonstrated more severe acute inflammation, more

severe chronic inflammation, and more erosion than the normal capacity cohort[70]; they also noted that mast cell counts between the 2 groups were roughly equal. The investigators concluded that these findings lend further support to the hypothesis that low bladder capacity serves as a reliable biomarker for differentiation of bladder-centric IC/BPS from IC/BPS as a manifestation of a systemic pain syndrome.[70]

Colaco and colleagues[68] explored this hypothesis on an even more basic level by searching for differential gene expression in the bladder tissue of IC/BPS with low bladder capacity (<400 mL) compared with patients with IC/BPS with normal bladder capacity (≥400 mL) and control subjects with normal bladder capacity. The investigators performed RNA extraction and microarray assay to determine differentially expressed RNA transcripts (DETs) between the groups.[68] In all, 193 DETs were identified between the low bladder capacity IC/BPS and control group, and fewer DETs between the normal bladder capacity IC/BPS and control groups. Most of the upregulated transcripts were involved in inflammatory cell signaling, whereas most downregulated transcripts were involved in epithelial integrity proteins, such as uroplakin.[68] Choi and colleagues[71] performed reverse transcription-polymerase chain reaction (RT-PCR) analysis of biopsy specimen from 25 patients with IC/BPS and 5 controls. Their goal was to assess expression of WNT family genes, which when downregulated are associated with fibrotic changes. The investigators found silencing of WNT11, WNT 2B, WNT 5A, and WNT 10A in patients with IC/BPS compared with controls.[71] These findings support that the epithelium of IC/BPS is more prone to fibrosis than that of healthy controls, perhaps contributing to decreased bladder capacity and improper response to mucosal injury or irritation.[71] Taken together, these data support the hypothesis that anesthetic bladder capacity is not only different between patients with IC/BPS and controls but may also represent distinct disease phenotypes within IC/BPS. Based on these findings low anesthetic bladder capacity offers promise as a biomarker for bladder-centric IC/BPS and more accurate stratification of patients along the IC/BPS spectrum of disease.

Given the longstanding "leaky epithelium" hypothesis of IC/BPS pathogenesis, it is unsurprising that alterations in proteins related to urothelial structural integrity and permeability have become attractive biomarkers of disease. Although the authors' literature review did not necessarily reveal novel urothelial barrier biomarkers, the studies included in their review highlight unique clinical scenarios or modalities of assessing for these biomarkers. Cho and colleagues[72] sought to compare urothelial uroplakin expression in patients with IC/BPS who were scheduled to undergo augmentation ileocystoplasty, an indication of severe disease. Uroplakin is a urothelial protein that helps for an impermeable plaque on the surface of healthy urothelium.[73] Bladder tissue samples were collected from 19 subjects with ulcerative subtype IC/BPS and 5 controls; tissue was specifically collected from nonulcerated urothelium from study subject. Presence of uroplakin was assessed by immunofluorescence staining, and degree of uroplakin expression was measure by western blot. The investigators found that uroplakin expression was elevated in study subjects compared with controls.[72] This finding is contrary to the prior reports of uroplakin as a biomarker for IC/BPS, in which uroplakin is decreased leading to hyperpermeable urothelium.[74–76] The investigators hypothesize that this may be the result of a positive feedback loop between the diseased, ulcerated tissue and the surrounding healthy tissue in which uroplakin is compensatorily upregulated.[77] As such, this finding would provide some specificity in differentiating between ulcerative and nonulcerative subtypes of IC/BPS beyond cystoscopic inspection and biopsy.

Lui and colleagues sought to measure differential expression of different biomarkers of varying physiologic origins in the bladder tissue of patients with IC/BPS. In this study the investigators compared 17 subjects with IC/BPS not only with 10 healthy controls but also with 15 patients with bladder outlet obstruction, 13 with ketamine cystitis (KC), 12 with spinal cord injury, and 12 with recurrent urinary tract infection (UTI).[78] Bladder biopsy specimens were analyzed for expression of E-cadherin, a urothelial junction protein, as well as mast cell activation and presence of apoptotic cells, all measures of inflammation.[79,80] Patients with IC/BPS were found to have significantly decreased E-cadherin expression compared with controls, again supporting the hypothesis of structurally deficient urothelium in these patients. Patients with KC and UTI also demonstrated decreased E-cadherin expression, implying that there may be a shared pathogenesis between these conditions and IC/BPS.[78] All subjects with lower urinary tract pathologic condition demonstrated greater mast cell activity and greater presence of apoptotic cells compared with healthy controls, highlighting the sensitive but not specific role of inflammation within the urothelium in these disease processes.[78]

Inflammatory Biomarkers

The pathophysiology of IC/BPS is characterized by chronic inflammation and urothelial dysfunction. During states of inflammation, detrusor smooth muscle cells and urothelial cells produce chemokines, which are measurable in the urine. Early studies have demonstrated an elevation of inflammatory proteins in patients with IC/BPS. Inflammatory biomarkers therefore represent an important area of investigation. Tonyali and colleagues[81] demonstrated elevated levels of urinary nerve growth factor (NGF) in patients with IC/BPS compared with controls. Furthermore, normalized NGF levels were significantly correlated with more severe symptoms in those with IC/BPS.[81] Similarly, Jiang and colleagues[82] analyzed the urinary specimens of 127 patients with IC/BPS compared with controls, testing 31 candidate cytokines. The investigators found 5 urinary cytokines with high diagnostic value, including eotaxin-1, CXCL10, RANTES, and MCP-1. Identifying urinary biomarkers with high sensitivity and specificity carries important diagnostic value. Equally important is identifying which inflammatory biomarkers are differentially expressed, because this provides better insight into the specific pathophysiology of IC/BPS. For instance, eotaxin is a chemoattractant for eosinophils and its differential expression in patients with IC/BPS suggests an immune response to allergy-related inflammation. Elevated NGF identified in the study by Tonyali and colleagues[81] points to the role of peripheral nerve proliferation in IC/BPS and may explain persistent hyperalgesia in the absence of inflammation.

Perhaps even more clinically important is the ability to distinguish between IC/BPS and conditions with similar symptomatic presentation. In a subsequent study, Jiang and colleagues[83] identified urinary macrophage inflammatory protein 1β (MIP-1β) as having high sensitivity for distinguishing between patients with IC/BPS and healthy controls.[83] Furthermore, the investigators identified several urinary cytokines as differentially expressed in IC/BPS samples compared with samples from patients with OAB, including 3 cytokines identified in their prior study: CXCL10, eotaxin, and RANTES. The investigators proposed a diagnostic algorithm wherein MIP-1β is used in initial screening and the latter 3 are used in confirmatory testing. Subsequent validation of this and similar diagnostic algorithms could generate a series of accepted urinary assays for diagnosis that would avoid more invasive diagnostic testing. Ma and colleagues[84] similarly identified serum MIP-

1β as a promising biomarker for IC/BPS, among others. The investigators also identified serum interleukin-4 (IL-4), tumor necrosis factor alpha, Tie2, and serum amyloid A (SAA) as promising biomarkers, with SAA demonstrating the greatest area under curve on receiver operating characteristic of 0.85.[84] All these proteins represent inflammatory cytokines or chemokines.[84] Vera and colleagues identified a urinary biomarker, macrophage migration inhibitory factor that is not only significantly elevated in patients with IC/BPS compared with controls but also differentially elevated in patients with IC/BPS with Hunner lesions, compared with patients with IC/BPS without Hunner lesions.[85] Although OAB and IC/BPS share similar symptoms, their pathophysiology and treatment are different. Identification of IC/BPS biomarkers distinct from OAB can help avoid misdiagnosis and inappropriate or delayed treatment.

Neurogenic/Neurologic Biomarkers

As previously discussed, neurogenic or neurologic alterations in patients with IC/BPS have garnered interest in the realm of biomarker discovery. Given the heterogeneous presentation of IC/BPS pain, which often extends beyond the bladder or pelvis and can often persist after elimination of stimuli, there is almost certainly a neurologic component of IC/BPS pain. A literature search by the authors yielded 1 study by Pang and Liao[86] that described a novel technique to assess abnormalities of functional connectivity within the prefrontal cortex (PFC) of patients with IC/BPS. Rather than resting state fMRI, the investigators used resting state functional near-infrared spectroscopy (rs-fNIRS). fNIRS is a noninvasive, portable, optic-based functional brain imaging technology with few physical movement restrictions that detects changes in oxyhemoglobin signals in areas of the brain.[86,87] Comparison studies between fMRI and fNIRS have demonstrated the reliably of fNIRS and thus suitability for use in studying patients with IC/BPS.[86–89] In their study, 10 patients with IC/BPS and 15 age- and gender-matched controls were asked to empty their bladder before initiation of rs-fNIRS data collection to collect "empty bladder" PFC activity. Next, subjects were asked to drink water until they felt a strong urge to void at which point they were assessed for urinary incontinence and PFC activity was recorded. Finally, subjects were allowed to void. In both the empty bladder and urge-to-void states, patients with IC/BPS demonstrated significantly decreased functional connectivity in the dorsolateral PFC, frontopolar area, and the pars triangularis regions of the

PFC compared with controls.[86] These areas are intimately involved in sensory integration, motivational drive, mood control, cognitive processing, and decision making.[86] With regard to lower urinary tract activity, they contribute to integration and regulation of the urge to void; once the urge is sensed, the PFC can either encourage or discourage voiding based on other sensory inputs.[86] Decreased functional connectivity (FC) in these regions was also demonstrated in similar fNIRS studies in patients with OAB and urge urinary incontinence (UUI) but not IC/BPS.[86,90,91] These findings are not only illustrative of the central nervous system's role in IC/BPS but also demonstrate the feasibility of a new technology in the investigation of IC/BPS.[86]

Genomic, Proteomic, Metabolomic Biomarkers

IC/BPS research has benefited greatly from the emergence of bioinformatics and omics research. Made possible by the large-scale storage and distribution of tissue and urine samples by the MAPP Network, sequencing and identification of differentially expressed genes (DEGs), proteins, and metabolites as candidate biomarkers for IC/BPS has helped elucidate IC/BPS pathophysiology. A review of the literature by the authors revealed several such studies both at single centers and as part of the MAPP Network using both urothelial biopsy tissue and urine samples from patients with IC/BPS.

Parker and colleagues[53] applied mass spectrometry-based global metabolite profiling to urine specimens from 40 female IC/BPS supplied by the MAPP Network and 40 age-matched controls. Among multiple metabolites that discriminated subjects with IC/BPS from controls, Etio-S, a sulfo-conjugated 5-β reduced isomer of testosterone, demonstrated better than 90% specificity for IC/BPS.[53] This is the first study to identify Etio-S as a urinary biomarker in IC/BPS, and its mechanistic implications are unclear. The investigators assert that high concentrations of Etio-S may stimulate acute-phase reactants and local inflammatory effects; alternatively, they cite evidence that changes in Etio-S may have GABAergic effects manifested as acute stress, depression, or nociception.[53,92,93] Further research is needed to elucidate the mechanism of Etio-S in IC/BPS but its specificity for disease is promising.

Saha and colleagues[94] completed a bioinformatics study in which preexisting Gene Expression Omnibus (GEO) datasets were mined for IC/BPS-associated genes. One dataset contained cell lines treated with and without APF as well as bladder tissue samples from patients with IC/BPS and normal controls. Two datasets contained gene expression profiles of bladder biopsy tissues from patients with IC/BPS and normal controls. One dataset contained the gene expression profiles of urine sediment from patients with IC/BPS and normal controls. DEGs that were significantly different between patients with IC/BPS and controls were retrieved from all datasets and included for analysis; these were CD5, CD38, ITGAL, IL7R, KRLB1, and PSMB9.[94] After identification of significant DEGs, the investigators then performed reverse transcription quantitative polymerase Chain Reaction (RT-qPCR) analysis for these DEGs on newly obtained tissue from patients with IC/BPS and controls. RT-qPCR results showed that all 6 genes were overexpressed in patients with IC/BPS compared with controls. PSMB9, ITGAL, and KLRB1 were most significantly overexpressed in patients with IC/BPS compared with controls making them the most promising candidate biomarkers among DEGs.[94] According to the investigators, these genes are commonly, albeit nonspecifically, associated with autoimmune processes.[94,95] Autoimmunity is one of the many proposed pathophysiological causes for IC/BPS, supported by the relatively strong association between IC/BPS and autoimmune conditions, such as Sjögren syndrome.[94] There is some evidence to suggest that autoantibodies to the muscarinic M3 receptor are contributory to Sjögren syndrome; the M3 receptor happens to also be expressed in detrusor cells of the bladder.[94,96] Wu and colleagues[97] performed a similar GEO-based study in which they analyzed a database containing 5 patients with IC/BPS patients and 6 controls for DEGs. In all the investigators identified 483 DEGs between patients with IC/BPS and controls: 216 upregulated and 276 downregulated genes; however, at conclusion of their analysis only 3 genes were considered possible core IC/BPS-related genes: CXCL8, CXCL1, and IL-6.[97] All 3 of these genes produce chemokine or cytokine proteins involved in the inflammatory response, furthering the concept of dysregulated lower urinary tract inflammation in IC/BPS.[97,98]

Finally, Bradley and colleagues[57] performed an epigenomic study of voided urine samples to identify differentially expressed methylated genes in IC/BPS. Much like DEGs, differences in methylation, usually caused by environmental exposures, can both shed light on IC/BPS pathophysiology and potentially serve as a noninvasive biomarker. Urine samples from 8 female patients with IC/BPS and 8 female age-matched controls were included for analysis. Genes were analyzed for addition of a methyl group to the 5′ carbon of a cytosine moiety, generating 5-methylcytosine (5-mC), which occurs predominantly in the context of cytosines that precede guanine (5′-CpG-3′) dinucleotides, or CpGs.[57,99] In all, more than 1000 differentially methylated CpG sites between patients with IC/BPS and controls were identified; however, the most prominent pathway enriched for genes with differential methylation was the mitogen-activated protein kinase (MAPK) pathway, which contained 22 differentially methylated sites. In addition, one of the MAPK pathway genes, MDS1 and EVI1 complex locus (MECOM), contained multiple differentially methylated sites, increasing the likelihood of its significance. Although not classically associated with IC/BPS, MAPK is associated with inhibition of cell growth, inflammation, and regulation of apoptosis.[57,100] The findings of Bradley and colleagues[57] not only implicate MAPK signaling in the pathophysiology of IC/BPS but also support the idea that environmental exposures can cause fundamental epigenetic changes in patients with IC/BPS. For example, changes secondary to chronic UTI have been thought to contribute to IC/BPS symptoms and altered epigenetic expression may be the mechanism by which these changes manifest.[57,101]

Biomarkers in Response to Therapy

Another area in which biomarkers prove useful is in assessing response to treatment. Numerous treatment modalities are available for IC/BPS. For patients who fail conventional therapies, several nonstandard treatments have been explored. These treatments have had mixed success, and their mechanisms for improving symptoms associated with IC/BPS are still poorly understood. Studies on biomarker changes in response to novel therapies help improve our understanding of the therapeutic mechanisms.

Jiang and colleagues[102] tested urinary biomarkers of 40 patients with IC/BPS symptoms refractory to conventional therapy who received 4 intravesical injections of autologous platelet-rich plasma (PRP). The investigators found significant decreases in urinary levels of VEGF, NGF, and matrix metalloproteinase-13 alongside symptomatic improvement. These results suggest that the therapeutic effects of PRP are likely due to its ability to alleviate inflammation and reduce atypical angiogenesis.[102] Similarly, Peng and colleagues[103] tested urinary markers of 21 patients with IC/BPS who had failed conventional therapy and went on to receive treatment with intravesical onabotulinumtoxinA injections every 6 months for 4 total treatments. These investigators also found a significant decrease in the expression of VEGF following treatment. Although these patients also experienced symptomatic improvement, clinical improvement did not directly correlate with VEGF expression.[103] Shen and colleagues[104] also found a significant difference in VEGF as well as urinary chemokines IL-4 and IL-6 in 13 patients treated with extracorporeal shockwave for IC/BPS.

Finally, Peters and colleagues[105] tested urinary markers in patients who experienced successful sacral neuromodulator device implant for refractory urinary symptoms associated with IC/BPS. In this study, success was defined as 50% symptomatic improvement on the Interstitial Cystitis Symptom and Problem Index (ICSPI). The investigators found a positive correlation between urinary levels of CXCL-1 and soluble interleukin-1 receptor antagonist (sIL-1ra) and ICSPI and pain score, suggesting the ability of these markers to reflect severity of disease.[105] Furthermore, the investigators demonstrated a reduction in urinary levels of MCP-1 and sIL-1ra after treatment, which was significantly associated with symptomatic response. sIL-1ra elevation in serum has been associated with pain and stiffness in patients with fibromyalgia and MCP-1 is a potent chemotactic protein that helps maintain an inflammatory state in tissue.[105] Unlike in prior studies, these investigators did not see a significant decrease in urinary levels of VEGF, suggesting that the mechanism by which sacral neuromodulation improves IC/BPS symptoms may differ from the therapeutic mechanisms of ESWL, PRP, and intravesical onabotulinumtoxinA. Changes in biomarkers following treatment are evidence to change in the actual bladder microenvironment, beyond subjective symptomatic improvement. In the future, biomarkers also have the potential to provide objective measures of improvement.

SUMMARY

IC/BPS remains a challenging disease for clinicians, researchers, and patients. The heterogeneity of disease presentation and the absence of reliable biomarkers of disease make patient counseling and disease management difficult. Impressively, the coordination of resources within the MAPP Network has expanded our understanding of IC/BPS over a relatively short period and has benefited IC/BPS investigators both within the MAPP Network and at individual centers. The authors' review of literature highlighted several novel biomarkers for IC/BPS as well as cutting-edge methodologies for biomarkers identification. Identification of PFC changes supports the hypothesis that there is a central nervous system component

to IC/BPS while omics work helps elucidate differences between patients with IC/BPS and controls at the genome level and beyond. Although there remains no perfect biomarker for IC/BPS that is noninvasive, sensitive, and specific, and serves as a measure of disease progression/remission, there is reason for optimism as research in this area continues to meaningfully progress.

CLINICS CARE POINTS

- IC/BPS is a challenging and heterogenous clinical entity. As there is no perfect biomarker for IC/BPS diagnosis, clinical assessment remains paramount in patient management. Presence of pain is important in distiguishing IC/BPS from OAB.

DISCLOSURES

None.

REFERENCES

1. Berry SH, Elliott MN, Suttorp M, et al. Prevalence of symptoms of bladder pain syndrome/interstitial cystitis among adult females in the United States. J Urol 2011;186(2):540–4.
2. Suskind AM, Berry SH, Ewing BA, et al. The prevalence and overlap of interstitial cystitis/bladder pain syndrome and chronic prostatitis/chronic pelvic pain syndrome in men: results of the RAND Interstitial Cystitis Epidemiology male study. J Urol 2013;189(1):141–5.
3. Liu B, Su M, Zhan H, et al. Adding a sexual dysfunction domain to UPOINT system improves association with symptoms in women with interstitial cystitis and bladder pain syndrome. Urology 2014;84(6):1308–13.
4. Cox A. Management of interstitial cystitis/bladder pain syndrome. Can Urol Assoc J 2018;12(6 Suppl 3):S157–60.
5. Rabin C, O'Leary A, Neighbors C, et al. Pain and depression experienced by women with interstitial cystitis. Women Health 2000;31(4):67–81.
6. Michael YL, Kawachi I, Stampfer MJ, et al. Quality of life among women with interstitial cystitis. J Urol 2000;164(2):423–7.
7. Rothrock NE, Lutgendorf SK, Kreder KJ, et al. Stress and symptoms in patients with interstitial cystitis: a life stress model. Urology 2001;57(3):422–7.
8. French LM, Bhambore N. Interstitial cystitis/painful bladder syndrome. Am Fam Physician 2011;83(10):1175–81.

9. Hanno PM, Erickson D, Moldwin R, et al. Diagnosis and treatment of interstitial cystitis/bladder pain syndrome: AUA guideline amendment. J Urol 2015;193(5):1545–53.

10. Cox A, Golda N, Nadeau G, et al. CUA guideline: Diagnosis and treatment of interstitial cystitis/bladder pain syndrome. Can Urol Assoc J 2016; 10(5–6):E136–55.

11. Tincello DG, Walker AC. Interstitial cystitis in the UK: results of a questionnaire survey of members of the Interstitial Cystitis Support Group. Eur J Obstet Gynecol Reprod Biol 2005;118(1):91–5.

12. Hanno P, Dmochowski R. Status of international consensus on interstitial cystitis/bladder pain syndrome/painful bladder syndrome: 2008 snapshot. Neurourol Urodyn 2009;28(4):274–86.

13. Hanno PM, Landis JR, Matthews-Cook Y, et al. The diagnosis of interstitial cystitis revisited: lessons learned from the National Institutes of Health Interstitial Cystitis Database study. J Urol 1999;161(2): 553–7.

14. Buffington CA. Comorbidity of interstitial cystitis with other unexplained clinical conditions. J Urol 2004;172(4 Pt 1):1242–8.

15. Warren JW, Howard FM, Cross RK, et al. Antecedent nonbladder syndromes in case-control study of interstitial cystitis/painful bladder syndrome. Urology 2009;73(1):52–7.

16. Warren JW, Brown V, Jacobs S, et al. Urinary tract infection and inflammation at onset of interstitial cystitis/painful bladder syndrome. Urology 2008; 71(6):1085–90.

17. Ratliff TL, Klutke CG, Hofmeister M, et al. Role of the immune response in interstitial cystitis. Clin Immunol Immunopathol 1995;74(3):209–16.

18. Rourke W, Khan SA, Ahmed K, et al. Painful bladder syndrome/interstitial cystitis: aetiology, evaluation and management. Arch Ital Urol Androl 2014;86(2):126–31.

19. Engelhardt PF, Morakis N, Daha LK, et al. Long-term results of intravesical hyaluronan therapy in bladder pain syndrome/interstitial cystitis. Int Urogynecol J 2011;22(4):401–5.

20. Daly DM, Collins VM, Chapple CR, et al. The afferent system and its role in lower urinary tract dysfunction. Curr Opin Urol 2011;21(4):268–74.

21. You S, Yang W, Anger JT, et al. 'Omics' approaches to understanding interstitial cystitis/painful bladder syndrome/bladder pain syndrome. Int Neurourol J 2012;16(4):159–68.

22. Elbadawi A. Interstitial cystitis: a critique of current concepts with a new proposal for pathologic diagnosis and pathogenesis. Urology 1997;49(5A Suppl):14–40.

23. Parsons CL, Hurst RE. Decreased urinary uronic acid levels in individuals with interstitial cystitis. J Urol 1990;143(4):690–3.

24. Mulholland SG, Hanno P, Parsons CL, et al. Pentosan polysulfate sodium for therapy of interstitial cystitis. A double-blind placebo-controlled clinical study. Urology 1990;35(6):552–8.

25. Hohlbrugger G. The vesical blood-urine barrier: a relevant and dynamic interface between renal function and nervous bladder control. J Urol 1995;154(1):6–15.

26. Hohlbrugger G. Leaky urothelium and/or vesical ischemia enable urinary potassium to cause idiopathic urgency/frequency syndrome and urge incontinence. Int Urogynecol J Pelvic Floor Dysfunct 1996;7(5):242–55.

27. Sant GR, Theoharides TC. The role of the mast cell in interstitial cystitis. Urol Clin North Am 1994;21(1): 41–53.

28. Frenz AM, Christmas TJ, Pearce FL. Does the mast cell have an intrinsic role in the pathogenesis of interstitial cystitis? Agents Actions 1994;(41 Spec No):C14–5.

29. Sant GR, Kempuraj D, Marchand JE, et al. The mast cell in interstitial cystitis: role in pathophysiology and pathogenesis. Urology 2007;69(4 Suppl):34–40.

30. Hohenfellner M, Nunes L, Schmidt RA, et al. Interstitial cystitis: increased sympathetic innervation and related neuropeptide synthesis. J Urol 1992; 147(3):587–91.

31. Lundeberg T, Liedberg H, Nordling L, et al. Interstitial cystitis: correlation with nerve fibres, mast cells and histamine. Br J Urol 1993;71(4):427–9.

32. Theoharides TC, Cochrane DE. Critical role of mast cells in inflammatory diseases and the effect of acute stress. J Neuroimmunol 2004;146(1–2):1–12.

33. Clemens JQ, Mullins C, Ackerman AL, et al. Urologic chronic pelvic pain syndrome: insights from the MAPP Research Network. Nat Rev Urol 2019; 16(3):187–200.

34. Lai HH, Jemielita T, Sutcliffe S, et al. Characterization of Whole Body Pain in Urological Chronic Pelvic Pain Syndrome at Baseline: A MAPP Research Network Study. J Urol 2017;198(3):622–31.

35. Landis JR, Williams DA, Lucia MS, et al. The MAPP research network: design, patient characterization and operations. BMC Urol 2014;14:58.

36. Griffith JW, Stephens-Shields AJ, Hou X, et al. Pain and Urinary Symptoms Should Not be Combined into a Single Score: Psychometric Findings from the MAPP Research Network. J Urol 2016;195(4 Pt 1):949–54.

37. Clemens JQ, Calhoun EA, Litwin MS, et al. Validation of a modified National Institutes of Health chronic prostatitis symptom index to assess genitourinary pain in both men and women. Urology 2009;74(5):983–7.

38. O'Leary MP, Sant GR, Fowler FJ Jr, et al. The interstitial cystitis symptom index and problem index. Urology 1997;49(5A Suppl):58–63.

39. Krieger JN, Stephens AJ, Landis JR, et al. Relationship between chronic nonurological associated somatic syndromes and symptom severity in urological chronic pelvic pain syndromes: baseline evaluation of the MAPP study. J Urol 2015;193(4):1254–62.

40. Lai HH, Qiu CS, Crock LW, et al. Activation of spinal extracellular signal-regulated kinases (ERK) 1/2 is associated with the development of visceral hyperalgesia of the bladder. Pain 2011;152(9):2117–24.

41. Rudick CN, Jiang M, Yaggie RE, et al. O-antigen modulates infection-induced pain states. PLoS One 2012;7(8):e41273.

42. Sutcliffe S, Bradley CS, Clemens JQ, et al. Urological chronic pelvic pain syndrome flares and their impact: qualitative analysis in the MAPP network. Int Urogynecol J 2015;26(7):1047–60.

43. Sutcliffe S, Colditz GA, Goodman MS, et al. Urological chronic pelvic pain syndrome symptom flares: characterisation of the full range of flares at two sites in the Multidisciplinary Approach to the Study of Chronic Pelvic Pain (MAPP) Research Network. BJU Int 2014;114(6):916–25.

44. Sutcliffe S, Colditz GA, Pakpahan R, et al. Changes in symptoms during urologic chronic pelvic pain syndrome symptom flares: findings from one site of the MAPP Research Network. Neurourol Urodyn 2015;34(2):188–95.

45. Friedlander JI, Shorter B, Moldwin RM. Diet and its role in interstitial cystitis/bladder pain syndrome (IC/BPS) and comorbid conditions. BJU Int 2012;109(11):1584–91.

46. Marinkovic SP, Moldwin R, Gillen LM, et al. The management of interstitial cystitis or painful bladder syndrome in women. BMJ 2009;339:b2707.

47. Nguan C, Franciosi LG, Butterfield NN, et al. A prospective, double-blind, randomized cross-over study evaluating changes in urinary pH for relieving the symptoms of interstitial cystitis. BJU Int 2005;95(1):91–4.

48. Bird ET, Parker BD, Kim HS, et al. Caffeine ingestion and lower urinary tract symptoms in healthy volunteers. Neurourol Urodyn 2005;24(7):611–5.

49. Jura YH, Townsend MK, Curhan GC, et al. Caffeine intake, and the risk of stress, urgency and mixed urinary incontinence. J Urol 2011;185(5):1775–80.

50. Bassaly R, Downes K, Hart S. Dietary consumption triggers in interstitial cystitis/bladder pain syndrome patients. Female Pelvic Med Reconstr Surg 2011;17(1):36–9.

51. Shorter B, Lesser M, Moldwin RM, et al. Effect of comestibles on symptoms of interstitial cystitis. J Urol 2007;178(1):145–52.

52. Dagher A, Curatolo A, Sachdev M, et al. Identification of novel non-invasive biomarkers of urinary chronic pelvic pain syndrome: findings from the Multidisciplinary Approach to the Study of Chronic Pelvic Pain (MAPP) Research Network. BJU Int 2017;120(1):130–42.

53. Parker KS, Crowley JR, Stephens-Shields AJ, et al. Urinary Metabolomics Identifies a Molecular Correlate of Interstitial Cystitis/Bladder Pain Syndrome in a Multidisciplinary Approach to the Study of Chronic Pelvic Pain (MAPP) Research Network Cohort. EBioMedicine 2016;7:167–74.

54. Schrepf A, Bradley CS, O'Donnell M, et al. Toll-like receptor 4 and comorbid pain in Interstitial Cystitis/Bladder Pain Syndrome: a multidisciplinary approach to the study of chronic pelvic pain research network study. Brain Behav Immun 2015;49:66–74.

55. Gillenwater JY, Wein AJ. Summary of the National Institute of Arthritis, Diabetes, Digestive and Kidney Diseases Workshop on Interstitial Cystitis, National Institutes of Health, Bethesda, Maryland, August 28-29, 1987. J Urol 1988;140(1):203–6.

56. Rosamilia A, Igawa Y, Higashi S. Pathology of interstitial cystitis. Int J Urol 2003;10(Suppl):S11–5.

57. Bradley MS, Burke EE, Grenier C, et al. A genome-scale DNA methylation study in women with interstitial cystitis/bladder pain syndrome. Neurourol Urodyn 2018;37(4):1485–93.

58. Goo YA, Tsai YS, Liu AY, et al. Urinary proteomics evaluation in interstitial cystitis/painful bladder syndrome: a pilot study. Int Braz J Urol 2010;36(4):464–78.

59. Keay S, Zhang CO, Marvel R, et al. Antiproliferative factor, heparin-binding epidermal growth factor-like growth factor, and epidermal growth factor: sensitive and specific urine markers for interstitial cystitis. Urology 2001;57(6 Suppl 1):104.

60. Keay S, Zhang CO, Trifillis AL, et al. Decreased 3H-thymidine incorporation by human bladder epithelial cells following exposure to urine from interstitial cystitis patients. J Urol 1996;156(6):2073–8.

61. Keay S, Warren JW. A hypothesis for the etiology of interstitial cystitis based upon inhibition of bladder epithelial repair. Med Hypotheses 1998;51(1):79–83.

62. Keay S, Zhang CO, Shoenfelt JL, et al. Decreased in vitro proliferation of bladder epithelial cells from patients with interstitial cystitis. Urology 2003;61(6):1278–84.

63. Kim J, Freeman MR. Antiproliferative factor signaling and interstitial cystitis/painful bladder syndrome. Int Neurourol J 2011;15(4):184–91.

64. Yang W, Chung YG, Kim Y, et al. Quantitative proteomics identifies a beta-catenin network as an element of the signaling response to Frizzled-8 protein-related antiproliferative factor. Mol Cell Proteomics 2011;10(6). M110 007492.

65. Kutch JJ, Yani MS, Asavasopon S, et al. Altered resting state neuromotor connectivity in men with

chronic prostatitis/chronic pelvic pain syndrome: A MAPP: Research Network Neuroimaging Study. Neuroimage Clin 2015;8:493–502.

66. Martucci KT, Shirer WR, Bagarinao E, et al. The posterior medial cortex in urologic chronic pelvic pain syndrome: detachment from default mode network-a resting-state study from the MAPP Research Network. Pain 2015;156(9):1755–64.

67. Lai HH, Krieger JN, Pontari MA, et al. Painful Bladder Filling and Painful Urgency are Distinct Characteristics in Men and Women with Urological Chronic Pelvic Pain Syndromes: A MAPP Research Network Study. J Urol 2015;194(6):1634–41.

68. Colaco M, Koslov DS, Keys T, et al. Correlation of gene expression with bladder capacity in interstitial cystitis/bladder pain syndrome. J Urol 2014;192(4):1123–9.

69. Plair A, Evans RJ, Langefeld CD, et al. Anesthetic Bladder Capacity is a Clinical Biomarker for Interstitial Cystitis/Bladder Pain Syndrome Subtypes. Urology 2021;158:74–80.

70. Schachar JS, Evans RJ, Parks GE, et al. Histological evidence supports low anesthetic bladder capacity as a marker of a bladder-centric disease subtype in interstitial cystitis/bladder pain syndrome. Int Urogynecol J 2019;30(11):1863–70.

71. Choi D, Han JY, Shin JH, et al. Downregulation of WNT11 is associated with bladder tissue fibrosis in patients with interstitial cystitis/bladder pain syndrome without Hunner lesion. Sci Rep 2018;8(1):9782.

72. Cho KJ, Lee KS, Choi JB, et al. Changes in uroplakin expression in the urothelium of patients with ulcerative interstitial cystitis/bladder pain syndrome. Investig Clin Urol 2020;61(3):304–9.

73. Lee G. Uroplakins in the lower urinary tract. Int Neurourol J 2011;15(1):4–12.

74. Aboushwareb T, Zhou G, Deng FM, et al. Alterations in bladder function associated with urothelial defects in uroplakin II and IIIa knockout mice. Neurourol Urodyn 2009;28(8):1028–33.

75. Hu P, Deng FM, Liang FX, et al. Ablation of uroplakin III gene results in small urothelial plaques, urothelial leakage, and vesicoureteral reflux. J Cell Biol 2000;151(5):961–72.

76. Hu P, Meyers S, Liang FX, et al. Role of membrane proteins in permeability barrier function: uroplakin ablation elevates urothelial permeability. Am J Physiol Ren Physiol 2002;283(6):F1200–7.

77. Kaga K, Inoue KI, Kaga M, et al. Expression profile of urothelial transcription factors in bladder biopsies with interstitial cystitis. Int J Urol 2017;24(8):632–8.

78. Liu HT, Jiang YH, Kuo HC. Alteration of Urothelial Inflammation, Apoptosis, and Junction Protein in Patients with Various Bladder Conditions and Storage Bladder Symptoms Suggest Common Pathway Involved in Underlying Pathophysiology. Low Urin Tract Symptoms 2015;7(2):102–7.

79. Shie JH, Kuo HC. Higher levels of cell apoptosis and abnormal E-cadherin expression in the urothelium are associated with inflammation in patients with interstitial cystitis/painful bladder syndrome. BJU Int 2011;108(2 Pt 2):E136–41.

80. Shie JH, Liu HT, Kuo HC. Increased cell apoptosis of urothelium mediated by inflammation in interstitial cystitis/painful bladder syndrome. Urology 2012;79(2):484 e7–13.

81. Tonyali S, Ates D, Akbiyik F, et al. Urine nerve growth factor (NGF) level, bladder nerve staining and symptom/problem scores in patients with interstitial cystitis. Adv Clin Exp Med 2018;27(2):159–63.

82. Jiang YH, Jhang JF, Hsu YH, et al. Urine cytokines as biomarkers for diagnosing interstitial cystitis/bladder pain syndrome and mapping its clinical characteristics. Am J Physiol Ren Physiol 2020;318(6):F1391–9.

83. Jiang YH, Jhang JF, Hsu YH, et al. Urine biomarkers in ESSIC type 2 interstitial cystitis/bladder pain syndrome and overactive bladder with developing a novel diagnostic algorithm. Sci Rep 2021;11(1):914.

84. Ma E, Vetter J, Bliss L, et al. A multiplexed analysis approach identifies new association of inflammatory proteins in patients with overactive bladder. Am J Physiol Ren Physiol 2016;311(1):F28–34.

85. Vera PL, Preston DM, Moldwin RM, et al. Elevated Urine Levels of Macrophage Migration Inhibitory Factor in Inflammatory Bladder Conditions: A Potential Biomarker for a Subgroup of Interstitial Cystitis/Bladder Pain Syndrome Patients. Urology 2018;116:55–62.

86. Pang D, Liao L. Abnormal functional connectivity within the prefrontal cortex in interstitial cystitis/bladder pain syndrome (IC/BPS): A pilot study using resting state functional near-infrared spectroscopy (rs-fNIRS). Neurourol Urodyn 2021;40(6):1634–42.

87. Duan L, Zhang YJ, Zhu CZ. Quantitative comparison of resting-state functional connectivity derived from fNIRS and fMRI: a simultaneous recording study. Neuroimage 2012;60(4):2008–18.

88. Cui X, Bray S, Bryant DM, et al. A quantitative comparison of NIRS and fMRI across multiple cognitive tasks. Neuroimage 2011;54(4):2808–21.

89. Geng S, Liu X, Biswal BB, et al. Effect of Resting-State fNIRS Scanning Duration on Functional Brain Connectivity and Graph Theory Metrics of Brain Network. Front Neurosci 2017;11:392.

90. Nardos R, Karstens L, Carpenter S, et al. Abnormal functional connectivity in women with urgency urinary incontinence: Can we predict disease presence and severity in individual women using Rs-fcMRI. Neurourol Urodyn 2016;35(5):564–73.

91. Zuo L, Zhou Y, Wang S, et al. Abnormal Brain Functional Connectivity Strength in the Overactive Bladder Syndrome: A Resting-State fMRI Study. Urology 2019;131:64–70.

92. Li P, Bracamontes J, Katona BW, et al. Natural and enantiomeric etiocholanolone interact with distinct sites on the rat alpha1beta2gamma2L GABAA receptor. Mol Pharmacol 2007;71(6):1582–90.

93. Wilmore DW. Are the metabolic alterations associated with critical illness related to the hormonal environment? Clin Nutr 1986;5(1):9–19.

94. Saha SK, Jeon TI, Jang SB, et al. Bioinformatics Approach for Identifying Novel Biomarkers and Their Signaling Pathways Involved in Interstitial Cystitis/Bladder Pain Syndrome with Hunner Lesion. J Clin Med 2020;9(6). https://doi.org/10.3390/jcm9061935.

95. Bosch PC. A Randomized, Double-blind, Placebo-controlled Trial of Certolizumab Pegol in Women with Refractory Interstitial Cystitis/Bladder Pain Syndrome. Eur Urol 2018;74(5):623–30.

96. Iizuka M, Wakamatsu E, Tsuboi H, et al. Pathogenic role of immune response to M3 muscarinic acetylcholine receptor in Sjogren's syndrome-like sialoadenitis. J Autoimmun 2010;35(4):383–9.

97. Wu H, Su QX, Zhang ZY, et al. Exploration of the core genes in ulcerative interstitial cystitis/bladder pain syndrome. Int Braz J Urol 2021;47(4):843–55.

98. Russo RC, Garcia CC, Teixeira MM, et al. The CXCL8/IL-8 chemokine family and its receptors in inflammatory diseases. Expert Rev Clin Immunol 2014;10(5):593–619.

99. Jaenisch R, Bird A. Epigenetic regulation of gene expression: how the genome integrates intrinsic and environmental signals. Nat Genet 2003;33(Suppl):245–54.

100. Marentette JO, Hauser PJ, Hurst RE, et al. Tryptase activation of immortalized human urothelial cell mitogen-activated protein kinase. PLoS One 2013;8(7):e69948.

101. Shin CM, Kim N, Jung Y, et al. Role of Helicobacter pylori infection in aberrant DNA methylation along multistep gastric carcinogenesis. Cancer Sci 2010;101(6):1337–46.

102. Jiang YH, Kuo YC, Jhang JF, et al. Repeated intravesical injections of platelet-rich plasma improve symptoms and alter urinary functional proteins in patients with refractory interstitial cystitis. Sci Rep 2020;10(1):15218.

103. Peng CH, Jhang JF, Shie JH, et al. Down regulation of vascular endothelial growth factor is associated with decreased inflammation after intravesical OnabotulinumtoxinA injections combined with hydrodistention for patients with interstitial cystitis–clinical results and immunohistochemistry analysis. Urology 2013;82(6):1452 e1-6.

104. Shen YC, Tyagi P, Lee WC, et al. Improves symptoms and urinary biomarkers in refractory interstitial cystitis/bladder pain syndrome patients randomized to extracorporeal shock wave therapy versus placebo. Sci Rep 2021;11(1):7558.

105. Peters KM, Jayabalan N, Bui D, et al. Effect of Sacral Neuromodulation on Outcome Measures and Urine Chemokines in Interstitial Cystitis/Painful Bladder Syndrome Patients. Low Urin Tract Symptoms 2015;7(2):77–83.

Urine-Based Markers for Detection of Urothelial Cancer and for the Management of Non–muscle-Invasive Bladder Cancer

Yair Lotan, MD*, Fady J. Baky, MD

KEYWORDS

- Bladder cancer • Detection • Surveillance • Urine markers • Hematuria

KEY POINTS

- The ideal use of urine markers would be to develop markers of sufficient performance that would improve clinical care of patients at risk for bladder cancer or undergoing surveillance of NMIBC.
- In the setting of hematuria, markers could be used to tailor evaluation of hematuria patients to those most likely to have disease while avoiding evaluating in low-risk patients.
- There is a need for randomized trials to demonstrate the benefits of using a urine marker to triage patients for hematuria evaluation.
- For patients with NMIBC, markers could reduce interval of cystoscopy in patients with low-grade disease, improve detection of high-grade disease or assist in patients with atypical cystoscopy ("red patches") or atypical cytology.

CONSULTANT

Nanorobotics: consultant starting 5/21. C2I genomics: consultant starting 10/20. Photocure: consultant/advisor, scientific study or trial. AstraZeneca: consultant/advisor. Merck: consultant/advisor. Fergene: consultant. Abbvie: consultant (starting 6/20). Cleveland Diagnostics: consultant 2020, not 2021). Nucleix: consultant. Ambu: consultant. Seattle Genetics: consultant (agreement 12/20). Hitachi: 1/20. Ferring Research: 2/20 (not 2021). Verity Pharmaceuticals. Virtuoso Surgical (started 3/21). Nanorobot (started 6/21). Stimit (started 7/21). Urogen (started 10/21). Vessi. CAPs Medical. xCures (4/22). BMS (2020, not 2021). Aura Biosciences, Inc. (3/22). Convergent Genomics (4/22). Research; Abbott: scientific study or trial completed 3/19. Cepheid: scientific study or trial. Pacific Edge: scientific study or trial. FKD: scientific study or trial (completed 2019). MDxHealth: scientific study or trial. Biocancell: scientific study or trial (ended 1/20). GenomeDx Biosciences, Inc.: scientific study or trial. Storz: scientific study.

INTRODUCTION

Bladder cancer is the fifth most common nonskin, solid cancer overall with 81,180 estimated new cases in the United States in 2022.[1] Bladder cancer is usually diagnosed after patients become symptomatic with hematuria or as part of an evaluation for microhematuria (MH). MH has a high prevalence in society (rate and references) with a rate of cancer

Department of Urology, UT Southwestern Medical Center, 2001 Inwood Road, West Campus Building 3, Floor 4, Dallas, Texas 75390-9110, USA
* Corresponding author.
E-mail address: Yair.Lotan@utsouthwestern.edu

Urol Clin N Am 50 (2023) 53–67
https://doi.org/10.1016/j.ucl.2022.09.009
0094-0143/23/© 2022 Elsevier Inc. All rights reserved.

that ranges from 1% to 5% driven by risk factors (age, sex, smoking, and carcinogen exposure).[2] Currently, evaluation for hematuria is driven by the AUA/SUFU guidelines, and urine markers are not recommended for routine evaluation.[3]

Bladder cancer is a disease characterized by a high recurrence rate that is impacted by stage and grade of disease as well as factors such as size, multiplicity, and prior therapies.[4] The use of urine markers within the guidelines is recommended for very specific indications such as atypical cystoscopic findings or atypical cytologic findings. Routine use is also not recommended for patients undergoing surveillance.

In many ways, urine-based tumor markers including cytology are ideal for the detection of urothelial carcinoma since urothelial tumors are in direct contact with the urine. However, the process of identifying markers requires a robust evaluation including discovering optimal markers, validating them in independent cohorts, and establishing clinical utility.[5]

Urine cytology is the most commonly used urine marker and plays an important role in the surveillance of non–muscle-invasive bladder cancer (NMIBC). The development of superior noninvasive testing via voided tumor markers has been explored to enhance both diagnosis and surveillance and to reduce the frequency of invasive diagnostic procedures. Many protein, DNA and RNA, and molecular biomarkers have been examined as an adjunct to cystoscopy and cytology in the diagnosis and surveillance of bladder cancer, and several FDA-approved tumor markers are now available. The role of biomarkers remains an important area of further study to enhance the diagnosis and surveillance of bladder cancer. Beyond this, tumor markers may also play an important role in risk stratification and prediction of treatment response, allowing for personalized care for patients with bladder cancer.

Broadly, urine tumor markers can be categorized as (1) protein-based, (2) DNA based—mutation and epigenetic, (3) RNA based, and (4) cell based. Protein-based tests detect tumor-specific proteins or elevated levels of certain urinary proteins which may be associated with bladder cancer. Immunohistochemical studies are modified cytologic studies that enhance the ability to detect atypical urothelial cells by binding to specific antigens, causing fluorescence. Genetic-based assays can be designed to detect specific DNA or RNA markers of disease.

This article reviews the urine biomarkers currently available in the diagnosis and surveillance of bladder cancer.

DIAGNOSIS

Although most patients with bladder cancer are diagnosed during evaluation for hematuria, this evaluation remains low yield. In their study evaluating a large cohort of hematuria patients using criteria from the updated AUA guidelines, Woldu and colleagues found a malignancy rate of 0.4%, 1.0%, 6.4% for low, intermediate, and high-risk hematuria, and an 11.1% malignancy rate for gross hematuria, respectively.[6] The AUA/SUFU guidelines recommend a discussion of the risks and benefits of cystoscopy in low-risk microhematuria patients and allow for surveillance as an alternative to cystoscopy. Urine tumor markers may enhance the ability to appropriately risk stratify patients. A negative urine-marker test may restratify patients without disease into a low-risk category and allow the patient to avoid cystoscopy if so preferred. Conversely, a positive test may move a patient into a high-risk category, ensuring they undergo cystoscopy rather than elect for surveillance. Furthermore, a positive test may serve as an adjunct in high-risk patients with normal initial evaluation prompting repeat evaluation or closer surveillance. Finally, urine tumor markers may help characterize unusual appearing tumors of unclear malignant potential.

In the diagnostic setting, an ideal tumor marker would limit the rate of false-positive results in a disease with low prevalence, even among patients with increased risk. As such a marker with high positive predictive value (PPV) and high specificity is suited to this purpose. Several tumor markers have been developed with this goal of improving detection of bladder cancer. It should be noted that some markers such as NMP22 BladderChek (Alere NMP22 Bladder, Abbott Laboratories, Chicago, IL, USA), BTA tests (Polymedco, USA), and UroVysion (Abbott Laboratories, Abbott Park, IL, USA) have been FDA approved and several others such as Cxbladder (Pacific Edge Diagnostics, USA) tests, Xpert Bladder Cancer Detection (Xpert; CE-IVD, Cepheid, Sunnyvale, CA, USA), and Bladder CARE (Pangea Laboratory LLC, CA, USA) are commercially available. There are also multiple markers under development (**Tables 1 and 2**).

Protein-Based Assays

Urine protein components have long been studied as possible diagnostic tests for several genitourinary (and non-genitourinary) disease processes. Despite the technical difficulties of protein handling and the large variability in urine protein concentrations, several candidate proteins have been studied as possible adjuncts to bladder

Table 1
Commercially available biomarkers for bladder cancer detection

Class	Marker	Molecule	Reference	Year	Sensitivity	Specificity
Protein	BladderChek (Alere NMP22 Bladder, Abbot Labs)	Nuclear Matrix Protein 22	Grossman et al,[9] 2015	2005	55.7%	85.7%
	Bladder Tumor Antigen (Polymedco, USA) – POC and ELISA	Human complement factor H-related protein	Guo et al,[40] 2014 (POC) Glas et al (ELISA)	2014 2003	67% 75%	75% 65%
	UBC	Cytokeratin	Lu et al	2018	59.3%	86.1%
Cell Based	UroVysion (Abbott Laboratories)	Fluorescence in situ Hybridization	Hajdinjak	2008	72%	83%
RNA	CxBladderTriage; CxBladderDetect; CxBladderResolve	IGF, HOXA, MDK, CDC, IL8R	Kavaliers O'Sullivan Raman	2015 2012 2021	95%[a] 82% 92.4%[b]	98%[a] 85% 93.8%[b]
	Xpert Bladder Detection (Xpert; Cepheid)	ABL1, CRH, IGF2, UPK1B, ANXA10	Van Valenberg	2020	78%	84%

No prospective trials for bladder cancer detection using Bladder CARE.
[a] In macrohematuria only.
[b] Designed to be used after CxT.
Adapted from Molecular Biomarkers in Urologic Oncology from the 1st ICUD-WUOF International Consultation October 2020 with permission of the Société Internationale d'Urologie https://www.siu-urology.org/society/siu-icud.

Table 2
Experimental biomarkers for bladder cancer detection

Class	Molecule	Reference	Year	Sensitivity	Specificity
DNA	Telomerase reverse transcriptase (TERT) Fibroblast growth factor receptor 3 (FGFR3)	Allory et al,[22] 2014	2014	70%	–
	Cell-free DNA (cfDNA) cMyc, BCAS1, HER2	Cadio et al	2012	70%	75%
	TaqMan Array (12 + 2 gene panel)	Mengual et al,[51] 2007	2016	89%	95%
Mutations: FGFR3, TERT, HRAS Methylation: OTX1, ONECUT2, TWIST1	Van Kessel et al	2020		97%	83%
RNA	CAIX	De Martino et al	2015	86.2%	95.1%
	Survivin	Shariat et al,[30] 2004	2007	64%	93%

Adapted from *Molecular Biomarkers in Urologic Oncology* from the 1st ICUD-WUOF International Consultation October 2020 with permission of the Société Internationale d'Urologie https://www.siu-urology.org/society/siu-icud.

cancer diagnosis and surveillance. Thus far, only 2 urine protein markers have been FDA approved for the detection and/or surveillance of bladder cancer.

Nuclear matrix protein 22

Perhaps the most classic protein-based assay for the diagnosis of bladder cancer is nuclear matrix protein (NMP) 22.[7] NMPs are a family of proteins involved in the structure of the nucleus and its role in genetic transcription and replication. Several NMPs have been demonstrated to be overexpressed in urothelial carcinoma and can be detected in urine. Of these, NMP 22 has been used in both the diagnosis and surveillance of urothelial carcinoma. Two NMP22-based tests are currently FDA approved for the diagnosis and surveillance of bladder cancer. The NMP22 Bladder Cancer ELISA-Test (Alere NMP22 Bladder, Abbott Laboratories, Chicago, IL, USA) is quantitative while the NMP22 BladderChek is a qualitative point-of-care test.[8] NMP22 BladderChek has been FDA approved for use in bladder cancer diagnosis. As NMP22 is shed in the process of cell turnover, it suffers from the same limitations as classic urine cytology, namely a lower sensitivity for low-grade disease. However, multiple studies have demonstrated that despite its limitations it outperforms cytology in the detection of low-grade tumors. In addition, other inflammatory conditions such as infection and urolithiasis may result in false positives. Grossman and colleagues studied the use of NMP22 during the evaluation of patients with hematuria. The study included 1331 patients at elevated risk for bladder cancer

provided voided urine for cytology and NMP22 before cystoscopy. Bladder cancer was found in 79 patients, 44 of whom had positive NMP22 assays for a sensitivity of 55.7% versus 15.8% for voided cytology. NMP22 had a specificity of 85.7% versus 99.2% for cytology.[9] In a meta-analysis on NMP22 in the detection setting, Chou and colleagues found a sensitivity of 69% and a specificity of 77% for the NMP22 Bladder Cancer ELISA-Test.[10]

NMP22 likely performs best in combination with other molecular markers or when combined with clinical patient factors. Lotan and colleagues incorporated a nomogram of patient demographic and risk factors as well as cytology and NMP22 resulting in an accuracy of 80% in predicting bladder cancer in patients with hematuria.[11]

Bladder tumor antigen

Bladder tumor antigen (BTA) (Polymedco, Cortlandt, NY, USA) is a commercially available POC test that uses monoclonal antibodies to detect human complement factor H. Human complement factor H, a protein involved in the regulation of the alternate pathway of complement immune response. Two BTA tests are available, the qualitative BTA stat test and a quantitative BTA TRAK. In a meta-analysis, Chou and colleagues assessed the performance of each test in the detection of bladder cancer.[10] Across 8 studies, BTA stat had a sensitivity of 76% and specificity of 78%. For the quantitative test, BTA TRAK, the sensitivity was also 76%, but the specificity was 53%; however, there were limited studies assessing BTA TRAK in this setting.

Cytokeratin

Cytokeratins are structural proteins found in the intracytoplasmic cytoskeleton of epithelial cells. They are a component of intermediate filaments that may be released during mechanical and oxidative stress.[12] A commercially available ELISA-based test and a point-of-care assay have been developed (UBC Rapid, IDL Biotech AB).[13] Several prospective studies of the UBC assay have shown a modest sensitivity of approximately 59.3% with a specificity of 86.1%. These studies have included both patients at primary diagnosis and patients under surveillance for both known low-grade and high-grade diseases. Detection rates were higher in the primary setting, particularly for high-grade tumors.

Cell-Based Tests

UroVysion

Fluorescence in situ hybridization (FISH)—in which fluorescent dye tagged DNA segments are used to identify corresponding targets in DNA samples—has been studied in the diagnosis of bladder cancer. UroVysion (Abbott Laboratories, Abbott Park, IL, USA) is a FISH assay devised for the detection of bladder cancer in exfoliated urothelial cells. Specifically, the assay detects aneuploidy of chromosomes 3, 7, and 17 or loss of the 9p21 locus. This has been demonstrated to have a sensitivity of 72% and specificity of 83%. The sensitivity for low-grade cancers remains much lower.[14] The assay has also been studied as an adjunct to cytology, and when used in combination may have a higher sensitivity than when used alone, without affecting the test's specificity.

RNA Assays

mRNA assays have shown the potential to identify mutations in particular genes that may detect cancer in patients with uncertain or negative cystoscopy. There are increasingly reliable and reproducible PCR techniques readily available at many institutions for quantifying RNA. For this reason, RNA assays have been increasingly studied as possible replacements or adjuncts to urine cytology. The major limitation of RNA is its relative instability, which makes obtaining and maintaining RNA samples more variable than other DNA or protein markers. These limitations may be circumvented by RNA amplification techniques and commercial test systems that use RNA stabilizing techniques.

Cxbladder

Cxbladder (Pacific Edge Diagnostics, USA) is an mRNA assay designed to measure the concentration of 5 genes in urine, which may outperform cytology in the detection of urothelial carcinoma. These genes include MDK, HOXA13, CDC2/CDK1, IGFBP5, and CXCR2. Four separate tests are commercially available that incorporate the genes and clinical data: CxbladderTriage (CxbT), CxbladderDetect (CxbD), and Cxbladder-Resolve (CxbR) designed for diagnosis and CxbladderMonitor (CxbM) designed for surveillance.[15] The CxbM will be discussed in the surveillance section.

The CxbT is used in patients with microhematuria and combines the results of the gene assay with patient clinical factors to provide a risk stratification to identify those patients who may not require invasive evaluation with cystoscopy. As this test is meant to select patients who may avoid the established workup for microhematuria (cystoscopy with or without cytology), the utility is dependent on a high negative predictive value (NPV). This was studied by O'Sullivan and colleagues in a cohort of 695 patients from 11 urologic departments in Australia and New Zealand.[16] When genotypic data attained by CxbT was combined with patient age, gender, frequency of macrohematuria, and smoking history, there was a 100% detection rate of high-grade cancer. Importantly, the test demonstrated an NPV of 98%. Eighty percent of patients with microhematuria and no cancer would have been correctly circumvented from a full urologic workup by the results of CxbT.

CxbladderDetect is designed for patients with a higher risk of urothelial carcinoma. In the study mentioned earlier, O'Sullivan and colleagues assessed the utility of CxbD in patients with high-risk macrohematuria without a history of urothelial carcinoma. CxbD detected 97% of high-grade tumors and 100% of pT1 tumors with a sensitivity of 82% and a specificity of 85%. In addition, CxbD outperformed urine cytology in the detection of low-grade tumors with a sensitivity of 91% (vs 68%).

CxbladderResolve is the newest Cxbladder test designed for use after CxbD or CxbT to identify those test-positive patients with a high likelihood of high-impact tumors (HIT)—high-grade tumors Ta, T1-T3, and Tis.[17] CxbR integrates the expression levels of genotypic biomarkers with patient age and smoking history through a novel algorithm to identify high-risk patients. CxbR subsequently stratifies patients into 3 risk categories "high priority," "physician-directed protocol" (PDP), or "observation." Raman and colleagues examined the performance of CxbR alone in 863 patients. Forty-seven of 49 patients with HIT were triaged to "high priority" with the other 2 placed in the

"PDP" category resulting in a 95.5% sensitivity. Of the 40 patients with low-impact tumors, 9 were classified as "high priority," 27 as "PDP," and 4 as "observation."

Using the same cohort, they also examined the CxbR in combination with CxbD and CxbT in 548 patients. These patients initially underwent CxbT with 52% having negative results, including 1 with a Ta low-grade tumor. CxbD was performed on the remaining 263 CxbT-positive samples indicating a low probability of disease in 164 patients, including 1 patient with Ta low-grade disease. Finally, CxbR was performed on the remaining 99 samples and triaged 31 to "observation," 45 to "PDP," and 23 to "high priority." Again 1 patient with Ta low-grade disease was triaged to observation. Of the 45 triaged to "PDP," 1 had low-grade disease and another had high-risk disease. Of the 23 triaged to "high priority," 9 had high-risk disease and 14 had no disease. Cumulatively, the Cxbladder tests excluded 87% of disease-free patients from evaluation and correctly triaged all patients with high-risk disease to "high priority" or "PDP."

Xpert bladder cancer detection

Xpert Bladder Cancer Detection (Xpert; CE-IVD, Cepheid, Sunnyvale, CA, USA) is an assay that quantitates the expression of mRNA from 5 genes which may be overexpressed in bladder cancer. A companion test, Xpert Bladder Cancer Monitor, for monitoring patients with known bladder cancer is discussed in the following section. In a study of 828 patients with gross or microscopic hematuria, Xpert had a sensitivity of 78% overall and 90% for high-grade tumors. The NPV was 98%.[18]

DNA Assays

Bladder cancer is known to carry a high mutational burden, meaning that each bladder cancer harbors many different mutations.[19] Many mechanisms to screen urine for common DNA mutations have been proposed as potential targets for bladder cancer detection and surveillance. No current DNA-based tests have been FDA approved for clinical use, but several studies have been developed to assess various mutational assays. As urine concentration is highly dependent on patient fluid status, some assays are performed on spun down urine which is separated into cell pellets and supernatant. Alternatively, some assays are performed on whole urine.[20]

Several proto-oncogenes have been studied as frequent contributors to bladder cancer development and therefore possible targets for bladder cancer identification. Among the most studied are FGFR3, PIK3CA, RAS, and TERT. Fibroblast growth factor receptor 3 (FGFR3) is a type of receptor tyrosine kinase—a class of cell surface receptors that respond to extracellular signals and induce a downfield cascade of cell proliferation. FGFR3 mutations are found in approximately two-thirds of NMIBC, but this number is much lower in muscle-invasive bladder cancer (MIBC).[21] RAS proteins are a class of GTPases that are activated by the phosphorylation of bound GDP to GTP. Activating mutations result in downfield proliferation and are common mutations in a variety of malignancies. Telomerase reverse transcriptase (TERT) mutations have been frequently noted in bladder tumors, with some studies citing a mutation in up to 70% of bladder tumors.[22] TERT plays a role in increasing telomere length, which is essential to protecting cell DNA during progressive DNA replication. PIK3CA (phosphatidylinositol-3-kinase catalytic subunit alpha) is a transcription factor activated by the RTK-RAS-MAPK pathway, and is mutated in approximately 20% of bladder cancers.

DNA methylation studies

DNA methylation plays an important role in the epigenetic silencing and activation of certain genes. When located on the promoter sequence of a gene, methylation typically acts as a silencer preventing transcription and downfield growth and cell division. Variable DNA methylation has been identified as a component of cancer development. Hypomethylation of proto-oncogenes, or conversely hypermethylation of tumor suppressor genes may be identified in cancer cells. Methylation status can be assessed through several novel genetic assays.

Bladder CARE (Pangea Laboratory LLC, CA, USA) is a commercially available at-home urine collection test that detects hypermethylation of 3 biomarkers (TRNA-Cys, SIM2, and NKX_{1-1}).[23] These 3 loci have previously been demonstrated to be hypermethylated in patients with both NMIBC and MIBC. Of 77 patients with known bladder cancer, Bladder CARE correctly identified 60 as 'Positive' and 12 as 'High Risk' resulting in a sensitivity of 93.5%. Of the 136 individuals without bladder cancer, only 9 were identified as 'High Risk' and 1 'Positive' resulting in a specificity of 92.6%. Bladder CARE also quantified the rate of hypermethylation into a number termed the Bladder CARE Index (BCI), which could be used to estimate the probability of having disease.

Renard and colleagues used methylation-specific polymerase chain reaction to study the methylation status of a 2 gene panel (TWIST1 and NID2) in patients with hematuria. They were able to achieve a high sensitivity (90%) and specificity (93%) in 466 urine samples from patients with hematuria. Unfortunately, 2 trials of external validity on larger multi-institutional cohorts failed to achieve similar results with a sensitivity of 79% and specificity of 63%.

Hentschel and colleagues studied the methylation status of a panel of potential genes and found that the methylation status of *GHSR* and *MAL* was 80% sensitive and 93% specific in the identification of bladder cancer. As expected, this assay was more sensitive in higher grade and higher stage tumors, but interestingly, it was also more sensitive in male than in female patients (92% vs 79%).[24]

TERT and FGFR3

TERT and *FGFR3* mutations have been detected in urine via SNaPshot analysis—a DNA primer extension mechanism used to detect single nucleotide polymorphisms. Using this technique in the evaluation of patients with hematuria, Allory and colleagues demonstrated a 62% sensitivity and 90% specificity for *TERT* mutations and a 36% sensitivity for *FGFR3* mutations. An assay of these genes together demonstrated a 70% sensitivity.[22]

Cell-free DNA

Circulating plasma or serum cell-free DNA (cfDNA) has been studied as a potential marker for several nongenitourinary solid organ malignancies, prompting the investigation of its study in urine samples to detect bladder cancer. Casadio and colleagues studied quantities of cfDNA in a population of 51 patients with bladder cancer, 46 patients with hematuria, and 32 healthy controls by PCR.[20] They limited their analysis to sequences longer than 250 bp of *cMyc*, *BCAS1*, and *HER2*. Using an area under the curve (AUC) analysis, they established a threshold cfDNA quantity that resulted in a 0.70 sensitivity and 0.75 specificity. Other studies have replicated this datum with the same or other gene targets; however, all have been limited to similarly small patient populations.

TaqMan array (12 + 2 gene panel)

TaqMan probes are hydrolysis probes that increase the specificity of quantitative PCR. Mengual and colleagues have identified a 12 + 2 gene panel TaqMan array for urothelial carcinoma identification.[25] By starting with bladder washings from 244 patients with pathology-confirmed urothelial carcinoma, 48 genes were identified that were overrepresented in urothelial carcinoma. Subsequently, 211 and voided samples were analyzed by TaqMan arrays using these 48 selected genes. Of note, a cDNA preamplification step was used to counteract the RNA degradation

which occurred more prominently in voided urine than in bladder washings. From this cohort, 12 genes were identified that were predictive of urothelial carcinoma. This assay had a sensitivity of 70% for voided urine and 98% for bladder washings. Two additional genes (ASAM and MCM10) were added to this gene panel to achieve a sensitivity and specificity of 79% and 92%, respectively, in discriminating between low- and high-grade tumors.

Carbonic anhydrase IX

Carbonic anhydrase IX (CAIX) has been studied as a biomarker in renal cell carcinoma as well as in nongenitourinary malignancies such as breast cancer.[26] CAIX produces a carbonic anhydrase, which regulates cell pH in response to hypoxia, and therefore is upregulated in cell proliferation and tumor progression. CAIX is overexpressed in most urothelial carcinomas, and interestingly appears to be more heavily expressed in less invasive and low-grade tumors than in invasive and high-grade tumors. As CAIX activity has been demonstrated in tumor pathogenesis, the presence of urinary CAIX mRNA has been assessed as a possible tumor marker for urothelial carcinoma.

Malentacchi and colleagues studied the utility of voided CAIX mRNA in various urologic oncological cancer entities including bladder cancer.[27] Voided urine from 93 patients with known bladder cancer and 89 healthy controls was assessed for quantity of CAIX mRNA. Quantity of the full length CAIX protein isoform was also measured to control for variable baseline expression of CAIX among subjects. Relative quantity of urinary CAIX mRNA was elevated in patients with malignancy. Martino and colleagues used CAIX expression with a TaqMan Gene expression in a population of patients with urothelial carcinoma and healthy controls.[28] They found a sensitivity and specificity of 86.2% and 95.1%, respectively, compared to 43.5% and 100% for cytology. Most notably, the diagnostic accuracy remained high in low-grade tumors, and as previously demonstrated, CAIX expression decreased in more invasive, higher-grade tumors.

Survivin

Survivin is an antiapoptotic protein, which inhibits apoptosis, induces/upregulates angiogenesis, and promotes cell proliferation.[29,30] As discussed in the following section, elevated levels of survivin have been associated with the presence of disease. Survivin mRNA has also been studied as a potential biomarker for urothelial carcinoma. Horstmann and colleagues analyzed voided urine samples for surviving mRNA via real-time PCR and identified a cut-off level of 10,000 mRNA copies which had a sensitivity of 53% and specificity of 88% in a small sample size (32 urothelial carcinoma patients).[31] Low-stage (pTa) tumors were poorly detected (35%); however, 100% of invasive (4 pT1 and 4 pT2) cancers were detected. Other inflammatory processes (concomitant cystitis) did not confound survivin measurements.

MicroRNA

MicroRNA (miRNA) is an exciting new class of potentially noninvasive biomarkers for various disease states. MiRNAs are short segments of single-stranded RNA that play an important role in the regulation of post-transcriptional gene expression via messenger RNA silencing. By selectively binding to specific mRNA, miRNAs can cause destabilization of the mRNA or prevent translation into proteins by ribosomes. As miRNAs may be increasingly active in states of cell proliferation, their utility as a circulating biomarker for malignancy has become an area of study.

In bladder cancer, the miRNA-200 family has been identified as a potential marker of malignancy.[32] These miRNAs are thought to be involved in tumor cell adhesion, cell migration, invasion, and metastasis. Single miRNA levels have not demonstrated sufficient sensitivity for the diagnosis of bladder cancer, and increasingly multi-miRNA assays have been studied. In their meta-analysis of various miRNA assays, Kutwin and colleagues found that median sensitivities for various miRNA assays ranged from 80% to 86.6%.[33] Specificity for multi-miRNA assays has ranged from 60% to 70%, suggesting that miRNA may be more suitable as a diagnostic tool to reduce the need for invasive workup. Currently, the heterogeneity of various miRNA assays and the limited number of small cohort studies limits the utility of miRNA as a screening tool for urothelial carcinoma and no miRNA assays are currently commercially available for bladder cancer diagnosis.

Combined assays

Several studies have paired DNA mutation and methylation assays, along with clinical factors, in the evaluation of patients with hematuria. In 2016, Roprech and colleagues paired FGFR mutation assessment with a methylation panel (HS3ST2, SLIT2, and SEPTIN9) with clinical parameters (age and smoking status) and achieved a sensitivity of 97% and specificity of 84%.[34] Also in 2016, Dahmcke and colleagues studied mutations in TERT, FGFR3 paired with methylation status of SALL3, ONECUT2, CCNA1, BCL2, EOMES, and VIM for a sensitivity of 97% and specificity of 77%.[35] Finally in 2016, Van Kessel and colleagues studied mutations in FGFR3, TERT and HRAS paired with methylation status of OTX1, ONECUT2, and TWIST1 and achieved a sensitivity of 97% and specificity of 83%. The following year they were able to validate these findings in a prospective, multi-institutional study with a sensitivity of 93% and specificity of 86%.[36]

SURVEILLANCE

For patients diagnosed with NMIBC following resection and/or intravesical therapy, surveillance requires invasive interval cystoscopy and expensive delayed phase imaging to rule out upper tract recurrence. Cystoscopy can be associated with pain, hematuria, and even urinary tract infection. Small tumors and carcinoma in situ (CIS) can be missed on white light cystoscopy, and in patients with benign or inflammatory lesions, further evaluation requires biopsies or transurethral resections to rule out recurrence. Urine biomarkers hold the promise of reducing discomfort and morbidity for patients under surveillance for bladder cancer, while also reducing the risk of delayed diagnosis of recurrence.

As patients with a prior treated bladder cancer are more likely to have disease, and are therefore approached with a higher index of suspicion, the ideal tumor marker in the surveillance setting would be one with a high NPV and high sensitivity (**Tables 3** and **4**).

Protein Studies

Nuclear matrix protein 22

The nuclear matrix protein 22 assays, NMP22 BladderChek and NMP22 Elisa (Alere/Abbott, USA), were introduced in the discussion on protein tumor markers used for the diagnosis of bladder cancer. Both tests are additionally FDA approved as adjuncts to cystoscopy during the surveillance of bladder cancer. NMP22 was studied in this setting in a multicenter study of 668 patients undergoing surveillance for a history of bladder cancer. NMP22 outperformed voided cytology as an adjunct to cystoscopy, detecting 8 of 9 cancers that were not visualized during initial cystoscopy. Voided cytology detected only 3 of these. Cystoscopy combined with NMP22 diagnosed 102 of 103 recurrent malignancies.[37] In a multicenter prospective cohort study of 803 patients under surveillance for bladder cancer, Lotan and colleagues compared Cxbladder (discussed earlier), cytology, and both NMP22 modalities. They found that both NMP22 assays

Table 3
Commercially available biomarkers for bladder cancer surveillance

Class	Marker	Molecule	Reference	Year	Sensitivity	Specificity
Protein	BladderChek (Alere NMP22 Bladder, Abbot Labs)	Nuclear Matrix Protein 22	Van Rhijn et al	2005	71%	73%
	Bladder tumor antigen (Polymedco, USA) – POC and ELISA	Complement Factor H-related protein	Van Rhijn et al	2005	58% (POC) 71% (ELISA)	73% (POC) 66% (ELISA)
Cell Based	Cytology	–	Freifeld et al	2019	40.8%	92.8%
	UroVysion (Abbott Laboratories)	Fluorescence in situ hybridization	Dimashkieh et al	2013	62.2%	86.2%
RNA	Cxbladder Monitor	*IGF, HOXA, MDK, CDC, IL8R*	Lotan et al,[11] 2009	2017	91%	–
	Xpert BC	*ABL1, CRH, IGF2, UPK1B, ANXA10*	Pichler et al	2018	84%	91%
DNA	Bladder EpiCheck (Nucleix)	Multigene methylation assay	Wasserstrom et al,[48] 2016	2016	90%	83%

Adapted from Molecular Biomarkers in Urologic Oncology from the 1st ICUD-WUOF International Consultation October 2020 with permission of the Société Internationale d'Urologie https://www.siu-urology.org/society/siu-icud

underperformed Cxbladder and neither significantly outperformed cytology in the detection of recurrent disease. The point of care NMP22 BladderChek had a sensitivity of 11% and NPV of 86%, which was only slightly improved in the NMP22 Elisa to 26% and 87%.[38]

Bladder tumor antigen (complement factor H-related protein)

As discussed earlier, bladder tumor antigen detects human complement factor H-related protein and

has been FDA approved for the surveillance of urothelial carcinoma recurrence in combination with cystoscopy. Similar to NMP22, there are 2 assays, a qualitative POC assay (BTA Stat) and a qualitative ELISA (BTA-TRAK). In published reviews, BTA-TRAK has a sensitivity of 66% to 77% and a specificity of 5% to 75%, BTA Stat has a sensitivity of 57% to 82% and a specificity of 68% to 93%. Similar to NMP22, this may represent a higher sensitivity than cytology, but again a higher false-positive rate. Like other urine tumor markers, BTA

Table 4
Experimental biomarkers for bladder cancer surveillance

Class	Marker	Molecule	Reference	Year	Sensitivity	Specificity
RNA	MicroRNA	miR16, miR200c, miR205, miR21, miR221, miR3	Sapre et al	2015	88%	48%
DNA	Telomerase reverse transcriptase	*TERT*	Critelli et al,[47] 2016	2016	67%	–
	Fibroblast growth factor receptor 3	*FGFR3*	Allory et al,[22] 2014	2014	50%	71%
	–	*SOX1, L1-MET, IRAK3*	Su et al,[49] 2014	2014	86%	80%
	–	Mutation: *FGFR3* Methylation: *HS3ST2m SLIT2, SEPTIN9*	Roperch et al,[34] 2016	2016	90%	65%

Adapted from Molecular Biomarkers in Urologic Oncology from the 1st ICUD-WUOF International Consultation October 2020 with permission of the Société Internationale d'Urologie https://www.siu-urology.org/society/siu-icud.

demonstrates a lower sensitivity in the setting of low-grade disease than high-grade disease.[39,40]

Cell-Based Tests

Cytology

The AUA guidelines currently recommend the use of cytology during the surveillance of patients with intermediate- or high-risk bladder cancer. Microscopic analysis of urine sediment in bladder cancer has been used in some form since 1945, and has the advantages of being easily obtained and widely reviewable.[41] Cytology is limited, however, by known low sensitivity in low-grade disease with some estimates as low as 10%. Even in high-grade disease, sensitivity ranges widely from 40% to 70%.[42] Furthermore, there is some variability based on the experience of the reviewing histopathologist.

UroVysion

As discussed earlier, UroVysion is a FISH assay that can identify malignant urothelial cells in the setting of diagnosis and surveillance of bladder cancer. Originally approved to assist in the diagnosis of bladder cancer in patients with hematuria, UroVysion was subsequently studied and approved as an adjunct to cystoscopy in the surveillance of patients with known bladder cancer. In a prospective study of 159 patients with a prior diagnosis of bladder cancer, UroVysion detected 30% of 27 total recurrences, but 70% of those with T1 or Tis tumors. Further UV detected all CIS and was predictive of 2 additional patients who went on to develop CIS. Overall specificity was 95%.[43] Current AUA guidelines support the possible use of UroVysion in patients undergoing BCG and in those with equivocal cytology, as discussed in the following section.

CellDetect

CellDetect (Zetiq, Ramat Gan, Israel) is a commercially available staining technique that uses natural dyes which react differently to various intracellular pH. This can be used to identify cytoplasm of neoplastic cells resulting in a red/purple stain, while in non-neoplastic cells the dye will result in a blue/green stain. CellDetect has been used in several malignancies and has been studied in the diagnosis of bladder cancer. Davis and colleagues studied the efficacy of CellDetect in detect urothelial cancer in the surveillance setting.[44] Two hundred seventeen patients being monitored for urothelial cancer were consecutively enrolled and provided voided urine for staining with CellDetect. Ninety-six patients were confirmed to have disease on biopsy, including 41 with low-grade disease, 52 with high-grade disease, and 3 with

undetermined grade. CellDetect had a sensitivity of 84%, including 78% for high-grade disease, and a specificity of 84%. Thirty-four patients with positive CellDetect but no disease on biopsy were subsequently followed for 9 months, 21% subsequently developed biopsy-proven recurrence. This was compared to a recurrence rate of 5% for those with negative biopsy and negative CellDetect.

RNA Assays

Cxbladder Monitor

Cxbladder Monitor (Pacific Edge Diagnostics, USA) is an mRNA assay designed to assist in the surveillance of recurrent bladder cancer. Kavaliers and colleagues published the results of their trial evaluating 763 bladder cancer surveillance patients with Cxbladder Monitor and found a sensitivity of 93% as well as an NPV of 97%.[45] These results were confirmed in a similar trial by Lotan and colleagues in a study of 803 patients (sensitivity 91% and NPV 96%).

Xpert BC

The Xpert BC monitor system (Cepheid, Sunnyvale, CA, USA) is a second mRNA assay using 5 target genes (CRH, UPK1B, ABL1, IGF2, and ANXA10) to detect bladder cancer in the surveillance setting. From 2017 to 2011, several studies have prospectively evaluated this system. Sharma and colleagues published the results of a pooled meta-analysis of 11 studies and 2896 patients. The pooled sensitivity and specificity were 73% and 77%, respectively. Xpert BC performed better at detecting high-grade tumors with a sensitivity of 86% (vs 58% for low-grade). They concluded that while Xpert BC may be able to replace cytology in the surveillance of bladder cancer—albeit at the cost of a reduced specificity—it was unlikely to be a suitable candidate to replace cystoscopy altogether.

MicroRNA

Compared to the diagnostic setting, there are limited studies of the utilization of miRNA expression levels in the surveillance of bladder cancer. Sapre and colleagues compared various miRNA assays using AUC analysis and selected an assay of 6 (miR16, miR200c, miR205, miR21, miR221, and miR3).[32] When used in an independent cohort, this assay had a sensitivity of 88% and a specificity of 48%. Yun and colleagues evaluated the utility of miR200a and mi145 in the surveillance setting, and lower levels of miR200a were demonstrated to independently predict recurrence in patients under surveillance following resection of bladder cancer (OR 0.449).[46]

DNA Assays

TERT and FGFR3

The most studied DNA mutations in the diagnosis of bladder cancer, *TERT* and *FGFR3,* have also been the most studied in the surveillance of patients with known disease. Critelli and colleagues analyzed the urine of patients with known NMIBC for mutations in *TERT* and *FGFR3* as well as *PIK3CA* and *RAS*.[47] They found that the combination of *TERT* and *FGFR3* resulted in a sensitivity of 67%, while all genes together resulted in only an additional 2% sensitivity (69%).

DNA methylation studies

Bladder EpiCheck (Nucleix, San Diego, CA, USA) is the only commercially available epigenetic assay designed to be used as an adjunct to cystoscopy in the surveillance of bladder cancer. This assay tests the methylation status of 15 genes and determines whether the methylation status is consistent with the presence or absence of bladder cancer. In a validation study, Bladder Epi-Check was used in 222 patients with a history of bladder cancer under surveillance. Bladder Epi-Check correctly diagnosed 36 of 40 patients with biopsy-confirmed recurrence (sensitivity 90%) and correctly ruled out 151 of 182 cancer-free patients (specificity of 83%).[48]

Su and colleagues studied a panel of 3 genes' methylation status, *SOX1, L1-MET,* and *IRAK3* in the urine samples of 90 patients following TURBT.[49] Patients had variable grade and stage on initial diagnosis (Tis, Ta, T1; low and high grades), and samples were collected from both voided urine and bladder washings. This panel correctly predicted recurrence in 80% of those who recurred and accurately predicted no recurrence in 74% of patients who did not recur over a 5- to 89-month follow-up interval. This greatly outperformed cytology in their cohort (35% sensitivity) and awaits external, prospective validation.

Combined assays

As discussed earlier, assays combining specific mutations with gene methylation studies may result in improved specificity. Roprech and colleagues studied an assay of mutations in *FGFR3* and methylation changes in *HS3ST2, SLIT2,* and *SEPTIN9* with clinical parameters (age and smoking status) in bladder cancer and achieved a sensitivity and specificity of 90% and 65%, respectively.[34] This was slightly lower than in the evaluation of hematuria. In 2017, Beukers and colleagues used a combination of mutation analysis in *FGFR3* and *TERT* with the presence of hypermethylation of *OTX1* resulting in a sensitivity and specificity of 57% and 59%, respectively, for

low-grade tumors and 72% and 55%, respectively, for high-grade tumors.[50]

PROGNOSIS

The 2020 AUA guidelines for the treatment of NMIBC suggest 2 indications for the use of urine tumor markers, first to adjudicate equivocal cytology or cystoscopy results and second to predict response to intravesical BCG.

Inflammation following BCG can confound the results of both cystoscopy and urine cytology. In this setting, urinary markers may predict persistent or recurrent disease. Several studies have assessed the utility of UroVysion in the surveillance of post-TUR patients with bladder cancer undergoing intravesical BCG treatment.[51,52] Kamat and colleagues conducted a prospective clinical trial, 126 patients underwent UroVysion analysis at baseline after TUR, and at 6 weeks, 3 months, and 6 months of standard BCG therapy.[53] Patients with positive UroVysion were 3 to 5 times more likely to recur and 5 to 13 times more likely to progress than those with negative tests. In 2019, Lotan and colleagues validated the use of UroVysion to predict recurrence in patients undergoing BCG.[54] In this multi-institutional study of 150 patients with a history of bladder cancer, a positive FISH assay was associated with a 3.35 HR of developing recurrent disease.

Equivocal urine cytology or cystoscopy leaves clinicians and patients with a challenging clinical scenario and can require extensive evaluation to rule out an occult malignancy. Similarly in some patients, atypical urine cytology may be present in the absence of an identifiable lesion. In both these scenarios, the AUA guidelines suggest urine tumor markers may assist in mediating these results. Both UroVysion and uCyt (ImmunoCyt) have been studied in this context. Odisho and colleagues studied the use of reflex uCyt in all atypical cytology for a mixed cohort of patients undergoing evaluation of hematuria or surveillance for bladder cancer. Cystoscopy was repeated within 90 days of cytology and reflex uCyt. Among the patients undergoing surveillance for a prior diagnosis of bladder cancer, reflex uCyt had a sensitivity of 73% for disease recurrence and a specificity of 49%. For patients undergoing hematuria evaluation, reflex uCyt had a sensitivity of 85% and a specificity of 59%.[55]

Similarly, Lotan and colleagues studied the utility of reflex FISH (UroVysion) in patients undergoing evaluation of hematuria or surveillance for bladder cancer. In a 2008 study of 50 patients under evaluation for hematuria and 70 patients undergoing cancer surveillance, reflex FISH was used to adjudicate atypical cytology or abnormal cystoscopic findings.[56] In surveillance patients with equivocal lesions on cystoscopy, FISH detected all high-grade tumors, although it did miss one low-grade tumor. Among those with a negative cystoscopy but positive FISH, 3 patients were ultimately diagnosed with cancer including 2 bladder CIS and 1 prostate cancer in situ. In patients undergoing evaluation of hematuria with equivocal or negative cystoscopy, positive reflex FISH diagnosed 2 high-grade tumors with a PPV of 50%. In 2009, Lotan and colleagues published a second study of 108 patients evaluated for hematuria and 108 patients under surveillance.[57] Positive FISH in patients with equivocal cystoscopy detected 4 additional high-grade cancers, again with a PPV of 50% and NPV of 100%. In patients with negative cystoscopy, 2 additional cancers were diagnosed with a PPV of 10% and NPV of 100%. In patients with no cancer history and equivocal or negative cystoscopy, positive FISH detected 4 additional cancers. While not included in the guidelines as of yet, a study found that the Cxbladder Monitor test may also have value in adjudicating abnormal cystoscopy or cytology.[58]

Several experimental markers have been suggested as potential predictors of disease prognosis. FGFR3 has been noted to have different mutation profiles in NMIBC and MIBC. Most NMIBCs have mutations in FGFR3, whereas only approximately 15% of MIBCs have such mutations. NMIBC driven by mutations is slower to progress to MIBC than those without FGFR3 mutations. Conversely, urine detection of FGFR3 mutations may predict tumor recurrence. Zuiverloon and colleagues found that detection of urine FGFR mutations predicted a 3.8-fold increase in recurrence over 3.5 years.[59] Christensen and colleagues also found that high levels of FGFR3 and PIK3CA mutations in the urine of patients with NMIBC were associated with disease progression and high levels of these mutations in the urine of patients following radical cystectomy predicted worse recurrence-free survival.[60]

Cytokines and other inflammatory markers can be detected in the urine of patients with bladder cancer. Kamat and colleagues have studied a panel of cytokines and their ability to predict response to intravesical therapy.[61] In this study, urine from 125 patients with NMIBC was taken before and during BCG therapy and evaluated for levels of 9 cytokines (IL-2, IL-6, IL-8, IL-18, IL-1, TRAIL, IFN-g, IL-12, and TNFa). A nomogram based on changes in this panel predicted BCG response with 85.5% accuracy.

Similarly, quantification of various tumor cell plasma proteins and inflammatory markers have been assembled into ELISA-based assays to predict recurrence and response to intravesical therapy. Rosser and colleagues studied a 10-protein (IL8, Matrix Metalloprotein 9 [MMP9], MMP10, serpin family A member 1 [SERPINA1], Vascular Endothelial Growth Factor A [VEGFA], angiogenin [ANG], Carbonic anhydrase IX [CA9], APOE, Serpin Family, E Member 1 [SERPINE1], and Syndecan 1 [SDC1]) assay in the urine of 125 patients under surveillance for NMIBC with a sensitivity of 79% and specificity of 88%.[62]

SUMMARY

The ideal use of urine markers would be to develop markers of sufficient performance that would improve clinical care of patients at risk for bladder cancer or undergoing surveillance of NMIBC. In the setting of hematuria, these markers would tailor evaluation of hematuria patients to those most likely to have disease while avoiding evaluating in low-risk patients. This would improve identification of patients with cancer whose MH may be currently ignored.

There is a need for randomized trials to demonstrate the benefits of use of a urine marker in this setting. One such trial is the Cxbladder Hematuria Clinical Utility Study (NCT03988309), which randomizes patients to standard evaluation versus a marker-based approach in which low- and intermediate-risk patients based on AUA risk criteria for hematuria who have a negative marker just get observed and positive marker patients get cystoscopy.[63]

For patients with NMIBC, markers could reduce interval of cystoscopy in patients with low-grade disease, improve detection of high-grade disease, or assist in patients with atypical cystoscopy ("red patches") or atypical cytology.

Despite a growing number of candidate molecules under study, few tumor markers have progressed to the point of clinical utility and commercial use in the diagnosis and surveillance of bladder cancer. Improvement in DNA and RNA amplification and the ability to perform molecular quantification will allow further study of a rapidly growing variety of assays. It is likely moving forward that tumor marker panels, rather than a single gene or molecule will allow for the necessary sensitivity and specificity to become clinically useful in diagnosis, surveillance, and management of disease. Furthermore, it is likely that different panels will be necessary for different patients in different clinical scenarios. The promise of urine tumor markers remains in their ability to unlock more personalized care with more or less frequent surveillance, and early or delayed medical and surgical intervention based on risk profiling. Simultaneously these markers could decrease the need for invasive and expensive procedures. While promising research in this domain continues, widespread clinical application will require large cohort prospective trials for validation.

CLINICS CARE POINTS

- The use of urine markers within the guidelines is recommended for very specific indications such as atypical cystoscopic findings or atypical cytologic findings.
- Routine use is also not recommended for patients undergoing surveillance or hematuria evaluation.
- There are several potential uses for urine markers for detection and surveillance but there is a need for prospective trial demonstrating a clinical benefit.

DISCLOSURE

Dr Baky has no conflicts. These are all conflicts for Dr Lotan.

REFERENCES

1. Siegel RL, Miller KD, Fuchs HE, et al. Cancer statistics, 2022. CA Cancer J Clin 2022;72(1):7–33.
2. Evaluation of the New American Urological Association Guidelines Risk Classification for Hematuria | J Urol. Available at: https://www-auajournals-org.foyer.swmed.edu/doi/10.1097/ju.0000000000001550?10.1097/ju.0000000000001550. Accessed April 25, 2022.
3. Barocas DA, Boorjian SA, Alvarez RD, et al. Microhematuria: AUA/SUFU Guideline. J Urol 2020;204(4):778–86.
4. Chang SS, Boorjian SA, Chou R, et al. Diagnosis and Treatment of Non-Muscle Invasive Bladder Cancer: AUA/SUO Guideline. J Urol 2016;196(4):1021–9.
5. Optimal Trial Design for Studying Urinary Markers ...: Find It! Options. Available at: https://resolver-ebscohost-com.foyer.swmed.edu/openurl/?cusid=s9008684&sid=Entrez:PubMed&id=pmid:31102625. Accessed April 25, 2022.
6. Woldu SL, Souter L, Boorjian SA, et al. Urinary-based tumor markers enhance microhematuria risk stratification according to baseline bladder cancer prevalence. Urol Oncol Semin Orig Investig 2021;39(11):787.e1–7.
7. Miyanaga N, Akaza H, Tsukamoto T, et al. Urinary nuclear matrix protein 22 as a new marker for the screening of urothelial cancer in patients with microscopic hematuria. Int J Urol 1999;6(4):173–7.
8. Wang Z, Que H, Suo C, et al. Evaluation of the NMP22 BladderChek test for detecting bladder cancer: a systematic review and meta-analysis. Oncotarget 2017;8(59):100648–56.
9. Grossman HB, Messing E, Soloway M, et al. Detection of Bladder Cancer Using a Point-of-Care Proteomic Assay. JAMA 2005;293(7):810–6.
10. Chou R, Gore JL, Buckley D, et al. Urinary Biomarkers for Diagnosis of Bladder Cancer: A Systematic Review and Meta-analysis. Ann Intern Med 2015;163(12):922–31.
11. Lotan Y, Elias K, Svatek RS, et al. Bladder cancer screening in a high risk asymptomatic population using a point of care urine based protein tumor marker. J Urol 2009;182(1):52–7 [discussion: 58].
12. Huang YL, Chen J, Yan W, et al. Diagnostic accuracy of cytokeratin-19 fragment (CYFRA 21-1) for bladder cancer: a systematic review and meta-analysis. Tumour Biol J Int Soc Oncodevelopmental Biol Med 2015;36(5):3137–45.
13. Schmitz-Dräger BJ, Droller M, Lokeshwar VB, et al. Molecular markers for bladder cancer screening, early diagnosis, and surveillance: the WHO/ICUD consensus. Urol Int 2015;94(1):1–24.
14. Hajdinjak T. UroVysion FISH test for detecting urothelial cancers: Meta-analysis of diagnostic accuracy and comparison with urinary cytology testing. Urol Oncol Semin Orig Investig 2008;26(6):646–51.
15. Maas M, Bedke J, Stenzl A, et al. Can urinary biomarkers replace cystoscopy? World J Urol 2019;37(9):1741–9.
16. O'Sullivan P, Sharples K, Dalphin M, et al. A multigene urine test for the detection and stratification of bladder cancer in patients presenting with hematuria. J Urol 2012;188(3):741–7.
17. Raman JD, Kavalieris L, Konety B, et al. The Diagnostic Performance of Cxbladder Resolve, Alone and in Combination with Other Cxbladder Tests, in the Identification and Priority Evaluation of Patients at Risk for Urothelial Carcinoma. J Urol 2021;206(6):1380–9.
18. van Valenberg FJP, Hiar AM, Wallace E, et al. Validation of an mRNA-based Urine Test for the Detection of Bladder Cancer in Patients with Haematuria. Eur Urol Oncol 2021;4(1):93–101.
19. Robertson AG, Kim J, Al-Ahmadie H, et al. Comprehensive Molecular Characterization of Muscle-Invasive Bladder Cancer. Cell 2017;171(3):540–56. e25.
20. Casadio V, Calistri D, Tebaldi M, et al. Urine cell-free DNA integrity as a marker for early bladder cancer

diagnosis: preliminary data. Urol Oncol 2013;31(8): 1744–50.

21. Tomlinson DC, Baldo O, Harnden P, et al. FGFR3 protein expression and its relationship to mutation status and prognostic variables in bladder cancer. J Pathol 2007;213(1):91–8.

22. Allory Y, Beukers W, Sagrera A, et al. Telomerase reverse transcriptase promoter mutations in bladder cancer: high frequency across stages, detection in urine, and lack of association with outcome. Eur Urol 2014;65(2):360–6.

23. Piatti P, Chew YC, Suwoto M, et al. Clinical evaluation of Bladder CARE, a new epigenetic test for bladder cancer detection in urine samples. Clin Epigenetics 2021;13(1):84.

24. Hentschel AE, Beijert IJ, Bosschieter J, et al. Bladder cancer detection in urine using DNA methylation markers: a technical and prospective preclinical validation. Clin Epigenetics 2022;14(1):19.

25. Gene expression signature in urine for diagnosing and assessing aggressiveness of bladder urothelial carcinoma - PubMed. Available at: https://pubmed. ncbi.nlm.nih.gov/20406841/. Accessed May 7, 2022.

26. Carbonic anhydrase IX in bladder cancer: a diagnostic, prognostic, and therapeutic molecular marker - PubMed. Available at: https://pubmed.ncbi. nlm.nih.gov/19195047/. Accessed May 7, 2022.

27. Urinary carbonic anhydrase IX splicing messenger RNA variants in urogenital cancers - PubMed. Available at: https://pubmed.ncbi.nlm.nih.gov/ 27005925/. Accessed May 7, 2022.

28. Carbonic anhydrase IX as a diagnostic urinary marker for urothelial bladder cancer - PubMed. Available at: https://pubmed.ncbi.nlm.nih.gov/ 26138037/. Accessed May 7, 2022.

29. Ku JH, Godoy G, Amiel GE, et al. Urine survivin as a diagnostic biomarker for bladder cancer: a systematic review. BJU Int 2012;110(5):630–6.

30. Shariat SF, Casella R, Khoddami SM, et al. Urine detection of survivin is a sensitive marker for the noninvasive diagnosis of bladder cancer. J Urol 2004;171(2 Pt 1):626–30.

31. Horstmann M, Bontrup H, Hennenlotter J, et al. Clinical experience with survivin as a biomarker for urothelial bladder cancer. World J Urol 2010;28(3): 399–404.

32. A urinary microRNA signature can predict the presence of bladder urothelial carcinoma in patients undergoing surveillance | British Journal of Cancer. Available at: https://www.nature.com/articles/ bjc2015472. Accessed May 7, 2022.

33. Kutwin P, Konecki T, Borkowska EM, et al. Urine miRNA as a potential biomarker for bladder cancer detection – a meta-analysis. Cent Eur J Urol 2018; 71(2):177–85.

34. Roperch JP, Grandchamp B, Desgrandchamps F, et al. Promoter hypermethylation of HS3ST2, SEPTIN9 and SLIT2 combined with FGFR3 mutations as a sensitive/specific urinary assay for diagnosis and surveillance in patients with low or high-risk non-muscle-invasive bladder cancer. BMC Cancer 2016;16:704.

35. Dahmcke CM, Steven KE, Larsen LK, et al. A Prospective Blinded Evaluation of Urine-DNA Testing for Detection of Urothelial Bladder Carcinoma in Patients with Gross Hematuria. Eur Urol 2016;70(6):916–9.

36. Evaluation of an Epigenetic Profile for the Detection of Bladder Cancer in Patients with Hematuria | J Urol. Available at: https://www.auajournals.org/doi/abs/ 10.1016/j.juro.2015.08.085. Accessed May 7, 2022.

37. Grossman HB, Soloway M, Messing E, et al. Surveillance for Recurrent Bladder Cancer Using a Point-of-Care Proteomic Assay. JAMA 2006;295(3): 299–305.

38. Lotan Y, O'Sullivan P, Raman JD, et al. Clinical comparison of noninvasive urine tests for ruling out recurrent urothelial carcinoma. Urol Oncol Semin Orig Investig 2017;35(8):531.e15–22.

39. Raitanen MP, FinnBladder Group. The role of BTA stat Test in follow-up of patients with bladder cancer: results from FinnBladder studies. World J Urol 2008; 26(1):45–50.

40. Guo A, Wang X, Gao L, et al. Bladder tumour antigen (BTA stat) test compared to the urine cytology in the diagnosis of bladder cancer: A meta-analysis. Can Urol Assoc J 2014;8(5–6):E347–52.

41. Urine Sediment Smears as a Diagnostic Procedure in Cancers of the Urinary Tract. Available at: https:// www.science.org/doi/10.1126/science.101.2629.519. Accessed May 8, 2022.

42. Yafi FA, Brimo F, Auger M, et al. Is the performance of urinary cytology as high as reported historically? A contemporary analysis in the detection and surveillance of bladder cancer. Urol Oncol Semin Orig Investig 2014;32(1):27.e1–6.

43. Gudjónsson S, Isfoss BL, Hansson K, et al. The Value of the UroVysion® Assay for Surveillance of Non–Muscle-Invasive Bladder Cancer. Eur Urol 2008;54(2):402–8.

44. Davis N, Shtabsky A, Lew S, et al. A Novel Urine-Based Assay for Bladder Cancer Diagnosis: Multi-Institutional Validation Study. Eur Urol Focus 2018; 4(3):388–94.

45. Performance Characteristics of a Multigene Urine Biomarker Test for Monitoring for Recurrent Urothelial Carcinoma in a Multicenter Study | J Urol. Available at: https://www.auajournals.org/doi/abs/ 10.1016/j.juro.2016.12.010. Accessed May 7, 2022.

46. Yun SJ, Jeong P, Kim WT, et al. Cell-free microRNAs in urine as diagnostic and prognostic biomarkers of bladder cancer. Int J Oncol 2012;41(5):1871–8.

47. Critelli R, Fasanelli F, Oderda M, et al. Detection of multiple mutations in urinary exfoliated cells from

male bladder cancer patients at diagnosis and during follow-up. Oncotarget 2016;7(41):67435–48.

48. Wasserstrom A, Frumkin D, Dotan Z, et al. Mp13-15 molecular urine cytology – bladder epicheck is a novel molecular diagnostic tool for monitoring of bladder cancer patients. J Urol 2016;195(4, Supplement):e140.

49. Su SF, de Castro Abreu AL, Chihara Y, et al. A Panel of Three Markers Hyper- and Hypomethylated in Urine Sediments Accurately Predicts Bladder Cancer Recurrence. Clin Cancer Res 2014;20(7):1978–89.

50. Beukers W, van der Keur KA, Kandimalla R, et al. FGFR3, TERT and OTX1 as a Urinary Biomarker Combination for Surveillance of Patients with Bladder Cancer in a Large Prospective Multicenter Study. J Urol 2017;197(6):1410–8.

51. Mengual L, Marín-Aguilera M, Ribal MJ, et al. Clinical Utility of Fluorescent in situ Hybridization for the Surveillance of Bladder Cancer Patients Treated with Bacillus Calmette-Guérin Therapy. Eur Urol 2007;52(3):752–9.

52. Kipp BR, Karnes RJ, Brankley SM, et al. Monitoring intravesical therapy for superficial bladder cancer using fluorescence in situ hybridization. J Urol 2005;173(2):401–4.

53. Kamat AM, Dickstein RJ, Messetti F, et al. Use of Fluorescence In Situ Hybridization to Predict Response to Bacillus Calmette-Guérin Therapy for Bladder Cancer: Results of a Prospective Trial. J Urol 2012;187(3):862–7.

54. Lotan Y, Inman BA, Davis LG, et al. Evaluation of the Fluorescence In Situ Hybridization Test to Predict Recurrence and/or Progression of Disease after bacillus Calmette-Guérin for Primary High Grade Non-muscle Invasive Bladder Cancer: Results from a Prospective Multicenter Trial. J Urol 2019;202(5):920–6.

55. Odisho AY, Berry AB, Ahmad AE, et al. Reflex ImmunoCyt Testing for the Diagnosis of Bladder Cancer in Patients with Atypical Urine Cytology. Eur Urol 2013;63(5):936–40.

56. Prospective Evaluation of the Clinical Usefulness of Reflex Fluorescence In Situ Hybridization Assay in Patients With Atypical Cytology for the Detection of Urothelial Carcinoma of the Bladder | J Urol. Available at: https://www.auajournals.org/doi/abs/10.1016/j.juro.2008.01.105. Accessed May 25, 2022.

57. Schlomer BJ, Ho R, Sagalowsky A, et al. Prospective Validation of the Clinical Usefulness of Reflex Fluorescence In Situ Hybridization Assay in Patients With Atypical Cytology for the Detection of Urothelial Carcinoma of the Bladder. J Urol 2010;183(1):62–7.

58. Badrinath K, Neal S, Andrew KK, et al. Yair Lotan. Evaluation of Cxbladder and Adjudication of Atypical Cytology and Equivocal Cystoscopy. Eur Urol 2019;76(2):238–43.

59. Zuiverloon TCM, Tjin SS, Busstra M, et al. Optimization of Nonmuscle Invasive Bladder Cancer Recurrence Detection Using a Urine Based FGFR3 Mutation Assay. J Urol 2011;186(2):707–12.

60. Christensen E, Birkenkamp-Demtröder K, Nordentoft I, et al. Liquid Biopsy Analysis of FGFR3 and PIK3CA Hotspot Mutations for Disease Surveillance in Bladder Cancer. Eur Urol 2017;71(6):961–9.

61. Kamat AM, Briggman J, Urbauer DL, et al. Cytokine Panel for Response to Intravesical Therapy (CyPRIT): Nomogram of Changes in Urinary Cytokine Levels Predicts Patient Response to Bacillus Calmette-Guérin. Eur Urol 2016;69(2):197–200.

62. Rosser CJ, Chang M, Dai Y, et al. Urinary Protein Biomarker Panel for the Detection of Recurrent Bladder Cancer. Cancer Epidemiol Biomarkers Prev 2014;23(7):1340–5.

63. Edge Limited Pacific. Use of a Multiplexed Molecular Biomarker Test Cxbladder. In: Real World Decision making to provide clinical utility using a randomized Design. clinicaltrials.gov; 2022. Available at: https://clinicaltrials.gov/ct2/show/NCT03988309. Accessed May 5, 2022.

Biological Stratification of Invasive and Advanced Urothelial Carcinoma

Moritz J. Reike, MD[a,b], Alberto Contreras-Sanz, PhD[a], Peter C. Black, MD[a,*]

KEYWORDS

• Bladder cancer • Molecular subtyping • Classifier • Genetic mutation

KEY POINTS

- Molecular characterisation of bladder cancer has revealed distinct subtypes of bladder cancer that have improved our understanding of the underlying biology.
- Bladder cancer can harbor genomic alterations in DNA damage repair (DDR) genes that are associated with a favorable prognosis after chemotherapy.
- Mutations in ARID1A and APOBEC mutational signatures are associated with an unfavourable prognosis.
- Biomarker-driven clinical trials are currently recruiting with a focus especially on the utilization of DDR gene alterations to guide bladder preservation after neoadjuvant therapy.

INTRODUCTION

Bladder cancer (BC) is one of the most frequently diagnosed cancers worldwide in men and women.[1] It is responsible for almost 386,000 new diagnoses and 150,000 deaths per year.[2] Most of these cases present as non–muscle-invasive bladder cancer (NMIBC), but a significant proportion (up to 30%) as muscle-invasive bladder cancer (MIBC) or even metastatic urothelial carcinoma (mUC) at the time of diagnosis, and more progress from NMIBC to MIBC over time.

MIBC shows a 5-year survival rate of only 50% to 60%.[3] It is typically treated with the combination of neoadjuvant chemotherapy (NAC) and radical cystectomy (RC). However, because only approximately 40% of patients with MIBC seem to benefit from NAC, the determination of predictive biomarkers to discern likely responders from nonresponders is an important field of research.[4] Locally advanced BC and mUC are treated with multiple lines of systemic therapy.[5] Optimal sequencing and combination of therapies depend on delineation of the underlying biological mechanisms of response and resistance to each therapy.

We have seen a rapid advance in our understanding of the heterogenous transcriptomic, genomic, and immunologic landscape of BC over the past several years. This knowledge provides the molecular framework to develop biological stratification of BC with the potential to use it to develop a precision oncology approach to BC. In this review the authors focus on the molecular mechanisms of progression from NMIBC to MIBC and mUC. They highlight the potential clinical translation of new molecular advances to guide patient treatment.

METHODS

A nonsystematic literature search was conducted in MEDLINE and PubMed using the key words "bladder cancer," "urothelial carcinoma," or "metastatic urothelial carcinoma" in combination with any of the following terms: "resistance," "cancer," "immunotherapy," "chemotherapy," "subtype," "genetics," and "variant." Original and review

[a] Department of Urologic Sciences, University of British Columbia, Gordon & Leslie Diamond Health Care Centre, Level 6, 2775 Laurel Street, Vancouver, BC V5Z 1M9, Canada; [b] Department of Urology, Marien Hospital Herne, Ruhr–University Bochum, Hölkeskampring 40, 44625 Herne, Germany
* Corresponding author.
E-mail address: pblack@mail.ubc.ca

Urol Clin N Am 50 (2023) 69–80
https://doi.org/10.1016/j.ucl.2022.09.007
0094-0143/23/© 2022 Elsevier Inc. All rights reserved.

articles on translational science published before February 2022 were reviewed.

PROGRESSION FROM NON–MUSCLE-INVASIVE BLADDER CANCER TO MUSCLE-INVASIVE BLADDER CANCER

MIBC is believed to develop from noninvasive precursors. The molecular underpinnings of this temporal evolution, however, remain unresolved, and ultimately most patients with MIBC present with MIBC without a known history of NMIBC. The risk of progression to MIBC in those diagnosed with NMIBC depends on multiple clinical and pathologic features that are applied in clinical risk models to guide standard treatment. For example, the risk of progression varies from greater than 5% in patients with a low-risk NMIBC to approximately 60% for those with a high-grade T1 tumor and concurrent carcinoma in situ (CIS).[6,7] Standard treatment of high-risk NMIBC consists of transurethral resection of the bladder tumor (TURBT) followed by intravesical instillation of Bacillus Calmette-Guerin (BCG).[7]

The molecular landscape of NMIBC has been profiled by multiple groups using different approaches applied to varied patient populations. Beyond the technical considerations of the selected assays, a critical consideration is the heterogeneity of the patient population studied, which varies from a broad focus on mixed MIBC and NMIBC to a narrower focus on NMIBC and the narrowest focus on one NMIBC subpopulation (eg, Ta only or T1 only). Furthermore, it is critical to consider the role of BCG treatment when correlating the molecular findings to the clinical outcomes. Within the context of these important clinical considerations, some recurrent findings have been reported across multiple studies.

The most extensive molecular analysis of NMIBC to date was conducted by the UROMOL consortium that identified 3 genomic and 4 transcriptomic subtypes.[8] The combination of these molecular subtypes with clinical risk parameters enhanced stratification with respect to progression-free survival (PFS) in a cohort of 535 patients who were predominantly treated without BCG. Within these so-called UROMOL2021 subtypes, class 2a tumors had the worst prognosis and demonstrated the most aggressive molecular pattern, including genomic alterations of the p53-pathway, loss of RB1, and presence of APOBEC-mutational signatures. These findings led the investigators of this analysis to suggest that this type of tumor should be considered for immediate RC instead of BCG instillations. However, the

potential response of class 2a tumors to BCG could not be assessed in this study.

The Lund group initially described their RNA and immunohistochemistry (IHC)-based taxonomy in a mixed population of NMIBC and MIBC, which revealed that most NMIBC were classified as Urobasal A or genomically unstable (GU) and only few were Urobasal B or infiltrated or squamous cell carcinoma (SCC)-like.[9,10] The Lund taxonomy classifies tumors independent of tumor stage, with tumor stage considered as an additional risk parameter in patient risk stratification. Nonetheless, in a subsequent analysis focusing on 156 patients with T1 disease, 116 of whom were treated with BCG; the same group demonstrated that patients with GU and SCC-like tumors had a higher risk of progression to MIBC.[11] This study by Patschan and colleagues and other similar studies suggest that biological stratification of BC depends on specific definitions and focused analysis of individual disease states to overcome the clinical heterogeneity of these tumors.[11]

This focused approach was also critical to Hurst and colleagues in their description of 2 genomic subtypes (GS1 and 2) among 140 primary grade 1 or 2 Ta tumors.[12] GS1 showed a high number of mutations in chromatin modifier genes, whereas GS2 was dominated by a loss of 9q including TSC1, increased Ki67, as well as upregulated glycolysis, DNA repair, and mTORC1 signaling. Hurst and colleagues subsequently expanded their analysis to include a multiomics analysis of Ta and T1 tumors combined and separately.[13] In the combined analysis, they defined 4 subtypes whose prognostic value was comparable to T-stage. The analysis of T1 tumors (63 of 104 were treated with BCG) separately linked TP53 and RB1 mutations to worse PFS, thus identifying a high-risk group within T1 tumors similar to the class 2a tumors in the UROMOL2021 classification. On the other hand, mutations of ERCC2 and ERBB2/3 were associated with a high tumor mutational burden (TMB) and a significantly better PFS. Similarly, a high immune infiltration was linked to a lower probability of recurrence or progression. The transcriptomic subtypes derived from this cohort aligned well with those defined by the UROMOL2021 classification.

Robertson and colleagues also focused on transcriptomic classification of T1 tumors treated according to the current standard of care with restaging TURBT and adequate intravesical BCG.[14] They identified 5 different expression subtypes that demonstrated heterogenous biology and differential recurrence rates after BCG. Most of the tumors were luminal papillary according to the Lund taxonomy, although the T1-Lum subtype had the highest luminal papillary score, the highest *FGFR3* expression, and the lowest recurrence rate. The T1-LumGU was associated with CIS, and the T1-Inflam subtype was infiltrated with immune cells. The socalled T1-Myc and T1-Early subtypes were associated with the highest rate of recurrence (47% within 24 months).

Bellmunt and colleagues similarly focused on high-grade T1 tumors treated with intravesical BCG, but analyzed the correlation of somatic mutation profiles with clinical outcomes.[15] Mutations in the DNA damage repair genes *ERCC2* and *BRCA2* as well as high TMB were associated with favorable outcome, whereas alterations in *TP53* (mutation), *ARID1A* (mutation), *CCNE1* (amplification), and *CDKN2A* (deletion) marked a more aggressive phenotype. The latter were associated with extensive lamina propria invasion, and the investigators suggested that these patients should be considered for early RC.

This analysis of Bellmunt and colleagues identified some individual genomic markers that have been correlated to outcome after BCG therapy in multiple studies, including a negative correlation with mutation in *ARID1A*[15–17] and *CCNE1* amplification[15–17] and a positive correlation with mutation in *ERCC2*[13,15–17] and TMB.[13,15,17] In these various analyses of high-risk NMIBC treated with BCG, it is impossible to distinguish the prognostic value of the individual biomarkers from their potential predictive value. True predictive markers can only be assessed by comparing patients managed with and without the treatment in question. In one series of patients treated without BCG, *ARID1A* mutations also correlated with a worse relapse-free survival but there was insufficient power to detect a difference in PFS,[18] which suggests that this is a prognostic biomarker, and a role in predicting response to BCG needs further study. In MIBC it has been established that high TMB is a favorable prognostic marker,[19] whereas mutation in *ERCC2* correlates with survival after neoadjuvant chemotherapy[20,21] but has no prognostic implications in the absence of chemotherapy, making it a predictive marker of response to chemotherapy.[19]

ERCC2 is of particular interest in the context of progression from NMIBC to MIBC. Pietzak and colleagues found that the rate of *ERCC2* mutations was significantly reduced in MIBC that had progressed from a previously treated NMIBC compared with primary MIBC, reinforcing that *ERCC2* mutations may also have sensitized to BCG response.[22] The lower rate of *ERCC2* mutations in patients with secondary MIBC was associated with a lower response rate to NAC; this highlights again that we need to consider the

impact of prior therapy when interpreting molecular analyses of bladder cancer.

Study of the tumor immune microenvironment has become the focus of a significant body of research related to systemic immune checkpoint inhibition (ICI). Some of these same principles may also be relevant in the study of BCG response in NMIBC. Hurst and colleagues found distinct immunologic features in their classification of Ta and T1 tumors, although it is premature to link these to patient outcomes and potential treatment effects.[13] Taber and colleagues demonstrated an increase in immune infiltration in higher disease stages and linked the expression of programmed cell death protein 1 and programmed cell death ligand 1 (PD-L1) with an increased risk of recurrence and progression in NMIBC.[23]

Most of these studies have described associations between molecular features of NMIBC and rates of recurrence or progression, but few studies have elucidated mechanisms of progression to MIBC. Heide and colleagues performed whole-exome sequencing in samples from multiple regions within the bladder of 10 patients undergoing RC for NMIBC (including CIS) or MIBC with the aim of inferring temporal evolution of bladder cancer invasion from the spatial distribution of genomic alterations.[24] Three patients harbored both invasive and papillary tumor elements, but there was evidence for the invasive tumor evolving from the papillary tumor in only one of them. In the other 2 cases the papillary and invasive tumor regions developed in parallel but separately from each other; this puts into question the commonly held belief that invasive tumors develop from papillary precursors. The investigators were able to compare MIBC and concurrent CIS in 4 additional bladders. In 3 cases most (>75%) of the genomic changes were shared between the CIS and the MIBC; this is consistent with the notion that MIBC develops from subclones of CIS, although analysis did not reveal obvious genomic changes that explained the progression from CIS to MIBC. In the fourth case, the CIS was located distant from the MIBC, and only 15% of changes were shared. Four cases of MIBC demonstrated a large number of clonal mutations and few regional private mutations, suggesting that these tumors formed as single clonal expansions.

Sjödahl and colleagues reported on molecular changes in a longitudinal study of 73 patients who started with NMIBC and progressed to MIBC.[25] Most NMIBC tumors were assigned to the luminal subtype based on RNA expression, and this subtype persisted after progression to MIBC. Hotspot mutations in *FGFR3*, *PIK3CA*, and *TERT* were consistent throughout progression in most cases, although a small number of cases showed wide variation between the NMIBC and MIBC. These genomic changes were not associated with subtype changes. A switch from wild-type to altered TP53 as determined by IHC was observed in only 24% of patients, and this was associated with a subtype switch, suggesting a possible causal relationship. Bacon and colleagues demonstrated a high clonal similarity between pre-BCG and post-BCG tumor samples, but patients with a relapse showed a high number of somatic clonal switches.[17] Progression to MIBC was associated with high genomic concordance between pre-BCG and post-BCG sample.

BIOLOGICAL STRATIFICATION OF MUSCLE-INVASIVE BLADDER CANCER

RNA-based molecular subtyping has provided an important framework for the study of MIBC and, pending validation, may also offer some guidance for treatment selection. The underlying premise is that MIBC is a heterogenous disease that can be subclassified into 2 or more subtypes based on gene expression. Several groups have reported variable approaches to subtyping that result in some commonalities but also important differences.[19,26–30] In an attempt to develop a common standard for subtyping, an international group constructed a consensus classification that differentiates 6 classes: luminal papillary, luminal non-specified, luminal unstable, stroma-rich, basal/squamous, and neuroendocrine-like (**Table 1**).[31]

The basal subtype is defined by the expression of markers expressed in the basal layer of the urothelium, including KRT5/6 and KRT14. These tumors are associated with high clinical stage and poor overall survival. Luminal tumors are enriched for markers of urothelial differentiation such as FOXA1, GATA3, and PPARG. These tumors are more heterogenous and can be divided into additional subtypes. Luminal papillary tumors, for example, which are characterized by a high rate of FGFR3 alterations and overexpression, are associated with a particularly favorable outcome. The neuroendocrine-like subtype is noteworthy because it resembles conventional urothelial carcinoma histologically but expresses typical neuroendocrine genes and proteins and has the worst prognosis of all subtypes.[10,19,31,32]

Response to neoadjuvant chemotherapy (NAC) may vary by subtype. Choi and colleagues[28] first reported that the p53-like subtype from the MD Anderson classification had a very poor response to NAC in 3 different patient cohorts. Seiler and colleagues[33] subsequently determined that patients with basal tumors had the largest relative

benefit from NAC compared with patients treated without NAC; this was corroborated by similar findings in a trial of patients treated with NAC plus bevacizumab.[34] In the Seiler series, patients with luminal tumors had the best prognosis regardless of their treatment. Lotan and colleagues subsequently reported that clinical stage T1-T2 luminal tumors are less likely to be upstaged to pathologic T3-T4 at the time of RC in the absence of NAC, suggesting that luminal tumors may be less aggressive. In a pooled analysis of 601 patients with MIBC from multiple centers,[35] this same group demonstrated that luminal tumors do not benefit from NAC, and the investigators suggested that NAC should be prioritized in nonluminal subtypes; this requires further validation before being implemented clinically. Both the GUSTO trial in the United Kingdom and the SUBTYP trial in the United States are designed to validate subtyping in this context.

Two more recent studies report quite different associations between subtype and response to NAC. Taber and colleagues reported in a mixed neoadjuvant and metastatic population that the basal/squamous subtype according to the consensus classification had the lowest response rate and the worst survival.[36] Some of the differences between this report and the Seiler series may relate to the mixed patient population with different biology, different endpoints, and different impact of TURBT in patients receiving NAC versus chemotherapy for metastatic BC.[37] Furthermore, this study did not compare them with patients not treated with chemotherapy, so that the true predictive value of subtyping cannot be determined. Nonetheless, Sjödahl and colleagues[38] also reported the worst response and survival after NAC in patients with basal/squamous tumors (Lund taxonomy). Some of the important differences here might be related to the different subtyping classifiers.[39]

The co-expression extrapolation (COXEN) model represents another approach to use tumor gene expression to predict response to NAC. In a multicenter trial, patients were randomized between gemcitabine/cisplatin (GC) and methotrexate-vinblastine-adriamycin-cisplatin (ddMVAC), and all patients were scored based by the COXEN model to predict the efficacy of each NAC regimen. The study did not meet the primary endpoint for either the GC or ddMVAC score to predict ypT0 or ypT≤1 after the corresponding NAC, but the GC score showed a significant association with downstaging after NAC regardless of chemotherapy regimen.[40]

Mutations in DNA damage repair (DDR) genes have also been associated with response to

Table 1
Overview of the consensus classes

MIBC Subtype	Differentiation	Oncogenic Mechanisms	Histology	Clinical	Median Over Survival (y)
Luminal papillary (LumP)	Luminal	PPARG alterations FGFR3 mutations CDKN2A deletions	Papillary morphology	T2+	4
Luminal nonspecified (LumNS)	Luminal	PPARG alterations ELF3 mutations	Micropapillary variant	Older patients (80+)	1.8
Luminal unstable (LumU)	Luminal	PPARG alterations ERBB2 amplifications ERCC2 mutations Genomic instability	—	Possibly better response to chemotherapy and immunotherapy	2.9
Stroma-rich	Basal and Luminal	—	—	Possibly more resistance to chemotherapy and immunotherapy	3.8
Basal/Squamous (Ba/Sq)	Basal and squamous	EGFR mutations	Squamous differentiation	T3/T4 Women	1.2
Neuroendocrine-like (NE-like)	Neuroendocrine	Loss of TP53 and RB1	Neuroendocrine differentiation	Worst prognosis	1

From left to right: names of the different MIBC subtypes, differentiation features associated with MIBC subtypes, dominant oncogenic mechanisms represented by each class, histopathologic characteristics of each subtype, notably clinical features associated with each subtype, median overall survival in years differentiated by subtype.
Adapted from Kamoun, A. et al. A Consensus Molecular Classification of Muscle-invasive Bladder Cancer. Eur Urol 77, 420-433, https://doi.org/10.1016/j.eururo.2019.09.006 (2020).

chemotherapy for mUC[41] and NAC for MIBC. The latter includes both the nucleotide excision repair gene ERCC2[20,21,42] and a panel of 3 genes: ATM, RB1, and FANCC.[43,44] These discoveries led to initialization of 3 different trials incorporating these biomarkers to test whether they can identify a subpopulation of patients who can avoid RC after NAC. Preliminary results have been reported in abstract form for 2 of these trials, although a report on the primary endpoint (metastasis-free survival) is pending. In the RETAIN trial, 33 of 71 patients had a DDR mutation, and 26 of these patients were observed without RC after NAC. Seventeen (65%) of these 26 recurred, including 1 with mUC and 6 with MIBC.[45] It is possible that some patients with recurrent/persistent MIBC could still have a favorable outcome after RC, and it will be impossible to tell in a single-arm trial what the outcome of these patients might have been with earlier RC. In the GU 16-257 trial (Hoosier Cancer Research Network), approximately half of the patients preserved their bladders after clinical complete response to NAC plus nivolumab regardless of DDR gene mutation.[46] Nine of thirty-one patients managed with bladder preservation recurred in the bladder, 7 underwent RC (3 had MIBC), and 1 metastasized. ERRC2 mutations and TMB were associated with pathologic response, but mutations in ATM, RB1, and FANCC were not.[46] Because this trial allows bladder preservation in patients with clinical complete response who harbor no DDR mutations, it will tell us the true impact of DDR mutation in this setting. The Alliance A031701 trial (NCT03609216) is currently accruing. In this trial patients who harbor any one of 9 deleterious DDR gene alterations will be offered bladder preservation if they achieve a clinical complete response to NAC.

Molecular subtyping has been tested also for its capacity to predict response to immunotherapy and trimodal therapy (TMT). Efstathiou and colleagues reported in a cohort of 136 patients treated with TMT that subtype was not associated with response and survival after treatment.[47] However, the favorable outcomes of the luminal infiltrated and basal subtypes were noteworthy in this study, as these subtypes did worse with RC only in the Seiler series. This report on TMT found that tumors with a high T-cell inflammation signature or high stromal signature did well with TMT and poorly with RC, suggesting that molecular signatures could assist treatment selection.

Multiple studies have investigated the impact of molecular subtyping on response to ICI with variable results[48] in the context of both mUC and neoadjuvant therapy for MIBC.[49] In the single-arm phase 2 trial testing atezolizumab in patients with platinum-refractory mUC (IMvigor210), response to ICI was highest in the genomically unstable (GU) subtype (Lund taxonomy), which corresponds to the luminal unstable subtype (consensus subtyping) which is also linked to high TMB.[50] However, with the same agent in the neoadjuvant setting, there was no correlation to subtype.[51,52] Although the objective response rate in IMvigor210 was particularly high in the neuronal subtype (TCGA subtyping),[53] this was not validated in patients treated with pembrolizumab in the neoadjuvant setting.[51,54] The heterogeneity of results here is likely due in part to the application of different classifiers and the profiling of remote archived primary tumor specimens in patients subsequently treated for platinum-refractory mUC.

BIOLOGICAL STRATIFICATION OF METASTATIC UROTHELIAL CARCINOMA

Molecular analysis of mUC is less mature because tissue samples for profiling are scarce. Many analyses are either based on the primary tumor or a very small sample size. In a pan-cancer analysis, mUC was described as having a high TMB and the highest number among all solid tumors of alterations in oncogenic driver genes.

An analysis of fresh metastatic biopsies of 116 patients with mUC who were mostly platinum-refractory (82%) revealed 2 subtypes based on mutational signature, including one driven by APOBEC and one related to reactive oxygen species.[55] The rate of significantly mutated genes did not differ between both subgroups. The APOBEC-driven tumors responded more favorably to treatment. Potentially targetable alterations were identified in 98% of patients. The investigators not only defined 5 new subtypes based on RNA sequencing but also applied the consensus subtyping. The new subtypes included 2 luminal subtypes, a stroma-rich and a basal/squamous subtype, which generally aligned with established MIBC subtyping. Correlations of a subtype to treatment response and prognosis were not reported.

Molecular subtyping of mUC has otherwise mostly been based on profiling of archived pathologic samples of the primary tumor, as described earlier for clinical trials testing ICI.[49,50,56,57] Sjödahl and colleagues demonstrated high concordance (82%) between MIBC samples from TURBT and lymph node metastasis from subsequent RC.[58] Most of the discordance was in primary basal/squamous tumors. Vandekerkhove and colleagues showed an enrichment of the stroma-rich subtype in patients with mUC, especially after chemotherapy and in tissue taken from metastatic sites (consensus subtyping).[59]

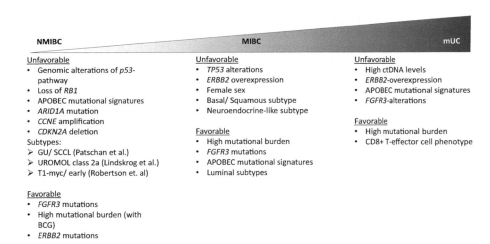

Fig. 1. Overview of the biological stratification of urothelial carcinoma with respect to risk of disease progression.

Other markers to predict response to ICI include PD-L1 IHC and TMB. Virtually every ICI clinical trial has included PD-L1 IHC, and the net conclusion from all of these trials is that PD-L1 expression currently has no clinical utility in the management of mUC. The phase 3 IMvigor211 trial with atezolizumab in patients with platinum-refractory mUC demonstrated that the VENTANA SP142 PD-L1 IHC assay had prognostic value that could not have been determined from the corresponding single-arm phase 2 trial (IMvigor210); this underscores the importance of testing biomarkers in comparative trials. TMB was associated with survival after treatment with atezolizumab in IMvigor210 but not in other trials.[49,57,59–61] Independent of organ of origin, solid tumors with high TMB or mismatch-repair deficiency are considered susceptible to ICI after exhaustion of other established treatment options.[62–64]

Intertumor (ie, between tumor sites in the same patient) heterogeneity[65] is particularly important in patients with mUC. Faltas and colleagues demonstrated a high degree of spatial and temporal heterogeneity by whole exome sequencing in a cohort of 32 patients with matched primary and metastatic tissue, 16 of whom had matched tissue before and after chemotherapy.[66] Only 28% of mutations on average were shared between prechemotherapy and postchemotherapy samples, for both primary and metastatic sites. Similar findings were made when the analysis was reduced to include only known oncogenic driver alterations. Interestingly, this study suggests that metastasis is an early event in the natural history of bladder cancer. In this study, as in most studies of mUC, the mutational landscape did not differ markedly from that of MIBC as reported in the TCGA. Thomsen and colleagues reported similar spatial and

temporal heterogeneity in a small cohort of patients with mUC.[67,68] Actionable alterations that could potentially be targeted by therapeutic agents were not observed in all tumor samples. These 2 studies have important implications for single targeted therapies such as erdafitinib (pan-FGFR-inhibitor) that would not be expected to be efficacious against all clones.

Some investigators have suggested that it is necessary to examine metastases to address the high degree of intertumor heterogeneity if the paradigm of precision oncology is to be applied successfully to mUC. Alternatively, circulating cell-free tumor (ct) DNA may offer a method to overcome the need for biopsy of metastatic sites and to enable molecular profiling of mUC in real time.[69–71] Vandekerkhove and colleagues demonstrated 83.4% concordance between circulating tumor DNA (ctDNA) and matched metastatic tissue using a panel of 60 genes known to be important in UC[59]; this suggests that ctDNA reflects the genomic landscape of metastatic sites, but it also implies a lower degree of intertumor heterogeneity in these patients, as the ctDNA is not revealing additional alterations not identified in sampled metastatic sites. Differences between the various reports may relate to the sequencing methodology, selected genes, and patient selection including the amount of prior treatment. ctDNA is also gaining traction as an assay to measure tumor burden independent of the genomic profile of the tumor. Multiple studies have demonstrated that the presence or amount of ctDNA is prognostic in the MIBC and mUC settings.[57,59,72,73]

Erdafitinib is the first approved targeted therapy in bladder cancer, and its use depends on the detection of specific FGFR3 or FGFR2 alterations in tumor tissue[74]; this has brought molecular stratification of mUC into routine clinical practice. Detection of similar alterations in ctDNA could also be relevant,[71] although there could be some risk of missing alterations.[75,76] Some reports suggest that patients with *FGFR3* alterations may have a lower response to platinum-based chemotherapy[77] but there is no clear link to survival across multiple studies.[59,77–79] Although there was some early indication that these patients might respond poorly to ICI, this has since been discounted.[80]

SUMMARY

The progression of NMIBC to MIBC and MIBC to mUC represents the critical steps that lead to poor outcomes in patients with BC. A better understanding of the molecular mechanisms underlying this serial progression is critical to develop better treatments for these patients. As multiple new treatment modalities have entered clinical practice in the last several years,[62,63,74,81] and as our molecular understanding of urothelial carcinoma increases, the role of biological stratification of invasive and advanced urothelial carcinoma to assess prognosis and guide treatment selection is gaining clinical relevance (**Fig. 1**). Many biomarkers are under investigation, including biomarker-driven clinical trials, but none has been adopted into routine clinical practice. The need for biomarkers will only increase, as we have more treatment options from which to choose but also as tumors are exposed to sequential treatment-related selection processes that affect the molecular landscape.

ACKNOWLEDGMENTS

Funded by the Deutsche Forschungsgemeinschaft (DFG, German Research Foundation), RE 4782/1-1.

CONFLICT OF INTEREST

M.J. Reike: none; Contreras-Sanz: none; P.C. Black has been a consultant for AbbVie, Astellas Pharma, EMD-Serono, Pfizer, Janssen Oncology, Bayer, Merck, Sanofi Canada, Biosyent, Ferring, Roche Canada, MDxHealth, AstraZeneca, UroGen Pharma, Bristol-Myers Squibb, Fergene, Prokarium, Protara, QED, STIMIT, Theralase, and Verity. He has received research funding from iProgen and shares a patent with Decipher Biosciences.

REFERENCES

1. Ferlay J, Soerjomataram I, Dikshit R, et al. Cancer incidence and mortality worldwide: sources, methods and major patterns in GLOBOCAN 2012. Int J Cancer 2015;136(5):E359–86. https://doi.org/10.1002/ijc.29210.
2. Jemal A, Bray F, Center MM, et al. Global cancer statistics. CA Cancer J Clin 2011;61(2):69–90. https://doi.org/10.3322/caac.20107.
3. Shah JB, McConkey DJ, Dinney CP. New strategies in muscle-invasive bladder cancer: on the road to personalized medicine. Clin Cancer Res 2011;17(9):2608–12. https://doi.org/10.1158/1078-0432.CCR-10-2770.
4. Grossman HB, Natale RB, Tangen CM, et al. Neoadjuvant Chemotherapy plus Cystectomy Compared with Cystectomy Alone for Locally Advanced Bladder Cancer. New Engl J Med 2003;349(9):859–66. https://doi.org/10.1056/NEJMoa022148.
5. Witjes JA, Bruins HM, Cathomas R, et al. European Association of Urology Guidelines on Muscle-invasive and Metastatic Bladder Cancer: Summary of the 2020 Guidelines. Eur Urol 2021;79(1):82–104. https://doi.org/10.1016/j.eururo.2020.03.055.
6. Sylvester RJ, Rodriguez O, Hernandez V, et al. European Association of Urology (EAU) Prognostic Factor Risk Groups for Non-muscle-invasive Bladder Cancer (NMIBC) Incorporating the WHO 2004/2016 and WHO 1973 Classification Systems for Grade: An Update from the EAU NMIBC Guidelines Panel. Eur Urol 2021;79(4):480–8. https://doi.org/10.1016/j.eururo.2020.12.033.
7. Babjuk M, Burger M, Capoun O, et al. European Association of Urology Guidelines on Non-muscle-invasive Bladder Cancer (Ta, T1, and Carcinoma in Situ). Eur Urol 2022;81(1):75–94. https://doi.org/10.1016/j.eururo.2021.08.010.
8. Lindskrog SV, Prip F, Lamy P, et al. An integrated multi-omics analysis identifies prognostic molecular subtypes of non-muscle-invasive bladder cancer. Nat Commun 2021;12(1):2301. https://doi.org/10.1038/s41467-021-22465-w.
9. Sjodahl G, Lauss M, Lovgren K, et al. A molecular taxonomy for urothelial carcinoma. Clin Cancer Res 2012;18(12):3377–86. https://doi.org/10.1158/1078-0432.CCR-12-0077-T.
10. Sjodahl G, Eriksson P, Liedberg F, et al. Molecular classification of urothelial carcinoma: global mRNA classification versus tumour-cell phenotype classification. J Pathol 2017;242(1):113–25. https://doi.org/10.1002/path.4886.
11. Patschan O, Sjodahl G, Chebil G, et al. A Molecular Pathologic Framework for Risk Stratification of Stage T1 Urothelial Carcinoma. Eur Urol 2015;68(5):824–32. https://doi.org/10.1016/j.eururo.2015.02.021. ; discussion 835-6.
12. Hurst CD, Alder O, Platt FM, et al. Genomic Subtypes of Non-invasive Bladder Cancer with Distinct Metabolic Profile and Female Gender Bias in KDM6A Mutation Frequency. Cancer Cell 2017;

32(5):701–715 e7. https://doi.org/10.1016/j.ccell.2017.08.005.

13. Hurst CD, Cheng G, Platt FM, et al. Stage-stratified molecular profiling of non-muscle-invasive bladder cancer enhances biological, clinical, and therapeutic insight. Cell Rep Med 2021;2(12). https://doi.org/10.1016/j.xcrm.2021.100472.

14. Robertson AG, Groeneveld CS, Jordan B, et al. Identification of Differential Tumor Subtypes of T1 Bladder Cancer. Eur Urol 2020;78(4):533–7. https://doi.org/10.1016/j.eururo.2020.06.048.

15. Bellmunt J, Kim J, Reardon B, et al. Genomic Predictors of Good Outcome, Recurrence, or Progression in High-Grade T1 Non-Muscle-Invasive Bladder Cancer. Cancer Res 2020;80(20):4476–86. https://doi.org/10.1158/0008-5472.CAN-20-0977.

16. Pietzak EJ, Bagrodia A, Cha EK, et al. Next-generation Sequencing of Nonmuscle Invasive Bladder Cancer Reveals Potential Biomarkers and Rational Therapeutic Targets. Eur Urol 2017;72(6):952–9. https://doi.org/10.1016/j.eururo.2017.05.032.

17. Bacon JVW, Muller DC, Ritch E, et al. Somatic Features of Response and Relapse in Non-muscle-invasive Bladder Cancer Treated with Bacillus Calmette-Guerin Immunotherapy. Eur Urol Oncol 2021. https://doi.org/10.1016/j.euo.2021.11.002.

18. Balbas-Martinez C, Rodriguez-Pinilla M, Casanova A, et al. ARID1A alterations are associated with FGFR3-wild type, poor-prognosis, urothelial bladder tumors. PLoS One 2013;8(5):e62483. https://doi.org/10.1371/journal.pone.0062483.

19. Robertson AG, Kim J, Al-Ahmadie H, et al. Comprehensive Molecular Characterization of Muscle-Invasive Bladder Cancer. Cell 2017;171(3):540–556 e25. https://doi.org/10.1016/j.cell.2017.09.007.

20. Liu D, Plimack ER, Hoffman-Censits J, et al. Clinical Validation of Chemotherapy Response Biomarker ERCC2 in Muscle-Invasive Urothelial Bladder Carcinoma. JAMA Oncol 2016;2(8):1094–6. https://doi.org/10.1001/jamaoncol.2016.1056.

21. Van Allen EM, Mouw KW, Kim P, et al. Somatic ERCC2 Mutations Correlate with Cisplatin Sensitivity in Muscle-Invasive Urothelial Carcinoma. Cancer Discov 2014;4(10):1140–53. https://doi.org/10.1158/2159-8290.Cd-14-0623.

22. Pietzak EJ, Zabor EC, Bagrodia A, et al. Genomic Differences Between "Primary" and "Secondary" Muscle-invasive Bladder Cancer as a Basis for Disparate Outcomes to Cisplatin-based Neoadjuvant Chemotherapy. Eur Urol 2019;75(2):231–9. https://doi.org/10.1016/j.eururo.2018.09.002.

23. Taber A, Prip F, Lamy P, et al. Immune Contexture and Differentiation Features Predict Outcome in Bladder Cancer. Eur Urol Oncol 2022;5(2):203–13. https://doi.org/10.1016/j.euo.2022.01.008.

24. Heide T, Maurer A, Eipel M, et al. Multiregion human bladder cancer sequencing reveals tumour evolution, bladder cancer phenotypes and implications for targeted therapy. J Pathol 2019;248(2):230–42. https://doi.org/10.1002/path.5250.

25. Sjodahl G, Eriksson P, Patschan O, et al. Molecular changes during progression from nonmuscle invasive to advanced urothelial carcinoma. Int J Cancer 2020;146(9):2636–47. https://doi.org/10.1002/ijc.32737.

26. Mo Q, Nikolos F, Chen F, et al. Prognostic Power of a Tumor Differentiation Gene Signature for Bladder Urothelial Carcinomas. J Natl Cancer Inst 2018;110(5):448–59. https://doi.org/10.1093/jnci/djx243.

27. Damrauer JS, Hoadley KA, Chism DD, et al. Intrinsic subtypes of high-grade bladder cancer reflect the hallmarks of breast cancer biology. Proc Natl Acad Sci U S A 2014;111(8):3110–5. https://doi.org/10.1073/pnas.1318376111.

28. Choi W, Porten S, Kim S, et al. Identification of distinct basal and luminal subtypes of muscle-invasive bladder cancer with different sensitivities to frontline chemotherapy. Cancer Cell 2014;25(2):152–65. https://doi.org/10.1016/j.ccr.2014.01.009.

29. Rebouissou S, Bernard-Pierrot I, Reyniès Ad, et al. EGFR as a potential therapeutic target for a subset of muscle-invasive bladder cancers presenting a basal-like phenotype. Sci Translational Med 2014;6(244):244ra91. https://doi.org/10.1126/scitranslmed.3008970.

30. Marzouka NA, Eriksson P, Rovira C, et al. A validation and extended description of the Lund taxonomy for urothelial carcinoma using the TCGA cohort. Sci Rep 2018;8(1):3737. https://doi.org/10.1038/s41598-018-22126-x.

31. Kamoun A, de Reynies A, Allory Y, et al. A Consensus Molecular Classification of Muscle-invasive Bladder Cancer. Eur Urol 2020;77(4):420–33. https://doi.org/10.1016/j.eururo.2019.09.006.

32. Batista da Costa J, Gibb EA, Bivalacqua TJ, et al. Molecular Characterization of Neuroendocrine-like Bladder Cancer. Clin Cancer Res 2019;25(13):3908–20. https://doi.org/10.1158/1078-0432.CCR-18-3558.

33. Seiler R, Ashab HAD, Erho N, et al. Impact of Molecular Subtypes in Muscle-invasive Bladder Cancer on Predicting Response and Survival after Neoadjuvant Chemotherapy. Eur Urol 2017;72(4):544–54. https://doi.org/10.1016/j.eururo.2017.03.030.

34. McConkey DJ, Choi W, Shen Y, et al. A Prognostic Gene Expression Signature in the Molecular Classification of Chemotherapy-naive Urothelial Cancer is Predictive of Clinical Outcomes from Neoadjuvant Chemotherapy: A Phase 2 Trial of Dose-dense Methotrexate, Vinblastine, Doxorubicin, and Cisplatin with Bevacizumab in Urothelial Cancer. Eur Urol 2016;69(5):855–62. https://doi.org/10.1016/j.eururo.2015.08.034.

35. Lotan Y, de Jong JJ, Liu VYT, et al. Patients with Muscle-Invasive Bladder Cancer with Nonluminal Subtype Derive Greatest Benefit from Platinum Based Neoadjuvant Chemotherapy. J Urol 2021. https://doi.org/10.1097/JU.0000000000002261. 101097JU0000000000002261.

36. Taber A, Christensen E, Lamy P, et al. Molecular correlates of cisplatin-based chemotherapy response in muscle invasive bladder cancer by integrated multi-omics analysis. Nat Commun 2020;11(1): 4858. https://doi.org/10.1038/s41467-020-18640-0.

37. Roumiguie M, Contreras-Sanz A, Kumar G, et al. Reconciling differences in impact of molecular subtyping on response to cisplatin-based chemotherapy. Nat Commun 2021;12(1):4833. https://doi.org/10.1038/s41467-021-24837-8.

38. Sjödahl G, Abrahamsson J, Holmsten K, et al. Different Responses to Neoadjuvant Chemotherapy in Urothelial Carcinoma Molecular Subtypes. Eur Urol 2021. https://doi.org/10.1016/j.eururo.2021.10.035.

39. De Jong JJ, Gibb EA. Re: Gottfrid Sjödahl, Johan Abrahamsson, Karin Holmsten, et al. Different Responses to Neoadjuvant Chemotherapy in Urothelial Carcinoma Molecular Subtypes. Eur Urol. 2022;81: 316-7.: Neoadjuvant Chemotherapy Response in Muscle-invasive Bladder Cancer: Differences in Intrinsic Biology or Subtyping Nomenclature? Eur Urol. Nov 12 2021;81(4):e90-e91. https://doi.org/10.1016/j.eururo.2021.12.033.

40. Flaig TW, Tangen CM, Daneshmand S, et al. A Randomized Phase II Study of Coexpression Extrapolation (COXEN) with Neoadjuvant Chemotherapy for Bladder Cancer (SWOG S1314; NCT02177695). Clin Cancer Res 2021;27(9): 2435–41. https://doi.org/10.1158/1078-0432.CCR-20-2409.

41. Teo MY, Bambury RM, Zabor EC, et al. DNA Damage Response and Repair Gene Alterations Are Associated with Improved Survival in Patients with Platinum-Treated Advanced Urothelial Carcinoma. Clin Cancer Res 2017;23(14):3610–8. https://doi.org/10.1158/1078-0432.CCR-16-2520.

42. Li Q, Damish AW, Frazier Z, et al. ERCC2 Helicase Domain Mutations Confer Nucleotide Excision Repair Deficiency and Drive Cisplatin Sensitivity in Muscle-Invasive Bladder Cancer. Clin Cancer Res 2019;25(3):977–88. https://doi.org/10.1158/1078-0432.CCR-18-1001.

43. Plimack ER, Dunbrack RL, Brennan TA, et al. Defects in DNA Repair Genes Predict Response to Neoadjuvant Cisplatin-based Chemotherapy in Muscle-invasive Bladder Cancer. Eur Urol 2015; 68(6):959–67. https://doi.org/10.1016/j.eururo.2015.07.009.

44. Miron B, Hoffman-Censits JH, Anari F, et al. Defects in DNA Repair Genes Confer Improved Long-term Survival after Cisplatin-based Neoadjuvant Chemotherapy for Muscle-invasive Bladder Cancer. Eur Urol Oncol 2020;3(4):544–7. https://doi.org/10.1016/j.euo.2020.02.003.

45. Geynisman DM, Abbosh P, Ross EA, et al. A phase II trial of risk enabled therapy after initiating neoadjuvant chemotherapy for bladder cancer (RETAIN BLADDER): Interim analysis. J Clin Oncol 2021; 39(6_suppl):397. https://doi.org/10.1200/JCO.2021.39.6_suppl.397.

46. Galsky MD, Daneshmand S, Chan KG, et al. Phase 2 trial of gemcitabine, cisplatin, plus nivolumab with selective bladder sparing in patients with muscle-invasive bladder cancer (MIBC): HCRN GU 16-257. J Clin Oncol 2021;39(15_suppl):4503. https://doi.org/10.1200/JCO.2021.39.15_suppl.4503.

47. Efstathiou JA, Mouw KW, Gibb EA, et al. Impact of Immune and Stromal Infiltration on Outcomes Following Bladder-Sparing Trimodality Therapy for Muscle-Invasive Bladder Cancer. Eur Urol 2019; 76(1):59–68. https://doi.org/10.1016/j.eururo.2019.01.011.

48. Sharma P, Retz M, Siefker-Radtke A, et al. Nivolumab in metastatic urothelial carcinoma after platinum therapy (CheckMate 275): a multicentre, single-arm, phase 2 trial. Lancet Oncol 2017;18(3): 312–22. https://doi.org/10.1016/s1470-2045(17)30065-7.

49. Rosenberg JE, Hoffman-Censits J, Powles T, et al. Atezolizumab in patients with locally advanced and metastatic urothelial carcinoma who have progressed following treatment with platinum-based chemotherapy: a single-arm, multicentre, phase 2 trial. Lancet 2016;387(10031):1909–20. https://doi.org/10.1016/s0140-6736(16)00561-4.

50. Mariathasan S, Turley SJ, Nickles D, et al. TGFbeta attenuates tumour response to PD-L1 blockade by contributing to exclusion of T cells. Nature 2018; 554(7693):544–8. https://doi.org/10.1038/nature25501.

51. Szabados B, Kockx M, Assaf ZJ, et al. Final Results of Neoadjuvant Atezolizumab in Cisplatin-ineligible Patients with Muscle-invasive Urothelial Cancer of the Bladder. Eur Urol 2022. https://doi.org/10.1016/j.eururo.2022.04.013.

52. Powles T, Kockx M, Rodriguez-Vida A, et al. Clinical efficacy and biomarker analysis of neoadjuvant atezolizumab in operable urothelial carcinoma in the ABACUS trial. Nat Med 2019;25(11):1706–14. https://doi.org/10.1038/s41591-019-0628-7.

53. Kim J, Kwiatkowski D, McConkey DJ, et al. The Cancer Genome Atlas Expression Subtypes Stratify Response to Checkpoint Inhibition in Advanced Urothelial Cancer and Identify a Subset of Patients with High Survival Probability. Eur Urol 2019;75(6): 961–4. https://doi.org/10.1016/j.eururo.2019.02.017.

54. Necchi A, Raggi D, Gallina A, et al. Impact of Molecular Subtyping and Immune Infiltration on

Pathological Response and Outcome Following Neoadjuvant Pembrolizumab in Muscle-invasive Bladder Cancer. Eur Urol 2020. https://doi.org/10.1016/j.eururo.2020.02.028.

55. Nakauma-González JA, Rijnders M, van Riet J, et al. Comprehensive Molecular Characterization Reveals Genomic and Transcriptomic Subtypes of Metastatic Urothelial Carcinoma. Eur Urol 2022. https://doi.org/10.1016/j.eururo.2022.01.026.

56. Galsky MD, Saci A, Szabo PM, et al. Nivolumab in Patients with Advanced Platinum-resistant Urothelial Carcinoma: Efficacy, Safety, and Biomarker Analyses with Extended Follow-up from CheckMate 275. Clin Cancer Res 2020;26(19):5120–8. https://doi.org/10.1158/1078-0432.CCR-19-4162.

57. Powles T, Assaf ZJ, Davarpanah N, et al. ctDNA guiding adjuvant immunotherapy in urothelial carcinoma. Nature 2021;595(7867):432–7. https://doi.org/10.1038/s41586-021-03642-9.

58. Sjodahl G, Eriksson P, Lovgren K, et al. Discordant molecular subtype classification in the basal-squamous subtype of bladder tumors and matched lymph-node metastases. Mod Pathol 2018;31(12):1869–81. https://doi.org/10.1038/s41379-018-0096-5.

59. Vandekerkhove G, Lavoie JM, Annala M, et al. Plasma ctDNA is a tumor tissue surrogate and enables clinical-genomic stratification of metastatic bladder cancer. Nat Commun 2021;12(1):184. https://doi.org/10.1038/s41467-020-20493-6.

60. Powles T, Durán I, van der Heijden MS, et al. Atezolizumab versus chemotherapy in patients with platinum-treated locally advanced or metastatic urothelial carcinoma (IMvigor211): a multicentre, open-label, phase 3 randomised controlled trial. Lancet 2018;391(10122):748–57. https://doi.org/10.1016/s0140-6736(17)33297-x.

61. Snyder A, Nathanson T, Funt SA, et al. Contribution of systemic and somatic factors to clinical response and resistance to PD-L1 blockade in urothelial cancer: An exploratory multi-omic analysis. Plos Med 2017;14(5):e1002309. https://doi.org/10.1371/journal.pmed.1002309.

62. Balar AV, Castellano D, O'Donnell PH, et al. First-line pembrolizumab in cisplatin-ineligible patients with locally advanced and unresectable or metastatic urothelial cancer (KEYNOTE-052): a multicentre, single-arm, phase 2 study. Lancet Oncol 2017;18(11):1483–92. https://doi.org/10.1016/s1470-2045(17)30616-2.

63. Bellmunt J, de Wit R, Vaughn DJ, et al. Pembrolizumab as Second-Line Therapy for Advanced Urothelial Carcinoma. N Engl J Med 2017;376(11):1015–26. https://doi.org/10.1056/NEJMoa1613683.

64. Powles T, Csőszi T, Özgüroğlu M, et al. Pembrolizumab alone or combined with chemotherapy versus chemotherapy as first-line therapy for advanced urothelial carcinoma (KEYNOTE-361): a randomised, open-label, phase 3 trial. Lancet Oncol 2021;22(7):931–45. https://doi.org/10.1016/s1470-2045(21)00152-2.

65. da Costa JB, Gibb EA, Nykopp TK, et al. Molecular tumor heterogeneity in muscle invasive bladder cancer: Biomarkers, subtypes, and implications for therapy. Urol Oncol 2018. https://doi.org/10.1016/j.urolonc.2018.11.015.

66. Faltas BM, Prandi D, Tagawa ST, et al. Clonal evolution of chemotherapy-resistant urothelial carcinoma. Nat Genet 2016;48(12):1490–9. https://doi.org/10.1038/ng.3692.

67. Thomsen MB, Nordentoft I, Lamy P, et al. Spatial and temporal clonal evolution during development of metastatic urothelial carcinoma. Mol Oncol 2016;10(9):1450–60. https://doi.org/10.1016/j.molonc.2016.08.003.

68. Thomsen MBH, Nordentoft I, Lamy P, et al. Comprehensive multiregional analysis of molecular heterogeneity in bladder cancer. Sci Rep 2017;7(1):11702. https://doi.org/10.1038/s41598-017-11291-0.

69. Bettegowda C, Sausen M, Leary RJ, et al. Detection of Circulating Tumor DNA in Early- and Late-Stage Human Malignancies. Sci Translational Med 2014;6(224):224ra24. https://doi.org/10.1126/scitranslmed.3007094.

70. Birkenkamp-Demtroder K, Nordentoft I, Christensen E, et al. Genomic Alterations in Liquid Biopsies from Patients with Bladder Cancer. Eur Urol 2016;70(1):75–82. https://doi.org/10.1016/j.eururo.2016.01.007.

71. Vandekerkhove G, Todenhofer T, Annala M, et al. Circulating Tumor DNA Reveals Clinically Actionable Somatic Genome of Metastatic Bladder Cancer. Clin Cancer Res 2017;23(21):6487–97. https://doi.org/10.1158/1078-0432.CCR-17-1140.

72. Christensen E, Birkenkamp-Demtroder K, Sethi H, et al. Early Detection of Metastatic Relapse and Monitoring of Therapeutic Efficacy by Ultra-Deep Sequencing of Plasma Cell-Free DNA in Patients With Urothelial Bladder Carcinoma. J Clin Oncol 20 2019;37(18):1547–57. https://doi.org/10.1200/JCO.18.02052.

73. Raja R, Kuziora M, Brohawn PZ, et al. Early Reduction in ctDNA Predicts Survival in Patients with Lung and Bladder Cancer Treated with Durvalumab. Clin Cancer Res 2018;24(24):6212–22. https://doi.org/10.1158/1078-0432.CCR-18-0386.

74. Loriot Y, Necchi A, Park SH, et al. Erdafitinib in Locally Advanced or Metastatic Urothelial Carcinoma. N Engl J Med 2019;381(4):338–48. https://doi.org/10.1056/NEJMoa1817323.

75. Siefker-Radtke AO, Loriot Y, Necchi A, et al. 751P Analysis of circulating tumor DNA (ctDNA) from the phase II BLC2001 trial of erdafitinib in locally

advanced or metastatic urothelial carcinoma (mUC) to identify markers of intrinsic resistance to fibroblast growth factor receptor (FGFR)-targeted therapy. Ann Oncol 2020;31doi. https://doi.org/10.1016/j.annonc.2020.08.823.

76. Crowley E, Di Nicolantonio F, Loupakis F, et al. Liquid biopsy: monitoring cancer-genetics in the blood. Nat Rev Clin Oncol 2013;10(8):472–84. https://doi.org/10.1038/nrclinonc.2013.110.

77. Teo MY, Mota JM, Whiting KA, et al. Fibroblast Growth Factor Receptor 3 Alteration Status is Associated with Differential Sensitivity to Platinum-based Chemotherapy in Locally Advanced and Metastatic Urothelial Carcinoma. Eur Urol 2020;78(6):907–15. https://doi.org/10.1016/j.eururo.2020.07.018.

78. Turo R, Harnden P, Thygesen H, et al. FGFR3 expression in primary invasive bladder cancers and matched lymph node metastases. J Urol 2015;193(1):325–30. https://doi.org/10.1016/j.juro.2014.06.026.

79. Tully KH, Jutte H, Wirtz RM, et al. Prognostic Role of FGFR Alterations and FGFR mRNA Expression in Metastatic Urothelial Cancer Undergoing Checkpoint Inhibitor Therapy. Urology 2021;157:93–101. https://doi.org/10.1016/j.urology.2021.05.055.

80. Wang L, Gong Y, Saci A, et al. Fibroblast Growth Factor Receptor 3 Alterations and Response to PD-1/PD-L1 Blockade in Patients with Metastatic Urothelial Cancer. Eur Urol 2019;76(5):599–603. https://doi.org/10.1016/j.eururo.2019.06.025.

81. Powles T, Sridhar SS, Loriot Y, et al. Avelumab maintenance in advanced urothelial carcinoma: biomarker analysis of the phase 3 JAVELIN Bladder 100 trial. Nat Med 2021;27(12):2200–11. https://doi.org/10.1038/s41591-021-01579-0.

The Association Between the Urinary Microbiome and Bladder Cancer

Ahmed A. Hussein, MD, PhD*, Gary Smith, PhD, Khurshid A. Guru, MD

KEYWORDS

• Bladder cancer • Urinary • Microbiome • Microbiota • Biofilms

KEY POINTS

- Urinary microbiome contributes to various urologic diseases, including bladder cancer.
- Differences exist in the urinary microbiome across different stages of bladder cancer.
- The bladder cancer-associated microbiome is different from the urinary microbiome.

INTRODUCTION

In the United States, approximately 81,180 new cases and 17,100 deaths from bladder cancer are estimated to occur in 2022.[1] Chemical carcinogenesis is thought to be associated with much of the burden of bladder cancer, including cigarette smoking (40%–60% of new cases), occupational exposure (10%–20%), chlorination of drinking water, contamination with Arsenic, and other more poorly characterized environmental causes. Urothelial cells lining the bladder and urinary tract are constantly exposed to potentially mutagenic environmental agents that are filtered into the urine by the kidneys and excreted in urine.[2] Interestingly, these factors are known to affect the composition of the microbiome, which includes symbiotic bacteria, fungi, parasites, and viruses that inhabit the epithelial surfaces of the human body.[3] It is believed that the microbiome is involved in various normal human physiologic functions, and possibly in the pathogenesis of various human diseases, including cancer.[4]

The urinary microbiome can be defined experimentally by the genomes of the urinary tract-associated microbial taxa (microbiota), in addition to the products of the microbiota and the abiotic constituents of the host environment.[5] Until recently, the bladder and urine—until reaching the urethra—have been considered sterile in healthy individuals. However, the inability to identify viable bacteria in the urinary tract was attributed to the shortcomings of the conventional microbiological culture methods that could neither isolate nor characterize the full spectrum of urinary bacterial species.[6] This dogma has been disproved, and it is now well established that the urinary microbiota exists and the specific taxa present can be identified using 16S ribosomal RNA (rRNA) sequencing. The diversity of taxa within the microbiome has been described in terms of alpha diversity (the diversity of bacterial populations within a sample), beta diversity (differences between bacterial populations across different samples) and differential abundance (differences in taxonomic composition between samples).[7]

Microbial dysbiosis has been implicated in many pathologic processes in various organs. In the gastrointestinal tract for instance, dysbiosis has been associated with various diseases, including irritable bowel syndrome, Crohn's disease, and colorectal cancer.[8–10] Similarly in the urinary tract, alterations of the urinary microbiome were described in patients with urge urinary incontinence, overactive bladder[11,12] as well as interstitial

Disclosures: None.
Department of Urology, Roswell Park Comprehensive Cancer Center, Elm and Carlton Street, Buffalo, NY 14263, USA
* Corresponding author.
E-mail address: Ahmed.Aly@RoswellPark.org

cystitis and neurogenic bladder dysfunction.[6,13,14] The relationship between various microorganisms and cancer is not new. For example, human papillomavirus (HPV) has been implicated in anal cancer[15] as well as cervical[16] and penile cancers.[17] Epstein Barr Virus (EBV) has been associated with Burkitt's lymphoma.[18] Hepatitis B and C were associated with hepatocellular carcinoma.[19] Helicobacter pylori has been associated with the development of gastric carcinoma[20] and Escherichia coli has been associated with colorectal carcinoma.[21] More recently, many studies investigated the alteration of the urinary microbiome in patients with bladder cancer, the focus of this article.

Clinical Relevance

Bladder cancer is the 6th most common cancer worldwide, and the 11th most common cause of cancer-specific mortality.[22] Approximately two-thirds of patients present with nonmuscle-invasive bladder cancer (NMIBC) while the remainder present with muscle-invasive disease (MIBC). Following the transurethral resection of bladder tumors (TURBT), NMIBC commonly recurs and can progress to MIBC. Consequently, adjuvant intravesical treatment with chemotherapy or Bacillus Calmette-Guerin (BCG) is recommended after TURBT. BCG, live attenuated mycobacterium that has been used as a vaccine for tuberculosis, is usually reserved for patients at higher risk of recurrence and progression. Nevertheless, more than 50% of patients with NMIBC who receive BCG exhibit disease recurrence, and up to one-third progress to MIBC within 5 years.[23] While clinical and pathologic variables (such as T stage, tumor size, grade, and multiplicity) have been proposed as predictors of disease recurrence and progression, there is limited understanding of why some NMIBC respond to BCG while others do not.

Whether the alteration of the urinary microbiome contributes to the development or progression of bladder cancer by altering the tumor microenvironment or affecting the response to intravesical treatment with BCG is unknown and warrants further investigation. If the urinary microbiome is mechanistically related to the risk of recurrence after BCG treatment, the microbiome has the potential to serve as a biomarker to identify the cancers that are less likely to respond to intravesical chemotherapy, and therefore that should be referred for early cystectomy.

DISCUSSION

The urinary microbiome may play a key role toward the maintenance of homeostasis of the urinary tract, including development, regulation of epithelial junctions of the urothelium, and protection of the urothelium against pathogens and harmful compounds.[5] Waste products of metabolism, smoking, and occupational exposure are filtered by the kidneys and transported to the bladder whereby they are temporarily stored. While in the bladder, such chemicals may alter the composition of the urinary microbiome and urinary tract homeostasis.[3,24] Microbial dysbiosis caused by such chemicals can predispose to malignancy through the release of antiapoptotic agents, genotoxins, or carcinogenic metabolites capable of induction of neoplastic mutations in the adjacent uroepithelial cells.[25] The microbiome also may induce changes in these procarcinogenic metabolites in urine (eg, conjugation or deconjugation), which in turn can promote carcinogenesis. **Fig. 1** summarizes the different proposed mechanisms by which the urinary microbiome may be associated with carcinogenesis or response to therapy.

Over the course of an individual's life, the composition of the urinary microbiome may be affected by several factors, including gender, age, diet, lifestyle, changes in the intestinal bacterial diversity, and other unknown factors. Further, the urinary microbiota is responsive to antibiotic therapy,[26] and may vary with hormonal changes associated with puberty and menopause, as well as other clinical factors such as constipation and urinary incontinence.[27]

Table 1 summarizes studies that investigated the association between the urinary microbiome and bladder cancer.

Bladder Cancer Versus Controls

Alpha diversity refers to the diversity of bacterial populations within a sample and is estimated by Observed, Chao1, Shannon, Simpson, and Ace diversity indices. Prior studies have reported conflicting results comparing urine samples from patients with bladder cancer versus healthy controls. Some studies *did not* show a significant difference in any of the alpha diversity measures,[28–30] while others observed statistically significant increases in the richness of the bacterial population as measured in 3 or more indices (Wu and colleagues, using Observed Species, Chao1, Shannon, and Ace indices and Zeng and colleagues using Observed Species, Chao1, and Ace indices).[31,32] Other studies have found a significant difference in alpha diversity but used only 1 index (Chao1 index[33] and Faith phylogenetic diversity index[34]). Oresta and colleagues observed *higher* evenness in the urine of patients with

Potential roles of the urinary microbiome in the urinary tract

Homeostatis & Carcinogenesis

Protection of the urothelium against
pathogens & harmful compounds

Waste products cause
microbial dysbiosis

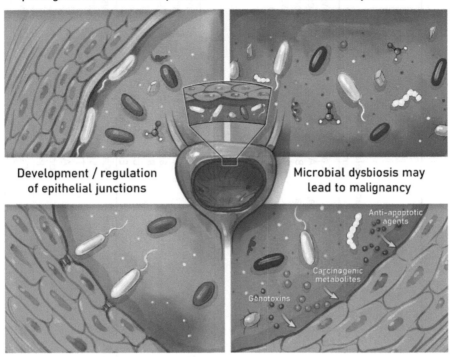

Development / regulation
of epithelial junctions

Microbial dysbiosis may
lead to malignancy

Fig. 1. Summarizes the different proposed mechanisms by which the urinary microbiome may be associated with carcinogenesis or response to therapy.

bladder cancer obtained by catheter.[35] It is worth noting that one study reported significantly *lower* diversity in bladder tissue (not urine) from patients with bladder cancer (Shannon index only).[36]

Beta diversity refers to differences between bacterial populations across different samples. It is usually estimated using the Bray–Curtis dissimilarity score paired with classical multidimensional scaling. Some studies showed a significant difference between urine from patients with bladder cancer versus controls, suggesting a difference among microbial communities between these groups,[30,31,33] while other studies did not observe such difference.[28,34,35]

Relative differential abundance measures the balance between specific microbial groups within a community that may be more relevant to the pathogenesis of bladder cancer. At the phylum level, a higher abundance of Actinobacteria and Proteobacteria were observed in the urine of patients with bladder cancer.[30,33,36] On the other hand, higher abundance of Firmicutes and Deinococcus-Thermus were observed in urine

samples from controls.[30] Liu and colleagues, reported higher abundance of Firmicutes and Bacteroidetes in control urines, but higher abundance of Deinococcus-Thermus in urines of patients with bladder cancer [36]. At the genus level, Hussein and colleagues, observed higher abundance of Actinomyces, Achromobacter, Brevibacterium, and Brucella in urines of patients with bladder cancer, while Salinococcus, Jeotgalicoccus, Escherichia-Shigella, Faecalibacterium, Thermus, and Lactobacillus were significantly more abundant in urine samples from healthy controls.[30] Actinomyces and Brucella were observed previously to be enriched in urine samples of patients with bladder cancer.[33,36] Previous studies also identified the enrichment of other genera, such as Pelomonas, Finegoldia, and Corynebacterium, Enterococcus, Campylobacter, and Ruminococcoca.[28,29,33,35,36] Some studies identified Veillonella to be more abundant in urine of patients with muscle invasive bladder cancer as well as in female patients with bladder cancer,[30,35] while others associated it with controls.[28]

Table 1
Summary of studies to date investigating urinary microbiome and bladder cancer

Study, Year	BCa N	Non-BCa N	Females, n (%)	Sample	Alpha-Diversity	Beta-Diversity	Relative Abundance of Phyla	Relative Abundance of Genera	Other
Hussein et al,[30] 2021	43	10	7	MSU Cath	NS	Different	BCa: Actinobacteria, Proteobacteria Non-BCa: Firmicutes, Deinococcus-Thermus	BCa: Actinomyces, Achromobacter, Brevibacterium, and Brucella Non-BCa: Salinococcus, Jeotgalicoccus, Escherichia-Shigella, Faecalibacterium, Thermus, and Lactobacillus	MIBC vs NMIBC BCG responders vs non responders Male vs females with BCa
Oresta et al,[35] 2021	51	10	0	Catheter	Eveness	NS		BCa: Increased Veillonella and Corynebacterium and decreased Ruminococcus 1 and unclassified genus of Enterobacteriaceae	High risk vs low risk MSU vs washouts (irrigation)
Zeng et al,[32] 2020	62	19	0	MSU	Observed Species, Chao1, Ace	NR	No significant difference	BCa: Sphingobacteriaceae, Thermoactinomycetes, Acinetobacter Controls: Serratia, Proteus, Laceyella	High vs low risk of recurrence
Chipollini et al,[34] 2020	27	10	13	MSU	Different, Faith phylogenetic	NS	NR	BCa: Bacteroides and Faecalibacterium Controls: Bacteroides, Lachnoclostridium, and Burkholderiaceae	Invasive vs superficial cancer

methodological factors (sample type [voided, midstream urine, bladder wash], storage conditions [use of preservative or frozen samples], processing and extraction techniques), as well as variations in bioinformatics analyses. Additionally, most of these studies were retrospective in nature with a relatively small number of cases, relatively short follow-up, and the lack of longitudinal follow-up, which can make it difficult to discern a complete and durable response to BCG. Another important limitation is that the 16S rRNA gene sequencing-based technology used allows the identification of bacteria at the genus level, but does not allow the identification of bacteria at the species level, or identification of nonbacterial microorganisms, such as viruses and fungi.

Whether bacteria adherent to the bladder mucosa (biofilms) are a more reliable representation of the critical tumor-associated microbiome is yet to be defined. Analysis of biopsy material for biofilms could avoid sample contamination with urethral microbiota in the urethra, especially in women.[44] Hence, profiling the microbiome of tumor, peritumor and nontumor tissues of patients with bladder cancer seem to be the appropriate way to ascertain the association between the pathogenic effect of microbial dysbiosis and the onset, progression, and relapse of cancer. This realization has led to a shift in focus to the characterization of the microbiome present in bladder tissues rather than in the urine, including both tumor and normal bladder mucosa. Nevertheless, obtaining bladder biopsies or suprapubic aspirates in healthy individuals remains an ethical challenge, and most studies included only tissues from patients with bladder cancer. Nadler and colleagues showed abundant bacterial aggregation on the surface epithelium in 2 patients with pT2 urothelial bladder cancer.[45] Another study showed that the genus Burkholderia was more abundant in neoplastic versus nonneoplastic bladder tissue. Importantly, their findings demonstrated that the urinary microbiome shares greater than 80% of the bacterial families present in paired bladder tissue, making the urinary microbiome a fair proxy of the tissue bacterial environment.[38] Another study that included 10 patients with bladder cancer (5 men and 5 women), identified 5 suspect genera (Akkermansia, Bacteroides, Clostridium sensu stricto, Enterobacter and Klebsiella) that were over-represented in bladder cancer tissue samples compared with the matched urine. They concluded that urine samples provide different results relative to tissue samples for the characterization of the bacteria involved in carcinogenesis.

Future Directions

Future studies should investigate the tumor-associated microbiome, as well as mapping the microbiome of the noninvolved bladder to define the extent of the dysbiotic microbiome in the bladder. Studies in colorectal cancer showed that the dysbiotic microbiome was present in normal-looking tissue close to the tumor. The use of other technologies that can characterize the microbiome down to the species level will allow the identification of specific strains of bacteria associated with bladder cancer.

SUMMARY

Variation in the urinary microbiome was noted between patients with bladder cancer and healthy controls, and also between cancers with different stages, between male and female patients, and between BCG responders and nonresponders. Optimizing urinary sampling, preservation, and other clinical factors that may affect the identification of components of the urinary microbiome will be key to better understanding the urinary microbiome and the initiation, progression, and response to the treatment of bladder cancers.

CLINICS CARE POINTS

- Variation in the urinary microbiome was noted between patients with bladder cancer and healthy controls.
- Variation in the urinary microbiome was noted across different bladder cancer stages, male and female patients, and in BCG responders versus nonresponders.
- Urinary microbiome may not represent the actual tumor-associated microbiome and therefore, it is vital to study the microbiome associated with bladder cancer tissue.
- The dysbiotic microbiome may extend beyond the location of the tumor to involve the surrounding tissues and may be associated with tumor multi-focality.
- Optimizing sampling, collection methods, timing, and other clinical factors that affect the characterization of the urinary microbiome is key to understanding the urinary microbiome. The exact association between the urinary microbiome and cancer is yet to be elucidated.

ACKNOWLEDGEMENTS

Roswell Park Alliance Foundation.

REFERENCES

1. Siegel RL, Miller KD, Fuchs HE, et al. Cancer statistics, 2022. CA Cancer J Clin 2022;72:7–33.
2. Saginala K, Barsouk A, Aluru JS, et al. Epidemiology of bladder cancer. Med Sci (Basel) 2020;8.
3. Costello EK, Stagaman K, Dethlefsen L, et al. The application of ecological theory toward an understanding of the human microbiome. Science 2012; 336:1255–62.
4. Dzutsev A, Goldszmid RS, Viaud S, et al. The role of the microbiota in inflammation, carcinogenesis, and cancer therapy. Eur J Immunol 2015;45:17–31.
5. Whiteside SA, Razvi H, Dave S, et al. The microbiome of the urinary tract–a role beyond infection. Nat Rev Urol 2015;12:81–90.
6. Fouts DE, Pieper R, Szpakowski S, et al. Integrated next-generation sequencing of 16S rDNA and metaproteomics differentiate the healthy urine microbiome from asymptomatic bacteriuria in neuropathic bladder associated with spinal cord injury. J Transl Med 2012;10:174.
7. Goodrich JK, Di Rienzi SC, Poole AC, et al. Conducting a microbiome study. Cell 2014;158:250–62.
8. Durban A, Abellan JJ, Jimenez-Hernandez N, et al. Structural alterations of faecal and mucosa-associated bacterial communities in irritable bowel syndrome. Environ Microbiol Rep 2012;4:242–7.
9. Ahn J, Sinha R, Pei Z, et al. Human gut microbiome and risk for colorectal cancer. J Natl Cancer Inst 2013;105:1907–11.
10. Petrov VA, Saltykova IV, Zhukova IA, et al. Analysis of gut microbiota in patients with parkinson's disease. Bull Exp Biol Med 2017;162:734–7.
11. Thomas-White KJ, Hilt EE, Fok C, et al. Incontinence medication response relates to the female urinary microbiota. Int Urogynecol J 2016;27:723–33.
12. Wu P, Chen Y, Zhao J, et al. Urinary Microbiome and Psychological Factors in Women with Overactive Bladder. Front Cell Infect Microbiol 2017;7:488.
13. Pearce MM, Hilt EE, Rosenfeld AB, et al. The female urinary microbiome: a comparison of women with and without urgency urinary incontinence. mBio 2014;5:e01283-14.
14. Siddiqui H, Lagesen K, Nederbragt AJ, et al. Alterations of microbiota in urine from women with interstitial cystitis. BMC Microbiol 2012;12:205.
15. Forman D, de Martel C, Lacey CJ, et al. Global burden of human papillomavirus and related diseases. Vaccine 2012;30(Suppl 5):F12–23.
16. Walboomers JM, Jacobs MV, Manos MM, et al. Human papillomavirus is a necessary cause of invasive cervical cancer worldwide. J Pathol 1999;189:12–9.
17. El-Omar EM, Oien K, El-Nujumi A, et al. Helicobacter pylori infection and chronic gastric acid hyposecretion. Gastroenterology 1997;113:15–24.
18. Buc E, Dubois D, Sauvanet P, et al. High prevalence of mucosa-associated E. coli producing cyclomodulin and genotoxin in colon cancer. PLoS One 2013;8: e56964.
19. Cambier S, Sylvester RJ, Collette L, et al. EORTC nomograms and risk groups for predicting recurrence, progression, and disease-specific and overall survival in non-muscle-invasive stage Ta-T1 urothelial bladder cancer patients treated with 1-3 years of maintenance bacillus calmette-guerin. Eur Urol 2016;69:60–9.
20. Babjuk M, Bohle A, Burger M, et al. EAU guidelines on non-muscle-invasive urothelial carcinoma of the bladder: update 2016. Eur Urol 2017;71:447–61.
21. Yatsunenko T, Rey FE, Manary MJ, et al. Human gut microbiome viewed across age and geography. Nature 2012;486:222–7.
22. Zhu L, Liu W, Alkhouri R, et al. Structural changes in the gut microbiome of constipated patients. Physiol Genomics 2014;46:679–86.
23. Bucevic Popovic V, Situm M, Chow CT, et al. The urinary microbiome associated with bladder cancer. Sci Rep 2018;8:12157.
24. Xu W, Yang L, Lee P, et al. Mini-review: perspective of the microbiome in the pathogenesis of urothelial carcinoma. Am J Clin Exp Urol 2014;2:57–61.
25. Hussein AA, Elsayed AS, Durrani M, et al. Investigating the association between the urinary microbiome and bladder cancer: An exploratory study. Urol Oncol 2021;39:370 e9–370 e19.
26. Wu P, Zhang G, Zhao J, et al. Profiling the urinary microbiota in male patients with bladder cancer in china. Front Cell Infect Microbiol 2018;8:167.
27. Zeng J, Zhang G, Chen C, et al. Alterations in urobiome in patients with bladder cancer and implications for clinical outcome: a single-institution study. Front Cell Infect Microbiol 2020;10:555508.
28. Bi H, Tian Y, Song C, et al. Urinary microbiota - a potential biomarker and therapeutic target for bladder cancer. J Med Microbiol 2019;68:1471–8.
29. Chipollini J, Wright JR, Nwanosike H, et al. Characterization of urinary microbiome in patients with bladder cancer: results from a single-institution, feasibility study. Urol Oncol 2020;38:615–21.
30. Oresta B, Braga D, Lazzeri M, et al. The microbiome of catheter collected urine in males with bladder cancer according to disease stage. J Urol 2021; 205:86–93.
31. Liu F, Liu A, Lu X, et al. Dysbiosis signatures of the microbial profile in tissue from bladder cancer. Cancer Medicine 2019;8:6904–14.
32. Lewis DA, Brown R, Williams J, et al. The human urinary microbiome; bacterial DNA in voided urine of

asymptomatic adults. Front Cell Infect Microbiol 2013;3:41.

33. Pederzoli F, Ferrarese R, Amato V, et al. Sex-specific alterations in the urinary and tissue microbiome in therapy-naive urothelial bladder cancer patients. Eur Urol Oncol 2020;3(6):784–8.

34. Matsumoto S, Hara T, Nagaoka M, et al. A component of polysaccharide peptidoglycan complex on Lactobacillus induced an improvement of murine model of inflammatory bowel disease and colitis-associated cancer. Immunology 2009;128:e170–80.

35. Naito S, Koga H, Yamaguchi A, et al. Prevention of recurrence with epirubicin and lactobacillus casei after transurethral resection of bladder cancer. J Urol 2008;179:485–90.

36. Zlotta AR, Drowart A, Van Vooren JP, et al. Evolution and clinical significance of the T cell proliferative and cytokine response directed against the fibronectin binding antigen 85 complex of bacillus Calmette-Guerin during intravesical treatment of superficial bladder cancer. J Urol 1997;157:492–8.

37. Kato I, Yokokura T, Mutai M. Correlation between increase in Ia-bearing macrophages and induction of T cell-dependent antitumor activity by Lactobacillus casei in mice. Cancer Immunol Immunother 1988; 26:215–21.

38. Chen F, Zhang G, Iwamoto Y, et al. BCG directly induces cell cycle arrest in human transitional carcinoma cell lines as a consequence of integrin cross-linking. BMC Urol 2005;5(8).

39. Nadler N, Kvich L, Bjarnsholt T, et al. The discovery of bacterial biofilm in patients with muscle invasive bladder cancer. APMIS 2021;129(5):265–70.

Combined Use of Magnetic Resonance Imaging and Biomarker Testing to Detect Clinically Significant Prostate Cancer

Nathan L. Samora, MD[a], Bashir Al Hussein Al Awamlh, MD[a],
Jeffrey J. Tosoian, MD, MPH[a,b,*]

KEYWORDS

- Prostatic neoplasms • Multiparametric MRI • Neoplasm grading biomarkers
- Early cancer detection • Biopsy • Risk stratification

KEY POINTS

- Literature on how best to combine mpMRI and biomarker testing for the detection of clinically significant prostate cancer are predominantly derived from retrospective analyses of clinical practice, posing significant limitations.
- In extant data comparing mpMRI-first to biomarker-first testing strategies, initial biomarker testing seems to offer a modest advantage in reducing the burden of testing while preserving the detection of clinically significant disease.
- For men presenting after an equivocal (PI-RADS 3) mpMRI, secondary biomarker testing seems helpful in identifying a proportion of men who can safely forego biopsy.
- For men presenting following a negative (PI-RADS 1–2) mpMRI, secondary biomarker testing could help identify patients at risk of false-negative imaging who stand to benefit from biopsy, particularly when the sensitivity of mpMRI is limited or unknown.
- Prospective studies in which all patients undergo mpMRI, biomarker testing, and biopsy are essential to better delineate the optimal combined use of these tools.

INTRODUCTION

Prostate cancer (PCa) is the most commonly diagnosed malignancy in men from the United States and a leading cause of death worldwide.[1–3] Widespread screening with prostate-specific antigen (PSA) in the 1990s contributed to a significant reduction in PCa mortality.[4–6] With the current understanding of the indolent nature of low-grade PCa; however, the poor specificity of PSA for high-grade cancer is increasingly problematic. Use of PSA as an isolated screening tool resulted in frequent negative biopsies and detection of low-grade cancers that do not stand to benefit from definitive treatment[7,8] and may, instead, incur harm.[9] There is a great need to incorporate emerging tools, such as multiparametric MRI

Competing Interests: J.J. Tosoian is a cofounder of LynxDx, Inc. The other authors declare no competing interests.
[a] Department of Urology, Vanderbilt University Medical Center, 1161 21st Ave., South A-1302 Medical Center North Nashville, TN 37232-2765, USA; [b] Vanderbilt-Ingram Cancer Center, 1301 Medical Center Drive, 1710 TVC, Nashville, TN 37232-5536, USA
* Corresponding author. Vanderbilt University Medical Center, 1161 21st Ave., South A-1302 Medical Center North Nashville, TN 37232-2765.
E-mail address: jeff.tosoian@vumc.org

urologic.theclinics.com

(mpMRI) and blood- or urine-based biomarker tests, into a more effective diagnostic pathway.

In response to this, the National Comprehensive Cancer Network (NCCN) clinical practice guidelines recommend mpMRI and/or biomarker testing in men with elevated PSA before immediate biopsy.[10] To varying degrees, these tools have been validated to better identify men most likely to harbor clinically significant PCa (defined as Grade Group ≥ 2, GG ≥ 2). Moreover, in patients with mpMRI-visible tumors, the use of targeted biopsies is known to improve the detection of GG ≥ 2 disease.[11,12] Still, in light of known limitations of mpMRI,[13] these guidelines offer that some may combine biomarkers with mpMRI to best determine the need for biopsy.

Despite a growing literature describing the use of mpMRI and biomarker tests, it remains unclear how to best combine these tools in clinical practice. We have previously presented validation data of clinically available biomarkers for detecting GG ≥ 2 PCa on biopsy.[14] To address the knowledge gap of combined diagnostic testing, the current report sought to review clinical studies describing the combined use of mpMRI and biomarker testing.

STUDY SELECTION

Our search included biomarker tests suggested for consideration by the NCCN Prostate Cancer Early Detection guidelines to further define the probability of high-grade cancer: 4Kscore, Prostate Health Index (phi), SelectMDx, MyProstateScore (MPS), ExoDx Prostate Intelliscore (EPI), and IsoPSA.[10] The PubMed and Embase databases were searched by test name and mpMRI in May of 2022. Resulting abstracts for each biomarker test were collected and reviewed to identify original research articles incorporating mpMRI and at least one biomarker test relative to a reference standard (ie, biopsy pathology). Review articles were not included, while their references were examined for additional eligible studies. There were no eligible reports of IsoPSA.

We placed emphasis on data directly applicable to clinical practice. Thus, we included studies that explicitly described a potentially adoptable testing approach and the outcomes observed under the testing approach. As such, nomogram-based predictive models and studies providing general measures of discriminative accuracy (ie, AUC) without potential clinical outcomes were not included. Unless otherwise described, patients with a negative mpMRI (PI-RADS 1–2) that proceeded to biopsy underwent systematic (standard 12-core template) prostate biopsies, and those with equivocal (PI-RADS 3) or positive (PI-RADS 4–5) mpMRI underwent systematic plus targeted biopsies.

FINDINGS
Blood-Based Biomarkers

4-Kallikrein score
The 4-kallikrein score (4Kscore) by OPKO Health (Miami, FL) is a blood-based assay that incorporates 4 kallikreins (PSA, free PSA [fPSA], intact PSA [iPSA], and human kallikrein 2 [hK2]) with clinical parameters (age, prior biopsy status, and digital rectal examination (DRE) [optional] findings) to predict the risk of detecting GG ≥ 2 PCa on prostate biopsy.[15] Uniquely, longer-term follow-up data have also shown that men with a 4Kscore less than 7.5% have a minimal (<1%) risk of developing metastatic PCa within 20 years.[16] The 4Kscore is reported as the percentage likelihood (0%–100%) of detecting GG ≥ 2 PCa on biopsy, and values < 7.5% are classified as low-risk. The 4Kscore test has been validated in pertinent clinical settings,[14] and the discriminatory value added by the 2 novel markers (iPSA, hK2) has been shown.[17] We identified 5 pertinent studies combining 4Kscore and mpMRI for the detection of GG ≥ 2 cancer.

4Kscore Performance with mpMRI
Punnen et al. PLoS One; 2018 In 2018, Punnen and colleagues retrospectively identified 300 consecutive men referred for PCa evaluation who underwent both mpMRI and 4Kscore testing.[18] Most patients were referred for evaluation due to elevated PSA, although some were due to abnormal DRE or mpMRI. Following mpMRI and 4Kscore testing, 149 men (49%) underwent prostate biopsy based on shared decision-making. Median PSA did not significantly differ between men who did versus did not undergo biopsy (6.3 vs 6.7 ng/mL, $P = .13$), while the biopsy group had a higher median 4Kscore (15% vs 7%, $P<.001$) and greater proportion of men with PI-RADS 4 to 5 mpMRI (100% vs 0%, $P<.001$). Among men that underwent biopsy, 67 (52%) were biopsy-naïve and 49 (33%) were found to have GG ≥ 2 cancer. The authors presented the proportion of biopsies avoided and GG ≥ 2 cancers missed under various applications of 4Kscore and mpMRI.

A strategy using 4Kscore alone (ie, biopsy if 4Kscore $\geq 7.5\%$) would have avoided 29% of biopsies while missing 12% of GG ≥ 2 cancers (ie, 88% sensitivity). Using mpMRI alone (ie, biopsy if PI-RADS ≥ 4) would have avoided 54% of biopsies while missing 23% of GG ≥ 2 cancers. A strategy using an initial 4Kscore test followed by mpMRI if

4Kscore ≥7.5%—in which biopsy was performed only if both tests were positive—would have avoided 29% of mpMRIs and 83% of biopsies while missing 33% of GG ≥ 2 cancers (ie, 67% sensitivity). A strategy in which both 4Kscore and mpMRI were obtained, and a biopsy was performed if either test was positive, would have avoided 15% of biopsies while missing 2% of GG ≥ 2 cancers (ie, 98% sensitivity) **(Table 1)**. Another strategy is described thus: obtain an mpMRI first. If it is positive, perform biopsy. If it is negative, perform 4Kscore testing and proceed to biopsy if 4Kscore ≥7.5%. This strategy also would have avoided 15% of biopsies and missed 2% of GG ≥ 2 cancers (ie, 98% sensitivity).

Marzouk et al. Urologic Oncology; 2019 Applying data from the 4Kscore US validation study and the PROMIS trial, Marzouk and colleagues sought to determine when, after initial 4Kscore testing, the use of mpMRI would change the decision to pursue biopsy.[19–21] The authors used an overall GG ≥ 2 PCa risk threshold of 7.5% (ie, based on both 4Kscore and mpMRI) to select for biopsy. They found that patients with a 4Kscore less than 5% would not have their risk of GG ≥ 2 cancer increase beyond 7.5% even if a subsequent mpMRI was positive (PI-RADS ≥3). In other words, initial 4Kscore values < 5% could be used to rule out the need for biopsy under this approach. By the same token, patients with 4Kscore ≥23% would not have their risk sufficiently reduced by a negative mpMRI to preclude biopsy (ie, to

<7.5% risk of GG ≥ 2 cancer). Using a strategy of initial 4Kscore testing, they found that 26% of men (those with 4Kscore <5%) would have avoided both mpMRI and biopsy, and 29% of men (those with 4Kscore >23%) would have proceeded directly to biopsy, and the remaining 45% (4Kscore 5%–23%) stood to benefit from additional risk stratification with mpMRI. While conceptual in nature, these data provide a clinically meaningful framework for clinicians to apply these tests in sequence.

Falagario et al. European Urology Oncology; 2020 Additional studies have explored combined and sequential uses of 4Kscore and mpMRI. Falagario and colleagues retrospectively assessed 266 biopsy-naïve patients that presented with clinical suspicion of PCa (PSA 3–20 ng/mL and/or abnormal DRE) and underwent mpMRI, 4Kscore, and biopsy.[22] On biopsy, 74 men (28%) were found to have GG ≥ 2 PCa.

The authors calculated PSA density (PSAD) and ERSPC risk calculator (ERSPC-RC)-based risk of GG ≥ 2 PCa for each patient. Performance measures of the diagnostic tools were calculated using different cutoff values, and decision curve analysis (DCA) was used to calculate the net clinical benefit of various testing approaches. Among 7 combined testing approaches, the authors presented the 3 best strategies in detail. Strategy 1 used an initial 4Kscore, and patients with 4Kscore ≥7.5% then proceeded to mpMRI. Biopsy was performed in patients with a positive mpMRI (ie, PI-RADS 3–5)

Table 1
Clinical outcomes of testing strategies using 4Kscore and/or mpMRI to guide the decision to perform prostate biopsy

Strategy	Biopsies Avoided N (%)	GG ≥2 Cancers Missed N (%)
Strategy 1: 4Kscore alone	43 (29%)	6 (12%)
Strategy 2: mpMRI alone	81 (54%)	11 (23%)
Strategy 3: 4Kscore → mpMRI (both positive)	124 (83%)	16 (33%)
Strategy 4: mpMRI ± 4Kscore (either positive)	23 (15%)	1 (2%)
Strategy 5: mpMRI and 4Kscore (either positive)	23 (15%)	1 (2%)

149 men underwent performances were determined in patients who underwent prostate biopsy, of which 49 (33%) had GG ≥2 cancer on biopsy.
  Strategy 1: Obtain 4Kscore alone. Biopsy if 4Kscore ≥7.5%.
  Strategy 2: Obtain mpMRI alone. Biopsy if mpMRI is positive (PI-RADS 4–5).
  Strategy 3: Obtain 4Kscore first. If less than 7.5%, do not perform biopsy. If ≥7.5%, obtain mpMRI, and perform biopsy if mpMRI positive (PI-RADS 4–5).
  Strategy 4: Obtain mpMRI first. If positive (PI-RADS 4–5), perform biopsy. If negative, obtain 4Kscore, and perform biopsy if 4Kscore ≥7.5%.
  Strategy 5: Obtain both 4Kscore and mpMRI. Biopsy if either 4Kscore ≥7.5% or mpMRI is positive (PI-RADS 4–5).
  Adapted from Punnen S, Nahar B, Soodana-Prakash N, et al. Optimizing patient's selection for prostate biopsy: A single institution experience with multi-parametric MRI and the 4Kscore test for the detection of aggressive prostate cancer. PLoS One 2018; 13:e0201384.

or 4Kscore greater than 18%. This approach would avoid 34% of mpMRI and biopsies, while missing 2.7% of GG $\geq$ 2 PCa. Strategies 2 and 3 used initial mpMRI, and biopsy was performed for positive mpMRI. Patients with negative mpMRI underwent second-line testing with 4Kscore (Strategy 2) or PSAD (Strategy 3), and biopsy was performed for elevated values (4Kscore $\geq$18%; PSAD $\geq$0.10 ng/ml^2). Both mpMRI-first approaches yielded a similarly low risk of missing GG $\geq$ 2 PCa ($\leq$2.7%), while avoiding slightly fewer biopsies than Strategy 1 (25% for 4Kscore, 28% for PSAD). The clinical outcomes of various sequential and combined testing approaches are included in **Table 2**.

De la Calle et al. Journal of Urology; 2021 Investigators at the University of California—San Francisco reported on the clinical use of 2 biomarkers (4Kscore test and EPI) and mpMRI in men referred for elevated PSA and/or abnormal DRE.[23] Similar to other such studies, the data were limited by the lack of a uniform approach to biomarker test selection and the fact that only patients deemed higher-risk, based on provider discretion, proceeded to biopsy (419/783, 54%). Men that underwent biopsy had a higher median PSA (6.6 vs 5.9 ng/mL, P<.001), 4Kscore (21.0 vs 8.0, P<.0001), and EPI (31.2 vs 14.5, P<.0001) than those that did not. Similarly, a greater proportion of biopsied men had PI-RADS 4 to 5 mpMRI (75% vs 31%, P<.001). Of the 419 men biopsied, 335 (80%) were biopsy-naïve, and 159 (38%) were diagnosed with GG $\geq$ 2 cancer on biopsy. While higher biomarker scores were generally associated with higher PI-RADS scores, mpMRI and biomarker test results were discordant in 39% of patients with 4Kscore and 41% of patients with EPI. Among 62 patients with both 4Kscore and EPI testing, these tests were discordant in 25 (40%).

The authors explored the clinical consequences of various testing approaches. Use of mpMRI alone (ie, biopsy if PI-RADS$\geq$3) would have avoided 40% of biopsies while missing 13% of GG $\geq$ 2 cancers (ie, 87% sensitivity). Using 4Kscore alone (ie, avoid biopsy if <7.5%) would have avoided 30% of biopsies while missing only 4% of GG $\geq$ 2 cancers (ie, 96% sensitivity). Sequential testing using 4Kscore first, then mpMRI if 4Kscore $\geq$7.5%—in which biopsy is performed if (1) initial 4Kscore $\geq$20% or (2) initial 4Kscore 7.5% to 20% and mpMRI was PI-RADS 3 to 5—would have avoided 30% of mpMRI and 39% of biopsies, while missing 5.6% of GG $\geq$ 2 cancers.

Using EPI alone (ie, avoid biopsy if < 15.6, as validated in biopsy-naïve men would have avoided

40% of biopsies while missing only 2 GG $\geq$ 2 cancers (4.8%).[24,25] A sequential approach using EPI first followed by mpMRI if EPI $\geq$15.6—in which biopsy is performed if (1) initial EPI $\geq$19 or (2) initial EPI 15.6 to 19 and subsequent mpMRI was positive (PI-RADS 3–5)—would have avoided 40% of mpMRIs and 43% of biopsies, while missing 4.8% of GG $\geq$ 2 cancers.

Employing an "*either/or*" strategy of ExoDx and mpMRI (ie, biopsy if EPI $\geq$15.6 *or* PI-RADS $\geq$3), 21% of biopsies would have been avoided while missing 2.6% of GG $\geq$ 2 cancers. Algorithms using mpMRI first followed by biomarker testing if negative rarely missed GG $\geq$ 2 cancer (<3%) but resulted in fewer biopsies avoided (17% for 4Kscore and 20% for EPI) than biomarker-first and biomarker-only approaches (see **Table 2**). Despite the limitations of a "convenience cohort," this analysis provided uniquely informative data.

Falagario et al. International Journal of Urology; 2021 While several studies have sought to determine the optimal sequential or combined use of biomarkers and mpMRI, Falagario and colleagues pursued a specific, clinically relevant question.[26] In patients with positive mpMRI (PI-RADS 3–5), the authors explored whether subsequent 4Kscore testing could allow for avoidance of systematic biopsy in favor of targeted biopsy only in select patients. They retrospectively evaluated 408 men with no PCa history who had undergone mpMRI, 4Kscore testing, and biopsy. Men with a positive mpMRI that underwent targeted plus systematic biopsy (n = 256) comprised the analytical cohort, of whom 179 (70%) were biopsy-naïve.

GG1 cancer was detected in 59 men (23%), and GG $\geq$ 2 cancer was detected in 94 men (37%). Of GG $\geq$ 2 cancers, 78% were detected on targeted biopsy ($\pm$ systematic biopsy), while 22% were detected only on systematic biopsy. Thus, forgoing systematic biopsy in all patients would have failed to detect 22% of GG $\geq$ 2 cancers. Using a model incorporating 4Kscore and mpMRI to avoid systematic biopsy in low-risk patients (ie, defer systematic biopsy if estimated risk <12.5%), 40% of systematic biopsies could be avoided, and GG1 cancer diagnoses would be reduced 34%, while missing 5% of GG $\geq$ 2 cancers. These findings provide promise that risk stratification with mpMRI and biomarker testing could reduce the burden of biopsy.

Prostate Health Index

The Prostate Health Index (phi) is a blood-based test from Beckman Coulter (Brea, CA) that combines the novel [-2] proPSA (p2PSA) with free and total PSA to predict the risk of GG $\geq$ 2 PCa

Table 2
Clinical outcomes of isolated, sequential, and combined testing strategies using mpMRI and biomarkers

Study, Year	N[b]	% GG ≥2	Initial Test	Perform Follow-Up if	Follow-Up Test	Perform Biopsy if	% mpMRI Avoided	% Biopsies Avoided	% GG ≥2 Missed
Falagario et al,[22] 2020	266	28%	4Kscore	≥7.5%	mpMRI	4Kscore >18% or PI-RADS 3–5	34%	34%	2.7%
			mpMRI	PI-RADS 1–2	4Kscore	MRI PI-RADS 3–5 or 4Kscore ≥18%	0%	25%	2.7%
			mpMRI	PI-RADS 1–2	PSAD	PI-RADS 3–5 or PSAD ≥0.10	0%	28%	2.7%
de la Calle et al,[23] 2021	338	33%	4Kscore	≥7.5%	mpMRI	4Kscore ≥20% or PI-RADS 3–5	30%	39%	5.6%
			mpMRI	PI-RADS 1–3	4Kscore	PI-RADS 4–5 or 4Kscore ≥20	0%	17%	2.4%
	113	32%	EPI	≥15.6	mpMRI	EPI ≥19 or PI-RADS 3–5	40%	43%	4.8%
			mpMRI	PI-RADS 1–3	EPI	PI-RADS 4–5 or EPI ≥19	0%	20%	2.4%
Maggi et al,[37] 2021	310	20%	SelectMDx	N/A		SelectMDx ≥-2.8	100%	54%	13%
			mpMRI	N/A		PI-RADS 4–5	0%	75%	39%
			mpMRI	PI-RADS 1–3	Select MDx	PI-RADS 4–5 or SelectMDx ≥-2.8	0%	46%	6%
				PI-RADS 1–2	SelectMDx	PI-RADS 3–5 or SelectMDx ≥-2.8	0%	40%	3%
Hendriks et al,[39] 2021	599	31%	SelectMDx	N/A		SelectMDx ≥-2.8	100%	38%	10%
			mpMRI	N/A		PI-RADS 3–5	0%	49%	5%
			SelectMDx	SelectMDx ≥-2.8	mpMRI	SelectMDx ≥-2.8 and PI-RADS 3–5	38%	60%	13%
			SelectMDx and mpMRI	N/A		Either SelectMDx ≥-2.8 or PI-RADS 3–5	0%	28%	2%

The clinical outcomes of various testing strategies (described later in discussion) are tabulated and reported for study participants who underwent mpMRI, biomarker testing, and prostate biopsy[a].

[a] All studies included only those patients who underwent all mpMRI, biomarker testing, and biopsy, except de la Calle et al. In their study, 442 men underwent 4Kscore and mpMRI, of whom 338 underwent biopsy; 179 men underwent EPI and mpMRI, of whom 113 underwent biopsy. These subsets with all 3 diagnostics (ie, including biopsy) were used to tabulate clinical outcomes.

[b] The overall study population in de la Calle et al. was 80% biopsy-naïve. The remainder of populations were 100% biopsy-naïve.

on biopsy. In contrast to the 4Kscore, phi does not include clinical variables. The phi output is a continuous value greater than zero, with higher values representing a higher likelihood of detecting any and GG $\geq$ 2 cancer on biopsy. phi has been validated in several studies, although various thresholds were assessed in each.[27–30] The test was approved by the FDA in 2012 for use in men 50 years and older, PSA 4 to 10 ng/mL, and with nonsuspicious DRE.[31] We identified 4 clinically pertinent studies combining phi and mpMRI for the detection of GG $\geq$ 2 cancer.

phi Performance with mpMRI

Gnanapragasam et al. Scientific Reports; 2016 Gnanapragasam and colleagues evaluated 279 men referred for repeat prostate biopsy due to ongoing suspicion of PCa or concern for under-staging of previously diagnosed PCa.[32] Most men had no previous PCa diagnosis, although 60 men (20%) had GG1 cancer and 5 men (2%) had GG2 cancer on previous biopsy. All men underwent mpMRI and subsequent phi testing before transperineal, mpMRI-fusion repeat biopsy. Of note, the study preceded PI-RADS version 2.0; instead, a Likert system was used, in which no lesions or Likert 1 to 2 lesions were categorized as negative, and Likert 3 to 5 lesions were categorized as positive mpMRI findings.

Overall, 94 men (35%) were found to have GG $\geq$ 2 cancer on repeat biopsy, including 21 of 94 men (22%) with negative mpMRI. Evaluating a strategy of mpMRI alone, the authors found that deferring biopsy in those with negative mpMRI would have avoided 34% of repeat biopsies and missed 21 (22%) GG $\geq$ 2 cancers (ie, 78% sensitivity). The authors then asked if there was a phi threshold above which biopsy would be warranted after a negative mpMRI. A strategy in which men with an initial negative mpMRI (n = 94) underwent follow-up phi testing, and proceeded to biopsy if phi $\geq$35, would have subjected 58% of men (63/ 94) to biopsy and detected 20 of 21 (95%) GG $\geq$ 2 cancers in this group (**Table 3**). A strategy in which both mpMRI and phi are obtained, and men proceed to biopsy if either is positive (ie, Likert 3–5 *or* phi $\geq$35), would have avoided 17% of unnecessary biopsies while missing 1% of GG $\geq$ 2 cancers.

Tosoian et al. Prostate Cancer and Prostatic Diseases; 2017 Tosoian and colleagues retrospectively assessed a consecutive series of 345 men with elevated PSA, concerning PSA kinetics, and/or abnormal DRE that underwent phi testing as part of clinical evaluation.[33] Of these, 121 (35%) also underwent mpMRI. Thus, 121 patients

(35%) had both mpMRI and phi testing, of whom 72 (60%) underwent prostate biopsy.

While limited by the lack of a uniform testing approach and criteria for biopsy, the findings reveal a significant increase in the risk of GG $\geq$ 2 PCa with increasing phi and PI-RADS scores. The authors specifically explored the use of previously established phi categories in 43 men with equivocal (PI-RADS 3) mpMRI who underwent biopsy. While GG $\geq$ 2 cancer was detected in eight of 43 men (19%) with PI-RADS 3 lesions, they found that zero of 15 men with phi less than 27 had GG $\geq$ 2 cancer, as compared with 8 of 28 men (29%) with phi $\geq$27. This implied a strategy in which men with initial, equivocal mpMRI underwent follow-up phi testing and proceed to biopsy only if phi $\geq$27 would have avoided 35% of biopsies in the PI-RADS 3 population while missing no GG $\geq$ 2 cancers (ie, 100% sensitivity).

Carbunaru et al. BJUI Compass; 2021 Carbunaru and colleagues evaluated 143 consecutive men referred for initial biopsy due to elevated PSA.[34] All men underwent mpMRI and phi testing followed by biopsy. In total, 55 men (38%) were found to have GG $\geq$ 2 cancer on biopsy, including 6 of 26 (23%) with PI-RADS 1 to 2, 9 of 47 (19%) with PI-RADS 3, and 40 of 70 (57%) with PI-RADS 4 to 5.

In men with a negative mpMRI, the authors assessed whether elevated biomarker levels could recapture patients with GG $\geq$ 2 cancer following false negative mpMRI. Use of PSAD $\geq$0.11 ng/ml^2 to rule-in biopsy would have detected all 6 GG $\geq$ 2 cancers while subjecting 31% of the group (8/26) to biopsy. Using phi $\geq$45 to rule-in biopsy also would have recaptured all 6 GG $\geq$ 2 cancers but subjected 58% of the group (15/26) to biopsy (see **Table 3**).

In patients with PI-RADS 4 to 5 mpMRI, they asked whether a low phi (<27) or low PSAD (<0.05 ng/ml^2) could have ruled out additional unnecessary biopsies in patients without GG $\geq$ 2 PCa that had a false positive mpMRI. This approach identified very few patients with PI-RADS 4 to 5 lesions that would avoid biopsy (2/70 [2.9%] for phi, 7/70 [10%] for PSAD) while maintaining 97.5% sensitivity in both cases (**Table 4**).

In patients with equivocal mpMRI (PI-RADS 3), the authors identified thresholds of phi and PSAD that seemed to improve risk stratification. Use of PSAD $\geq$0.07 to prompt biopsy detected 8 of 9 (89%) of GG $\geq$ 2 cancers while avoiding 28% of biopsies, and the use of phi $\geq$49 detected 100% of GG $\geq$ 2 cancers (9 of 9) while avoiding 45% of

Table 3
Clinical outcomes of secondary biomarker testing to rule-in biopsy after a negative (PI-RADS 1–2) mpMRI

Study	N	N (%)[a] GG ≥2 PCa	Secondary Biomarker Test to Rule-In Biopsy	N (%) Negative mpMRI Directed to Biopsy Due to Biomarker Test	N (%) of GG ≥2 Missed by False Negative mpMRI Recaptured by Biomarker Test
Gnanapragasam et al,[32] 2016	94[b]	21 (22%)	phi ≥35	63 of 94 (67%)	20 of 21 (95%)
Carbunaru et al,[34] 2021	26	6 (23%)	phi ≥45 PSAD ≥0.11 ng/mL²	15 of 26 (58%) 8 of 26 (31%)	6 of 6 (100%) 6 of 6 (100%)
Maggi et al,[37] 2021	178	10 (5.6%)	SelectMDx ≥−2.8 PSAD ≥0.15ng/mL²	53 of 178 (30%) 48 of 178 (27%)	8 of 10 (80%) 4 of 10 (40%)

Clinically, most men with PI-RADS 1 to 2 mpMRI will not proceed to biopsy. These studies assessed men with PI-RADS 1 to 2 mpMRI findings that did proceed to biopsy. This likely represents a subgroup of patients with other high-risk features directing them toward biopsy and may not represent the overall mpMRI-negative population. Relative to a clinical approach in which patients with PI-RADS 1 to 2 mpMRI forego biopsy, the table includes clinical outcomes that would have been observed if a secondary biomarker test was used to *rule-in* performing biopsy after a negative mpMRI.
[a] False negative rate of mpMRI (100% - sensitivity).
[b] Gnanapragasam et al. [32] used a Likert scale that preceded PI-RADS version 2.0.

Table 4
Clinical outcomes of secondary biomarker testing to rule-out biopsy after a positive (PI-RADS 4–5) mpMRI

Study	N	N (%) GG ≥2 PCa	Secondary Biomarker Test to Rule Out Biopsy	N (%) Positive mpMRI to Avoid Biopsy Based on Biomarker Test	N (%) GG ≥2 PCa Among pts with Positive mpMRI Who Deferred Biopsy Due to Secondary Biomarker Test
Carbunaru et al,[34] 2021	70	40 (57%)	phi <27	2 of 70 (2.9%)	1 of 2 (50%)
			PSAD <0.05 ng/mL^2	7 of 70 (10%)	1 of 7 (14%)
Fan et al,[35] 2021	108	52 (48%)	phi <27	8 of 108 (7.4%)	1 of 8 (12.5%)
Maggi et al,[37] 2021	78	38 (49%)	SelectMDx < - 2.8	24 of 78 (31%)	4 of 24 (17%)
			PSAD <0.15 ng/mL^2	28 of 78 (36%)	10 of 28 (36%)
Busetto et al,[38] 2021	12	6 (50%)	SelectMDx < −2.8	2 of 12 (17%)	0 of 2 (0%)
			PSAD < 0.15 ng/mL^2	1 of 12 (8.3%)	0 of 1 (0%)

Clinically, the vast majority of men with PI-RADS 4 to 5 mpMRI proceed to prostate biopsy. Relative to that clinical pathway, the table includes clinical outcomes that would have been observed if a secondary biomarker test was used to *rule-out* biopsy after a positive mpMRI.

biopsies (**Table 5**). Although models including PSAD outperformed phi across the overall population (AUC 0.85 with PSAD vs 0.81 with phi), these data demonstrated better performance with phi testing in the PI-RADS 3 population likely to benefit from additional risk stratification.

Fan et al. Scientific Reports; 2021 Fan and colleagues evaluated data from 164 men with at least one PI-RADS ≥3 lesion who underwent cognitive MRI-TRUS fusion-targeted biopsy.[35] All men had PSA ≥4 ng/mL and/or suspicious DRE and underwent phi testing before biopsy. Of the 164 patients, 118 (72%) were biopsy naïve. Overall, 68 men (41%) were found to have GG ≥ 2 cancer on biopsy, including 16 of 56 men (29%) with PI-RADS 3, and 52 of 108 men (48%) with PI-RADS 4 to 5 mpMRI findings. Stratified by mpMRI result, the authors evaluated the proportion of biopsies avoided and GG ≥ 2 cancers missed using several phi thresholds.

Consistent with previous reports,[34] there was limited improvement afforded by phi testing in patients with PI-RADS 4 to 5 mpMRI. For example, forgoing biopsy in patients with phi less than 27 would have missed 2% of GG ≥ 2 cancers (ie, 98% sensitivity) but only prevented 7% of biopsies (**Table 4**). In the PI-RADS 3 population (n = 56, of whom 16 [29%] had GG ≥ 2 PCa), a strategy of performing biopsy in patients with phi ≥50.1 (selected by maximizing Youden index) would have avoided 69% of biopsies while missing only 6% of GG ≥ 2 cancers (ie, 94% sensitivity) (**Table 5**). While the limited size of the PI-RADS 3 subgroup precluded the assessment of multiple cutoffs, findings based on the proposed threshold of 50.1 were encouraging.

Urine-based biomarkers

SelectMDx
The SelectMDx urine-based test (MDxHealth, Irvine, CA) incorporates post-DRE urinary mRNA expression (HOXC6 and DLX1) and clinical variables (age, PSA, prostate volume [optional], and DRE) to produce a continuous score (−6 to +6) that is converted into a percent likelihood of detecting GG ≥ 2 PCa on biopsy. In a biopsy-naïve referral cohort with PSA less than 10 ng/mL, a threshold of −2.8 was validated to offer 95% NPV, 89% sensitivity, and 53% specificity (ie, unnecessary biopsies avoided). In a separate model that did not include prostate volume, the threshold provided 92% NPV, 87% sensitivity, and 38% specificity.[36] We identified four clinical studies evaluating the use of SelectMDx and mpMRI for the detection of GG ≥ 2 cancer.

SelectMDx Performance with mpMRI
Maggi et al. Cancers; 2021 Maggi and colleagues analyzed data from 310 consecutive, biopsy-naïve men undergoing biopsy for PSA greater than 3 ng/mL and/or abnormal DRE.[37] All men underwent SelectMDx testing and mpMRI and then proceeded to biopsy. In total, 62 men (20%) were found to have GG ≥ 2 PCa on biopsy, including 10 of 178 men (5.6%) with PI-RADS 1 to 2, 14 of 54 men (26%) with PI-RADS 3, and 38 of 78 men (49%) with PI-RADS 4 to 5 mpMRI.

Using the previously proposed thresholds of −2.8 for SelectMDx and 0.15 ng/ml^2 for PSAD, the authors presented the clinical consequences of various testing strategies. For example, using SelectMDx alone to guide biopsy (ie, biopsy if SelectMDx ≥ -2.8) would have avoided 54% of biopsies while missing 13% of GG ≥ 2 cancers (ie, 87% sensitivity). Using mpMRI alone (ie, biopsy if PI-RADS ≥4) would have avoided 75% of biopsies while missing 39% of GG ≥ 2 cancers (ie, 61% sensitivity). An approach of upfront mpMRI followed by SelectMDx if mpMRI was negative (PI-RADS 1–3)−in which biopsy is performed if (1) mpMRI was positive or (2) follow-up SelectMDx was positive−would have avoided 46% of biopsies while missing 6% of GG ≥ 2 cancers (ie, 94% sensitivity). Applying this same approach while defining positive mpMRI as PI-RADS 3 to 5 would have avoided 40% of biopsies and missed only 3% of GG ≥ 2 cancers (ie, 97% sensitivity) (see **Table 2**).

The authors also investigated SelectMDx and PSAD as a secondary test in men with known mpMRI results. In men with PI-RADS 1 to 2 mpMRI, performing biopsy in patients with SelectMDx ≥ −2.8 would have subjected 30% of mpMRI-negative men (53/178) to biopsy while recapturing 80% of GG ≥ 2 cancer (8/10 cases) that would otherwise have been missed. Use of PSAD instead (ie, biopsy if ≥ 0.15 ng/ml^2) would have subjected 27% of men to biopsy while recapturing 4 of 10 (40%) GG ≥ 2 cancers (see **Table 3**).

In the 78 men with PI-RADS 4 to 5 mpMRI (38 [49%] with GG ≥ 2 PCa), foregoing biopsy if SelectMDx was less than −2.8 would have avoided 24 of 78 (31%) biopsies, while missing four of 38 (11%) of GG ≥ 2 cancers detected under a standard approach whereby all mpMRI-positive patients are biopsied. Using PSAD less than 0.15 ng/ml^2 to avoid biopsy in these men would have avoided 28 of 78 (36%) of biopsies while missing 10 of the 38 (26%) GG ≥ 2 cancers (see **Table 4**).

In the 54 men with equivocal (PI-RADS 3) findings, deferring biopsy if SelectMDx is less than −2.8 would have avoided 18 biopsies (33%)

Table 5
Clinical outcomes of secondary biomarker testing to rule-out biopsy after an equivocal (PI-RADS 3) mpMRI

Author, Year	Test	Threshold[a]	N	GG ≥2 PCa	Biopsies Avoided (%)	GG ≥2 Cancers Missed (%)[b]	Unnecessary Biopsies Avoided (%)[c]	NPV (%)
Carbanaru et al,[34] 2021	phi	49	47	19%	45%	0%	55%	100%
	PSAD	0.07			28%	11%	32%	92%
Fan et al,[35] 2021	phi	50.129	56	29%	68%	6%	92%	97%
Maggi et al,[37] 2021	Select MDx	−2.8	54	26%	33%	14%	40%	89%
	PSAD	0.15			NR	71%	NR	NR
Hendriks, et al[39] 2021	Select MDx	−2.8	38	24%	42%	22%	50%	83%
Morote et al,[40] 2022	Select MDx	13%	62	9.7%	47%	33%	48%	93%
	PSAD	0.007			47%	17%	50%	97%
Tosoian et al,[42] 2021	MPS	25	121	13%	39%	6%	44%	98%
	MPS	29.1			55%	6%	NR	NR
	PSAD	0.0745			17%	6%	NR	NR

Traditionally, most patients with PI-RADS 3 mpMRI have proceeded to biopsy. Secondary testing has been proposed to identify which patients can safely defer biopsy. Relative to a clinical approach in which patients with PI-RADS 3 mpMRI undergo biopsy, the table includes clinical outcomes that would have been observed if a secondary biomarker test was used to rule-out biopsy after a PI-RADS 3 mpMRI.

Abbreviation: NR, not reported or not calculable.

[a] Carbanaru et al.[34] applied multiple phi and PSAD thresholds values (ie, not predefined a priori). Fan et al.[35] applied phi thresholds based on maximum Youden index. Maggi et al.[37] applied the validated SelectMDx threshold of −2.8[36]. PSAD thresholds were based on previous publications [50]. Hendriks et al.[39] applied the validated SelectMDx threshold of −2.8.[36] According to the authors, Morote et al.[40] applied SelectMDx and PSAD thresholds that "maximized sensitivity" for GG ≥2 PCa detection, including the "0.007 ng/ml/cm3" PSAD threshold described in their letter. Tosoian et al.[42] explored MPS thresholds from 10 to 30 by increments of 5, of which we presented the threshold of 25 the authors proposed for future study. They also compared MPS and PSAD performance at thresholds based on a 10% probability of detecting GG ≥2 cancer (ie, MPS 29.1, PSAD 0.0745 ng/mL[2]).

[b] 100%−sensitivity

[c] Specificity.

while missing 2 of 14 (14%) GG $\geq$ 2 cancers. Conversely, deferring biopsy for men with PSAD less than 0.15 ng/ml^2 would have missed 10 of the 14 (71%) GG $\geq$ 2 cancers (see **Table 5**).

Busetto et al. World Journal of Urology; 2021 Busetto and colleagues evaluated 52 consecutive, biopsy-naïve men referred for biopsy due to elevated PSA and/or abnormal DRE.[38] All men underwent both mpMRI and SelectMDx testing and then proceeded to biopsy. In total, 7 cases of GG $\geq$ 2 cancer (13%) were identified on biopsy, including zero of 29 men (0%) with PI-RADS 1 to 2, one of the 11 men (9%) with PI-RADS 3, and six of 12 men (50%) with PI-RADS to 5 mpMRI findings.

As in previous reports, the authors used the thresholds of -2.8 for SelectMDx and 0.15 ng/ml^2 for PSAD.[37] They determined the clinical consequences of using these biomarkers to guide biopsy in men with known mpMRI results. Among the 29 men with PI-RADS 1 to 2 mpMRI, using a subsequent SelectMDx positive result to prompt biopsy would subject one additional patient (1/29 or 3.4%) to biopsy while there would be no additional GG $\geq$ 2 cancers to detect. Using PSAD instead (ie, biopsy if $\geq$ 0.15 ng/ml^2) would have subjected eight men (28%) to biopsy. Among men with PI-RADS 4 to 5 mpMRI, foregoing biopsy if SelectMDx was less than -2.8 would have avoided two of 12 biopsies (17%) without failing to detect any of the 6 GG $\geq$ 2 cancers. PSAD testing would have prevented one biopsy (8.3%) and also would not have missed any GG $\geq$ 2 cancers.

Among men with equivocal mpMRI, deferring biopsy when SelectMDx was less than -2.8 would have avoided three of 11 biopsies (27%) without missing the only case of GG $\geq$ 2 cancer (ie, 100% sensitivity). The use of PSAD instead (ie, defer biopsy if < 0.15 ng/ml^2) also would have prompted biopsy in the one case of GG $\geq$ 2 cancer, while insufficient data were provided to determine the proportion of biopsies avoided in this approach. This study was limited by the small sample size and low event rate.

Hendriks et al. Prostate Cancer and Prostatic Diseases; 2021 Hendriks and colleagues considered 699 consecutive, biopsy-naïve men referred due to PSA $\geq$ 3.0 ng/mL.[39] The analytical cohort included 599 men who had mpMRI and SelectMDx testing before biopsy, which included in-bore MR-guided biopsy for those with suspicious mpMRI (PI-RADS 3–5). GG $\geq$ 2 cancer was found in 183 men (31%) on biopsy, including 9 of 38 men (24%) with PI-RADS 3 mpMRI findings.

The authors reported the clinical consequences of multiple testing strategies using the SelectMDx cutoff of -2.8. Using SelectMDx alone (ie, avoid biopsy if SelectMDx negative) would have avoided 38% of biopsies while missing 10% of GG $\geq$ 2 cancers (ie, 90% sensitivity). Using mpMRI alone (ie, biopsy if PI-RADS $\geq$3) would have avoided 49% of biopsies while missing 5% of GG $\geq$ 2 cancers (ie, 95% sensitivity). An approach of SelectMDx testing first, followed by mpMRI if SelectMDx was positive—in which biopsy is performed only if SelectMDx and mpMRI were positive (PI-RADS 3–5)—would have avoided 60% of biopsies while missing 13% of GG $\geq$ 2 cancers (ie, 87% sensitivity) (see **Table 2**). An approach in which all men receive both SelectMDx and mpMRI and undergo biopsy if either test is positive would have avoided 28% of biopsies while missing 2% of GG $\geq$ 2 cancers (ie, 98% sensitivity).

In conjunction with decision curve analysis that indicated mpMRI alone conferred the greatest benefit, the authors concluded that if mpMRI availability is limited, it may be suitable to limit imaging to men with positive SelectMDx results. Lastly, the authors evaluated SelectMDx in 38 men with equivocal mpMRI (PI-RADS 3). In these men (9 [24%] with GG $\geq$ 2 PCa), deferring biopsy if SelectMDx was less than -2.8 would have avoided 42% of biopsies while missing 2 (22%) GG $\geq$ 2 cancers (ie, 78% sensitivity) (see **Table 5**).

Morote et al. European Urology; 2022 In a brief research letter, Morote and colleagues evaluated data from 62 consecutive men with PI-RADS 3 mpMRI who presented for biopsy.[40] All men received SelectMDx testing before biopsy. In total, 74% of the cohort was biopsy-naïve, and 6 men (10%) were found to have GG $\geq$ 2 cancer on biopsy.

The authors evaluated the proportion of biopsies avoided and GG $\geq$ 2 cancers missed using SelectMDx and PSAD at several thresholds. Result thresholds that "maximized sensitivity" for GG $\geq$ 2 cancer were 13% for SelectMDx (which coincides with the previously validated SelectMDx continuous score of -2.8), "0.007 ng/ml/cm^3" [sic; it is likely the authors meant 0.07 ng/ml/cm^3] for PSAD, and 5.5% for a model incorporating both SelectMDx and PSAD. Using SelectMDx alone (ie, avoid biopsy if GG $\geq$ 2 cancer risk on SelectMDx <13%) would have avoided 47% of biopsies while missing 33% GG $\geq$ 2 cancers (ie, 67% sensitivity). Using PSAD alone (ie, avoid biopsy if PSAD "<0.007 ng/ml/cm^3" [sic; as above]) also would have avoided 47% of biopsies, while missing fewer (n = 1 [17%]) GG $\geq$ 2 cancers (ie, 83% sensitivity) (see **Table 5**). Finally, using a model incorporating SelectMDx and PSAD—in which biopsy is performed if the model-estimated risk of GG $\geq$ 2 cancer is $\geq$ 5.5%—would have avoided 36% of biopsies and missed 0 GG $\geq$ 2 cancers (ie, 100% sensitivity).

MyProstateScore

The MyProstateScore (MPS) urine-based test (LynxDx, Ann Arbor, MI) incorporates levels of post-DRE urinary mRNA (PCA3 and the TMPRSS2:ERG gene fusion) with serum PSA to provide a continuous risk score for GG $\geq$ 2 PCa on biopsy (range 0–100). MPS was initially shown to provide significant improvement relative to PSA-based risk calculators, and the value added by each cancer-specific marker (PCA3, TMPRSS2:ERG) was demonstrated.[41] More recently, in men referred for initial prostate biopsy, the MPS threshold of 10 was validated to provide 98% NPV and 97% sensitivity, while ruling-out 33% of unnecessary biopsies (ie, 33% specificity).[42] We identified one published report combining the use of MPS and mpMRI.

MyProstateScore Performance with mpMRI

Tosoian et al. Urology; 2021 Tosoian and colleagues evaluated 540 consecutive patients presenting with elevated PSA and/or abnormal DRE who provided prebiopsy urine specimens and underwent diagnostic mpMRI and biopsy.[43] The decision to biopsy was made clinically through shared decision-making, thus the cohort was likely enriched for patients with visible lesions on mpMRI (PI-RADS 3–5). MPS was calculated retrospectively and was not available for clinical decision-making. The median PSA was 7.4 ng/mL, and 232 patients (43%) were biopsy-naïve. In all, 263 men (49%) were found to have GG $\geq$ 2 cancer on biopsy, including 16 of 121 men (13%) with PI-RADS 3, 131 of 234 men (56%) with PI-RADS 4, and 114 of 131 men (87%) with PI-RADS 5 mpMRI findings.

The authors found that MPS was significantly higher in patients with GG $\geq$ 2 cancer even after stratification by PI-RADS score, suggesting that MPS and mpMRI offer complementary information. Clinical consequences of MPS and PSAD testing were assessed in the PI-RADS 3 population (n = 121), in which median PSA (7.4 vs 7.1, P = .5) and PSAD (median 0.14 vs 0.12, P = .11) did not significantly differ by GG $\geq$ 2 cancer findings. MPS was significantly higher in those with versus without GG $\geq$ 2 cancer (median 43.2 vs 28.4, P = .003).

On decision curve analysis (DCA), MPS provided higher net benefit than PSAD across all relevant threshold probabilities. For example, at a threshold probability of 10%, MPS testing would have avoided 36 biopsies per 100 patients (36%) without missing a single GG $\geq$ 2 cancer, while PSAD would have avoided only 8 biopsies (8%). While the optimal MPS threshold was 29.1, in light of the limited sample size, the authors proposed the MPS threshold of 25—which would have avoided 44% of unnecessary biopsies and missed one (6%) GG $\geq$ 2 cancer (ie, sensitivity 94%)—for further assessment and clinical consideration (see **Table 5**).

ExoDx Prostate Intelliscore

The ExoDx Prostate Intelliscore (ExoDx or EPI) test (Exome Diagnostics, Waltham, MA) incorporates the expression of 3 urinary biomarkers (PCA3, ETS transcription factor [ERG], and SAM pointed domain containing ETS transcription factor [SPDEF]) to produce a continuous score (range 0–100) reflecting the likelihood of detecting GG $\geq$ 2 PCa on biopsy. In biopsy-naïve men, an EPI threshold of 15.6 was validated in 2 reports to provide 89% to 91% NPV, 92% to 93% sensitivity, and rule out 26% to 34% of unnecessary biopsies (ie, 26%–34% specificity).[24,25] There was one published report that assessed patients with EPI (and/or 4Kscore), mpMRI, and biopsy data.[23] The study from de la Calle and colleagues was described above with 4Kscore data.

DISCUSSION

Acknowledging the clinical heterogeneity of prostate cancer, an ideal diagnostic approach would reduce unnecessary prostate biopsies (ie, negative biopsies and those detecting GG1 PCa) while preserving the detection of clinically significant PCa. Available data indicate that both mpMRI and noninvasive biomarkers improve upon conventional risk stratification, but a critical question remains: if both tools are clinically available—what is the optimal approach to testing with mpMRI and biomarkers?

In addition to considering cost-effectiveness, the optimal answer to this question would come from a prospective study design, in which all patients undergo mpMRI, biomarker testing, and proceed to biopsy regardless of test results. While such trials are currently underway (NCT03784924; NCT03730324), several retrospective studies can provide some insight. Among other shortcomings, however, analyses based on "real-world" clinical data are limited by the fact that only those patients with higher-risk findings proceed to biopsy. With that in mind, the current review focused on reports providing clinically meaningful data. For clinicians, this includes potential thresholds to trigger biopsy and the clinical outcomes (ie, biopsies avoided, GG ≥ 2 cancers detected) observed under that testing strategy.

Sequential Testing

Based on clinical and practical factors, we have previously proposed that initial biomarker testing with a highly sensitive test (ie, to rule out the need for biopsy in those testing negative), followed by mpMRI in those testing positive, could be most sensible. The limitations of retrospective analyses notwithstanding, the current findings seem to support the validity of a biomarker-first approach. For example, Falagario and colleagues found that using an initial 4Kscore followed by mpMRI resulted in avoiding mpMRI and biopsy in 34% of patients and detected 97% of GG ≥ 2 cancers[22] (see **Table 2**). Meanwhile, a mpMRI-first approach avoided no mpMRI (0%) and fewer biopsies (25%) at the same sensitivity. Similarly, de la Calle and colleagues found that the use of 4Kscore before mpMRI would have avoided 30% of mpMRI and 39% of biopsies, while failing to detect 5.6% of GG ≥ 2 cancers.[23] By contrast, the mpMRI-first approach avoided no mpMRI and 17% of biopsies, while failing to detect 2.4% of GG ≥ 2 cancers. In this same study, an EPI-first testing approach would have avoided 40% of mpMRI and 43% of biopsies, with 4.8% of GG ≥ 2 cancers missed. The corresponding mpMRI-first approach would not have avoided any mpMRI and avoided 19% of biopsies, with 2.4% of GG ≥ 2 cancers missed.

Biomarker Testing after mpMRI

While we await prospective trial data to better inform sequential testing approaches, existing data can inform a related clinical question. Namely, is there a role for biomarker testing in patients who have *already* undergone mpMRI? As the answer to this question varies by mpMRI result, we assessed available data in negative (PI-RADS 1–2), positive (PI-RADS 4–5), and equivocal (PI-RADS 3) mpMRI groups.

PI-RADS 1 to 2 Population

For patients who have undergone a negative (PI-RADS 1–2) mpMRI, a pertinent clinical question is whether a secondary biomarker test could identify patients who do in fact harbor GG ≥ 2 PCa (ie, false negative mpMRI). Addressing this question first requires knowledge of the NPV for mpMRI, which is known to vary widely by practice and radiologists.[13] For most patients, NPV ≥95% (ie, ≤5% implied risk of GG ≥ 2 PCa) will be sufficient to confidently forego biopsy.[44] If the NPV of mpMRI

is low (eg, <92%, implied risk of GG ≥ 2 PCa >8%), however, the persistent risk of significant cancer merits the consideration of secondary testing. We assessed available biomarker data in the negative mpMRI population (see **Table 3**). Notably, however, most of the studies included only those patients who proceeded to biopsy *despite* a negative mpMRI—implying that such patients harbored other high-risk factors and may not represent the "at-large" PI-RADS 1 to 2 population.

Gnanapragasam and colleagues assessed 94 patients, of which 21 (22%) had GG ≥ 2 cancer on biopsy (ie, 22% false negative rate for mpMRI).[32] Using a phi threshold ≥35, 63 of these 94 men (67%) would have undergone biopsy, and 20 (95%) of the 21 GG ≥ 2 cancers missed by mpMRI would have been detected. Similarly, in the setting of a 23% false negative rate of mpMRI, Carbunaru and colleagues found that phi≥45 would have triggered biopsy in 15 of 26 men with negative mpMRI (58%), thereby capturing all 6 cases of GG ≥ 2 missed by mpMRI.[34] Maggi and colleagues analyzed 178 mpMRI-negative patients, of which 10 (6%) had GG ≥ 2 cancer (ie, 6% false negative rate). SelectMDx testing would have led to biopsy in 53 men (30%) while capturing 8 GG ≥ 2 cancers (80%).[37]

Thus, in the 2 studies with a false negative rate greater than 20% of PI-RADS 1 to 2 mpMRI, GG ≥ 2 cancer was detected in 33% of biopsies performed due to high biomarker values.[32,34] When mpMRI was highly sensitive (6% false negative rate), only 15% of biopsies detected GG ≥ 2 PCa.[37] Logically, it appears that secondary biomarker testing is most beneficial at clinical sites or settings in which mpMRI has limited sensitivity. Validation of optimal biomarker thresholds in this setting will better inform potential clinical applications.

PI-RADS 4 to 5 Population

Following a positive (PI-RADS 4–5) mpMRI, in which all patients typically undergo biopsy, 4 studies asked whether a low biomarker result could identify patients with false positive mpMRI (see **Table 4**). Overall, secondary biomarker testing strategies that maintained high sensitivity (≥95%) for GG ≥ 2 cancer would have avoided a limited proportion (<20%) of biopsies. Conversely, testing approaches that ruled out a substantial proportion of biopsies (>30%) came at the expense of failing to detect ≥10% of GG ≥ 2 cancers. Thus, consistent with the high positive predictive value of PI-RADS 4 to 5 lesions, the yield of secondary testing to preclude biopsy after positive mpMRI seems limited.

PI-RADS 3 Population

Equivocal mpMRI (ie, PI-RADS 3) findings are prevalent (14%–39%)[45–47] and have traditionally triggered biopsy, but the majority do not harbor GG $\geq$ 2 cancer (4%–27%)[45,48,49]—yielding the post-mpMRI cohort most likely to benefit from secondary testing before biopsy. We reviewed six studies in the PI-RADS 3 population (see **Table 5**).

Three studies explored the SelectMDx threshold (−2.8) previously validated in the biopsy referral population. Relative to an approach in which all patients with PI-RADS 3 undergo biopsy, secondary testing with SelectMDx would have avoided 33% to 47% of biopsies, while failing to detect 14% to 33% of GG $\geq$ 2 cancers. In two additional studies, secondary phi testing (threshold ~50) would have avoided 45% to 68% of biopsies, while missing $\leq$6% of GG $\geq$ 2 cancers. Our group assessed MPS and PSAD thresholds associated with a 10% probability of detecting GG $\geq$ 2 cancer (29.1 and 0.0745, respectively). While the use of either test would have missed only 6% of GG $\geq$ 2 cancers, MPS would have avoided 55% of biopsies compared with only 17% for PSAD. Given the limited number of outcomes, we proposed a more conservative MPS threshold of 25 for potential clinical application in men with PI-RADS 3 mpMRI findings.

Notably, proposed thresholds for phi and MPS outperformed PSAD, while the SelectMDx threshold (−2.8) validated in the overall population biopsy did not. While additional validation is needed, these findings appear to support the identification and validation of testing applications specific to the clinical population in question. Regardless, secondary biomarker testing seems to have a favorable yield in men with PI-RADS 3 mpMRI.

Limitations

This review has notable limitations. As described, clinical cohorts in which test results inform the decision to biopsy are skewed toward higher risk patients. While this would be expected to have limited impact in PI-RADS 3 to 5 men that have traditionally undergone biopsy, PI-RADS 1 to 2 patients proceeding to biopsy likely represent a subset of men with strong family history, worrisome PSA kinetics, or other high-risk factors. Furthermore, the overall number of patients and events was limited. As such, we aimed to provide specific numbers for sample size and outcomes to highlight the preliminary nature of these data. Moreover, other potentially informative studies were excluded due to lacking key elements required for meaningful interpretation (eg, cohort selection, stratified outcomes). While inclusion criteria were outlined a priori, ambiguous reporting in some cases obscured study appropriateness for inclusion. Ultimately, this report summarizes published studies providing sufficient context for clinical interpretation—a limited but growing body of data.

SUMMARY

Although limited in quantity and quality, published data exploring the combined use of mpMRI and biomarkers seem to provide modest support for a biomarker-first testing approach, in which only those patients with a positive biomarker test proceed to mpMRI and biopsy. In patients who have already undergone mpMRI, there seems to be a role for biomarker testing to inform the need for biopsy in the PI-RADS 3 population and in a subgroup of men with negative mpMRI—particularly when the sensitivity of mpMRI is limited or unknown. Acknowledging the limitations of these data, the current report outlines the performance of various testing approaches assessed in the literature. Prospective studies in which all patients undergo biomarker testing, mpMRI, and biopsy are anticipated to provide more definitive results.

CLINICS CARE POINTS

- Literature on how best to combine mpMRI and biomarker testing for the detection of clinically significant prostate cancer are predominantly derived from retrospective analyses of clinical practice, posing significant limitations.

- In extant data comparing mpMRI-first to biomarker-first testing strategies, initial biomarker testing seems to offer a modest advantage in reducing the burden of testing while preserving the detection of clinically significant disease.

- For men presenting after an equivocal (PI-RADS 3) mpMRI, secondary biomarker testing seems helpful in identifying a proportion of men who can safely forego biopsy.

- For men presenting following a negative (PI-RADS 1–2) mpMRI, secondary biomarker testing could help identify patients at risk of false-negative imaging who stand to benefit from biopsy, particularly when the sensitivity of mpMRI is limited or unknown.

- Prospective studies in which all patients undergo mpMRI, biomarker testing, and biopsy are essential to better delineate the optimal combined use of these tools.

ACKNOWLEDGMENTS

The authors would like to thank Rachel Walden MLIS (reference and instruction librarian, Vanderbilt University School of Medicine) for her contribution to the database search strategies.

REFERENCES

1. Siegel RL, Miller KD, Fuchs HE, et al. Cancer Statistics, 2021. CA Cancer J Clin 2021;71:7–33.
2. Rawla P. Epidemiology of Prostate Cancer. World J Oncol 2019;10:63–89.
3. Fitzmaurice C, Abate D, Abbasi N, et al. Global, Regional, and National Cancer Incidence, Mortality, Years of Life Lost, Years Lived With Disability, and Disability-Adjusted Life-Years for 29 Cancer Groups, 1990 to 2017: A Systematic Analysis for the Global Burden of Disease Study. JAMA Oncol 2019;5: 1749–68.
4. Hugosson J, Roobol MJ, Mansson M, et al. A 16-yr Follow-up of the European Randomized study of Screening for Prostate Cancer. Eur Urol 2019;76: 43–51.
5. Schroder FH, Hugosson J, Roobol MJ, et al. Prostate-cancer mortality at 11 years of follow-up. N Engl J Med 2012;366:981–90.
6. Schroder FH, Hugosson J, Roobol MJ, et al. Screening and prostate cancer mortality: results of the European Randomised Study of Screening for Prostate Cancer (ERSPC) at 13 years of follow-up. Lancet 2014;384:2027–35.
7. Fenton JJ, Weyrich MS, Durbin S, et al. Prostate-Specific Antigen-Based Screening for Prostate Cancer: Evidence Report and Systematic Review for the US Preventive Services Task Force. JAMA 2018;319: 1914–31.
8. Loeb S, Bjurlin MA, Nicholson J, et al. Overdiagnosis and overtreatment of prostate cancer. Eur Urol 2014; 65:1046–55.
9. Loeb S, Vellekoop A, Ahmed HU, et al. Systematic review of complications of prostate biopsy. Eur Urol 2013;64:876–92.
10. National Comprehensive Cancer Network. Prostate Cancer Early Detection Guidelines. 2022. Available at: https://www.nccn.org/guidelines/guidelines-detail? category=2&id=1460. Accessed July 22, 2022.
11. Drost FH, Osses DF, Nieboer D, et al. Prostate MRI, with or without MRI-targeted biopsy, and systematic biopsy for detecting prostate cancer. Cochrane Database Syst Rev 2019;4:CD012663.
12. Bass EJ, Pantovic A, Connor MJ, et al. Diagnostic accuracy of magnetic resonance imaging targeted biopsy techniques compared to transrectal ultrasound guided biopsy of the prostate: a systematic review and meta-analysis. Prostate Cancer Prostatic Dis 2022;25:174–9.
13. Sathianathen NJ, Omer A, Harriss E, et al. Negative Predictive Value of Multiparametric Magnetic Resonance Imaging in the Detection of Clinically Significant Prostate Cancer in the Prostate Imaging Reporting and Data System Era: A Systematic Review and Meta-analysis. Eur Urol 2020;78:402–14.
14. Eyrich NW, Morgan TM, Tosoian JJ. Biomarkers for detection of clinically significant prostate cancer: contemporary clinical data and future directions. Transl Androl Urol 2021;10:3091–103.
15. McDonald ML, Parsons JK. 4-Kallikrein Test and Kallikrein Markers in Prostate Cancer Screening. Urol Clin North Am 2016;43:39–46.
16. Stattin P, Vickers AJ, Sjoberg DD, et al. Improving the Specificity of Screening for Lethal Prostate Cancer Using Prostate-specific Antigen and a Panel of Kallikrein Markers: A Nested Case-Control Study. Eur Urol 2015;68:207–13.
17. Vickers A, Vertosick EA, Sjoberg DD, et al. Value of Intact Prostate Specific Antigen and Human Kallikrein 2 in the 4 Kallikrein Predictive Model: An Individual Patient Data Meta-Analysis. J Urol 2018;199: 1470–4.
18. Punnen S, Nahar B, Soodana-Prakash N, et al. Optimizing patient's selection for prostate biopsy: A single institution experience with multi-parametric MRI and the 4Kscore test for the detection of aggressive prostate cancer. PLoS One 2018;13:e0201384.
19. Parekh DJ, Punnen S, Sjoberg DD, et al. A multi-institutional prospective trial in the USA confirms that the 4Kscore accurately identifies men with high-grade prostate cancer. Eur Urol 2015;68: 464–70.
20. Ahmed HU, El-Shater Bosaily A, Brown LC, et al. Diagnostic accuracy of multi-parametric MRI and TRUS biopsy in prostate cancer (PROMIS): a paired validating confirmatory study. Lancet 2017;389: 815–22.
21. Marzouk K, Ehdaie B, Vertosick E, et al. Developing an effective strategy to improve the detection of significant prostate cancer by combining the 4Kscore and multiparametric MRI. Urol Oncol 2019;37: 672–7.
22. Falagario UG, Martini A, Wajswol E, et al. Avoiding Unnecessary Magnetic Resonance Imaging (MRI) and Biopsies: Negative and Positive Predictive Value of MRI According to Prostate-specific Antigen Density, 4Kscore and Risk Calculators. Eur Urol Oncol 2020;3:700–4.
23. de la Calle CM, Fasulo V, Cowan JE, et al. Clinical Utility of 4Kscore((R)), ExosomeDx and Magnetic Resonance Imaging for the Early Detection of High Grade Prostate Cancer. J Urol 2021;205:452–60.
24. McKiernan J, Donovan MJ, O'Neill V, et al. A Novel Urine Exosome Gene Expression Assay to Predict High-grade Prostate Cancer at Initial Biopsy. JAMA Oncol 2016;2:882–9.

25. McKiernan J, Donovan MJ, Margolis E, et al. A Prospective Adaptive Utility Trial to Validate Performance of a Novel Urine Exosome Gene Expression Assay to Predict High-grade Prostate Cancer in Patients with Prostate-specific Antigen 2-10ng/ml at Initial Biopsy. Eur Urol 2018;74:731–8.

26. Falagario UG, Lantz A, Jambor I, et al. Using biomarkers in patients with positive multiparametric magnetic resonance imaging: 4Kscore predicts the presence of cancer outside the index lesion. Int J Urol 2021;28:47–52.

27. de la Calle C, Patil D, Wei JT, et al. Multicenter Evaluation of the Prostate Health Index to Detect Aggressive Prostate Cancer in Biopsy Naive Men. J Urol 2015;194:65–72.

28. Nordstrom T, Vickers A, Assel M, et al. Comparison Between the Four-kallikrein Panel and Prostate Health Index for Predicting Prostate Cancer. Eur Urol 2015;68:139–46.

29. Seisen T, Roupret M, Brault D, et al. Accuracy of the prostate health index versus the urinary prostate cancer antigen 3 score to predict overall and significant prostate cancer at initial biopsy. Prostate 2015; 75:103–11.

30. Chiu PK, Ng CF, Semjonow A, et al. A Multicentre Evaluation of the Role of the Prostate Health Index (PHI) in Regions with Differing Prevalence of Prostate Cancer: Adjustment of PHI Reference Ranges is Needed for European and Asian Settings. Eur Urol 2019;75:558–61.

31. United States Food and Drug Administration. 2022. Available at: https://www.accessdata.fda.gov/scripts/cdrh/cfdocs/cfpma/pma.cfm?id=P090026. Accessed July 22, 2022.

32. Gnanapragasam VJ, Burling K, George A, et al. The Prostate Health Index adds predictive value to multiparametric MRI in detecting significant prostate cancers in a repeat biopsy population. Sci Rep 2016;6: 35364.

33. Tosoian JJ, Druskin SC, Andreas D, et al. Use of the Prostate Health Index for detection of prostate cancer: results from a large academic practice. Prostate Cancer Prostatic Dis 2017;20:228–33.

34. Carbunaru S, Stinson J, Babajide R, et al. Performance of prostate health index and PSA density in a diverse biopsy-naive cohort with mpMRI for detecting significant prostate cancer. BJUI Compass 2021;2:370–6.

35. Fan YH, Pan PH, Cheng WM, et al. The Prostate Health Index aids multi-parametric MRI in diagnosing significant prostate cancer. Sci Rep 2021; 11:1286.

36. Haese A, Trooskens G, Steyaert S, et al. Multicenter Optimization and Validation of a 2-Gene mRNA Urine Test for Detection of Clinically Significant Prostate Cancer before Initial Prostate Biopsy. J Urol 2019;202:256–63.

37. Maggi M, Del Giudice F, Falagario UG, et al. SelectMDx and Multiparametric Magnetic Resonance Imaging of the Prostate for Men Undergoing Primary Prostate Biopsy: A Prospective Assessment in a Multi-Institutional Study. Cancers (Basel) 2021;13.

38. Busetto GM, Del Giudice F, Maggi M, et al. Prospective assessment of two-gene urinary test with multiparametric magnetic resonance imaging of the prostate for men undergoing primary prostate biopsy. World J Urol 2021;39:1869–77.

39. Hendriks RJ, van der Leest MMG, Israel B, et al. Clinical use of the SelectMDx urinary-biomarker test with or without mpMRI in prostate cancer diagnosis: a prospective, multicenter study in biopsy-naive men. Prostate Cancer Prostatic Dis 2021;24: 1110–9.

40. Morote J, Diaz F, Celma A, et al. Behavior of SelectMDx and Prostate-specific Antigen Density in the Challenging Scenario of Prostate Imaging-Reporting and Data System Category 3 Lesions. Eur Urol 2022;81:124–5.

41. Tomlins SA, Day JR, Lonigro RJ, et al. Urine TMPRSS2:ERG Plus PCA3 for Individualized Prostate Cancer Risk Assessment. Eur Urol 2016;70: 45–53.

42. Tosoian JJ, Trock BJ, Morgan TM, et al. Use of the MyProstateScore Test to Rule Out Clinically Significant Cancer: Validation of a Straightforward Clinical Testing Approach. J Urol 2021;205:732–9.

43. Tosoian JJ, Singhal U, Davenport MS, et al. Urinary MyProstateScore (MPS) to Rule out Clinically-Significant Cancer in Men with Equivocal (PI-RADS 3) Multiparametric MRI: Addressing an Unmet Clinical Need. Urology 2022;164:184–90.

44. Vickers AJ, Van Calster B, Steyerberg EW. Net benefit approaches to the evaluation of prediction models, molecular markers, and diagnostic tests. BMJ 2016;352:i6.

45. Schoots IG, Osses DF, Drost FH, et al. Reduction of MRI-targeted biopsies in men with low-risk prostate cancer on active surveillance by stratifying to PI-RADS and PSA-density, with different thresholds for significant disease. Transl Androl Urol 2018;7: 132–44.

46. Filson CP, Natarajan S, Margolis DJ, et al. Prostate cancer detection with magnetic resonance-ultrasound fusion biopsy: The role of systematic and targeted biopsies. Cancer 2016;122:884–92.

47. Pokorny MR, de Rooij M, Duncan E, et al. Prospective study of diagnostic accuracy comparing prostate cancer detection by transrectal ultrasound-guided biopsy versus magnetic resonance (MR) imaging with subsequent MR-guided biopsy in men without previous prostate biopsies. Eur Urol 2014;66:22–9.

48. Venderink W, van Luijtelaar A, Bomers JGR, et al. Results of Targeted Biopsy in Men with

Magnetic Resonance Imaging Lesions Classified Equivocal, Likely or Highly Likely to Be Clinically Significant Prostate Cancer. Eur Urol 2018;73: 353–60.

49. Schoots IG. MRI in early prostate cancer detection: how to manage indeterminate or equivocal PI-RADS 3 lesions? Transl Androl Urol 2018;7: 70–82.

50. Stevens E, Truong M, Bullen JA, et al. Clinical utility of PSAD combined with PI-RADS category for the detection of clinically significant prostate cancer. Urol Oncol 2020;38(11):846.e9–16.

Circulating Tumor Cells and Circulating Tumor DNA in Urologic Cancers

Ikenna Madueke, MD, PhD*, Richard J. Lee, MD, PhD,
David T. Miyamoto, MD, PhD

KEYWORDS

- Circulating tumor cells • Circulating tumor DNA • Genitourinary cancer

KEY POINTS

- Liquid biopsies including circulating tumor cells (CTCs) and circulating tumor DNA (ctDNA) have potential as non-invasive biomarkers in urologic cancers.
- CTCs and ctDNA levels in the blood have been correlated with prognosis and stage in prostate, urothelial, and renal cancers.
- CTC and ctDNA analyses may also have value as predictive biomarkers and to monitor for minimal residual disease and disease recurrence after therapy.

KEY/ESSENTIAL HEADINGS
Introduction/History/Definitions/Background

The liquid biopsy field has been increasing in clinical relevance over the last 2 decades as the promise of precision medicine continues to be realized.[1] Liquid biopsy refers to the analysis of tumor components in the blood, saliva, urine, CSF, or other bodily fluids that can serve as prognostic and predictive biomarkers, as well as markers of disease evolution. Many urologic cancers exhibit tumor heterogeneity, and invasive tissue biopsies may not adequately capture the full spectrum of pathology.[2] Furthermore, cancers can evolve as they progress to more aggressive stages or under the selective pressures of therapy. In this regard, liquid biopsies offer the possibility of real-time noninvasive and dynamic monitoring of patients with respect to diagnosis, prognosis, treatment response, and treatment resistance. The main components of liquid biopsy include circulating tumor cells (CTC), circulating tumor DNA (ctDNA), and exosomes.[3] CTCs are cells that are shed into circulation from primary foci or from metastatic deposits.[4] On the other hand, ctDNA are circulating by-products of dying tumor cells.[4] In this brief review, we focus specifically on CTCs and ctDNA in urologic cancers.

History and biology of circulating tumor cells and circulating tumor DNA: The presence of CTCs was first postulated by Ashworth in 1869 when he proposed that these rare cells circulating in the blood were necessary to promote metastasis.[5] Mandel and Metais are credited with being the first to report the presence of cell-free DNA (cfDNA) in the plasma of diseased and nondiseased persons.[6] However, ctDNA refers to the mutated fraction of cfDNA that arises from cancer cells.[7–9] The emergence of CTCs and ctDNA in the circulation occurs through active and passive mechanisms. CTCs can be excreted, secreted, and undergo epithelial to mesenchymal transition (EMT).[10–12] The bulk of ctDNA is likely contributed by tumor cell necrosis and apoptosis.[13]

Detection of circulating tumor cells and circulating tumor DNA: CTCs are rare, and to be detected in circulation have to be enriched from a background of red and white blood cells.[14] The half-life of ctDNA is approximately 2 hours with rapid hepatic, splenic, and renal clearance.[15,16] The half-life of CTCs in circulation is similar at about 1 to 2.5 h.[17] CTC isolation and detection

Massachusetts General Hospital Cancer Center, Harvard Medical School, 55 Fruit Street, Boston, MA 02114, USA
* Corresponding author.
E-mail address: icmadueke@mgh.harvard.edu

Urol Clin N Am 50 (2023) 109–114
https://doi.org/10.1016/j.ucl.2022.09.010
0094-0143/23/© 2022 Published by Elsevier Inc.

techniques are based on physical properties as well as the expression of several markers. Regarding cell surface markers, assays are designed based on epithelial cellular adhesion molecule (EpCAM)-dependent and EpCAM-independent properties.[18] EpCAM-dependent assays use anti-EpCAM antibody-coated magnetic beads to isolate CTCs. Cellsearch is the only US Food and Drug Administration (FDA)-cleared CTC detection assay.[19] Another EpCAM-dependent assay is CellCollector, which is the first assay to isolate and enrich CTCs *in vivo*.[20] The volume limitation of Cellsearch (7.5 mL) is circumvented by this *in vivo* assay. Many CTCs undergo EMT and as such do not highly express EpCAM or cytokeratins. As a result, EpCAM-independent assays are necessary to isolate and enrich this subset of CTCs. EPithelial Immuno SPOT (EPISPOT) is an assay in this space, in which CTCs are identified based on the proteins that they express, which differ depending on the type of cancer. Other examples of EpCAM-independent assays include the CTC-iChip,[21] which isolates CTCs based on negative selection and depletion of hematopoietic cells from whole blood, and the Parsortix system,[22] which captures CTCs based on size and deformability.

With regard to ctDNA, given the small fraction of ctDNA compared with total cfDNA, highly sensitive techniques including PCR-based technologies and next-generation sequencing (NGS) are needed to analyze ctDNA and to detect genomic alterations. High sensitivity assays such as droplet digital polymerase chain reaction (ddPCR) can detect point mutations with sensitivities from 0.001% to 1%.[23] NGS can also detect genomic alterations, but at a lower sensitivity than PCR-based techniques, although primary tumor sequencing may not be necessary.[24] NGS assays include targeted gene panels as well as nontargeted assays such as whole-genome sequencing (WGS). Detection of epigenetic alterations in ctDNA has also been shown to have potential clinical significance. Newer techniques for analyzing methylation profiles of ctDNA are emerging, and may prove to be better approaches than somatic gene alteration profiling as methylation marks number in the millions compared with somatic mutations in the thousands.[25]

We will now discuss how these liquid biopsy techniques have been applied in prostate, urothelial, and renal cancers.

DISCUSSION

Prostate cancer: Prostate cancer (PCa) remains the most diagnosed male malignancy and second leading cause of cancer-related deaths in the Western world.[26] Prostate specific antigen (PSA) has improved screening and reduced mortality from the disease, although problems with specificity are well known as PSA can also be elevated in benign and inflammatory conditions. To this end, biomarker discovery for improved detection of clinically significant disease is a robustly active field. The importance of CTC and ctDNA as biomarkers in PCa has borne the most significance in the metastatic space. Although there is some evidence for CTCs and ctDNA in localized PCa, their translation to clinical application has been limited by small numbers in circulation. This is evident in work by Hennigan and colleagues, where they demonstrated a low abundance of ctDNA using ultra-low-pass whole-genome sequencing, which was unable to detect ctDNA in 112 patients with localized PCa regardless of grade.[27] In advanced prostate cancer, however, CTCs and ctDNA have been shown to have prognostic significance. CTCs were shown to predict improved overall survival (OS), with favorable groups represented by < 5 CTC in 7.5 mL blood.[28] In parallel with the increasing use of PSMA-based diagnostic imaging, the potential utility of CTC analyses has also been demonstrated. PSMA-positive CTCs have been shown to be an independent predictor of poorer treatment response, shorter progression-free survival (PFS), and OS.[29,30] Disease progression after the initiation of androgen deprivation therapy (ADT) is secondary to a multitude of mechanisms affecting the androgen receptor signaling pathway. Expression of androgen receptor splice variants is one such mechanism, and AR-V7 positive CTCs detected by the Johns Hopkins and EPIC AR-V7 assays have been shown to be associated with shorter PFS and OS in men treated with abiraterone or enzalutamide.[31] Similarly, the COU-AA-301 trial of abiraterone plus prednisone versus prednisone alone showed that CTC stratification combined with LDH level was a discriminatory surrogate marker to predict OS at 12 weeks.[32] Other studies have also shown that baseline CTC levels in metastatic castrate-resistant PCa can predict OS.[33]

Results from ctDNA studies in the metastatic PCa space have also revealed impactful findings. Wyatt and colleagues profiled the ctDNA genomic landscape of patients on enzalutamide treatment and were able to detect AR amplifications and AR mutations,[34] which may serve as potential biomarkers for treatment escalation or change. A recent study performed deep whole-genome sequencing of ctDNA before and after progression on AR pathway inhibitors, demonstrating AR augmentation as the dominant genomic driver of treatment resistance.[39]

There is also promise for CTCs and ctDNA to be used as predictive biomarkers. Drug approval in mPCa is usually based on OS and/or radiographic progression-free survival (rPFS) endpoints.[36] Results from the TOPARP-B trial showed that CTC kinetics were associated with rPFS with use of olaparib in mPCa with DNA damage repair (DDR) gene aberrations.[37] Additionally, CTC decrease greater than 30% from baseline following treatment has been shown to be associated with a survival benefit in castration-resistant PCa OS.[38] In the TOPARP-A trial, DDR mutations were detectable in ctDNA and decreased in mPCa patients responding to olaparib, while DDR gene in-frame reversion mutations emerged in patients with disease progression.[35]

Urothelial Cancer: The majority of urothelial carcinomas are located in the bladder, with about 5% to 10% originating in the upper tracts.[26] The mainstay of diagnosis involves invasive biopsy. Most urothelial carcinoma (UC) of the bladder are non-muscle invasive bladder cancer (NMIBC), and are treated with surgical resection with the addition of intravesical therapy for high-grade disease.[40] The majority of patients with NMIBC will recur within 5 years of diagnosis, with up to 15% progressing to invasive or metastatic disease.[41] For nonmetastatic muscle invasive bladder cancer (MIBC), treatment options include either radical cystectomy with bilateral pelvic lymphadenectomy with or without neoadjuvant chemotherapy, or bladder-sparing trimodality therapy.[41] Survival outcomes are essentially unchanged despite advancements in surgical technique, imaging modalities, and systemic therapies. Improved or novel biomarkers are thus necessary to improve risk stratification and monitoring residual or disease recurrence after definitive therapy. CTCs and ctDNA are biomarkers undergoing much evaluation in this space. CTC detection in patients with NMIBC was associated with decreased time to recurrence and time to disease progression.[42] Furthermore, among localized MIBC patients, those with detectable CTCs who have undergone definitive therapy with radical cystectomy have a higher risk of recurrence and reduced OS.[43,44] Not surprisingly, patients with metastatic UC have been shown to harbor significantly higher CTCs in several studies.[45,46]

Regarding ctDNA, it has been detected in plasma and urine of NMIBC and MIBC before disease progression is clinically apparent.[47] Additionally, ctDNA has shown prognostic value in localized UC as presurgery ctDNA levels are significantly associated with recurrence-free survival and OS.[48] Recent studies have also demonstrated that ctDNA may be useful in monitoring for minimal residual disease and early relapse following radical cystectomy.[49] In the metastatic space, NGS using the commercially available Guardant360 panel of 73 genes has been able to detect at least 1 GA in up to 95% of patients with mUC.[50]

Renal cancer: There is currently no recommended screening guideline for the general population for kidney cancer.[51] Symptomatology from renal cell cancer (RCC) manifests only in advanced disease stages. Up to 35% of patients diagnosed with RCC will have nonlocalized tumors and up to 40% of patients who undergo curative intent surgery will eventually relapse.[52] Adjunct biomarkers for improved risk-stratification of patients with renal cancer are thus needed.

In the metastatic setting, there have been studies that have linked the presence of CTCs with poor treatment response and shortened PFS. Bluemke and colleagues showed that the detection of CTCs was correlated with positive lymph nodes and synchronous metastasis at the time of radical nephrectomy.[53] Furthermore, CTCs in metastatic RCC (mRCC) showed variable plasticity with CTCs showing stem-cell-like characteristics associated with shorter PFS.[54] As with other urologic malignancies, patients with mRCC have been found to have higher levels of ctDNA than patients with localized RCC.[55] In RCC, cfDNA has been shown to be prognostic as patients with localized RCC that recurred had higher prenephrectomy cfDNA than those who did not, even though cfDNA levels were not associated with grade.[55,56] It should be noted, however, that although cfDNA levels in RCC are comparable to other solid GU tumors, the ctDNA fraction is significantly lower, and this has been borne out in several studies.[57,58] Concordance of genomic alterations in ctDNA for RCC and primary tumors have also been found to be notoriously low.[59,60]

SUMMARY

The prognostic and predictive potential of CTCs and ctDNA in urologic cancers is increasingly evident. However, there are several limitations that do not lend their use to broad-based clinical practice currently. Concordance for CTCs/ctDNA with tissue biopsy can vary greatly for several reasons postulated. The most likely is that CTCs and ctDNA represent subclones that may not be captured by the tissue biopsy. Selection pressures of treatment or disease progression may also spur mutations which are only representative in these liquid biopsies. Furthermore, there are discrepancies in CTC enumeration in the same patients depending on the assay used. These limitations suggest that more work is needed before CTCs and ctDNA are specific enough to be used for early cancer detection or available for prime-time clinical use.

Whether CTCs or ctDNA represent a better liquid biopsy component has also been debated. Each component has unique benefits, and the choice of liquid biopsy ultimately depends on the clinical question being investigated. Isolation of viable CTCs can allow for the generation of patient-derived xenografts, transcriptome analysis, and proteomic studies. On the other hand, ctDNA has the advantage of being able to be isolated from stored plasma or serum which can be stored for long periods of time across various spectrums of disease stages or evolution of disease in the same patient. This can allow for the standardization of techniques, especially across multiple institutions in the clinical trial setting.

Ultimately, the explosion of research into the molecular characterization and clinical significance of CTCs and ctDNA enhances personalized medicine. The ongoing multitude of prospective clinical trials investigating CTCs/ctDNA in various urologic cancers will provide us with better insights in the near future. Whether data from these clinical studies change how patients are risk-stratified, treated, and monitored will depend on if improvements in clinical outcomes are consistently shown.

CLINICS CARE POINTS

- Liquid biopsy methods are under active investigation in urologic cancers, but high-level evidence for their incorporation into clinical use is currently lacking.

ACKNOWLEDGEMENT

DTM acknowledges research funding from the Radiation Oncology Institute and the NIH (1R01CA259007-01A1).

DISCLOSURE

The authors have nothing to disclose.

REFERENCES

1. Zhang W, Xia W, Lv Z, et al. Liquid Biopsy for Cancer: Circulating Tumor Cells, Circulating Free DNA or Exosomes? Cell Physiol Biochem 2017;41(2): 755–68.

2. McGranahan N, Swanton C. Biological and therapeutic impact of intratumor heterogeneity in cancer evolution. Cancer Cell 2015;27(1):15–26.

3. Aghamir SMK, Heshmat R, Ebrahimi M, et al. Liquid Biopsy: The Unique Test for Chasing the Genetics of Solid Tumors. Epigenet Insights 2020;13. https://doi.org/10.1177/2516865720904052. 2516865720904052.

4. Kidess E, Jeffrey SS. Circulating tumor cells versus tumor-derived cell-free DNA: rivals or partners in cancer care in the era of single-cell analysis? Genome Med 2013;5(8):70.

5. Ashworth TR. A Case of Cancer in Which Cells Similar to Those in the Tumours Were Seen in the Blood after Death. Med J Aust 1869;14:146–7.

6. Mandel P, Metais P. Nuclear Acids In Human Blood Plasma. C R Seances Soc Biol Fil 1948;142(3–4): 241–3. Les acides nucleiques du plasma sanguin chez l'homme.

7. Anker P, Stroun M, Maurice PA. Spontaneous release of DNA by human blood lymphocytes as shown in an in vitro system. Cancer Res 1975; 35(9):2375–82.

8. Jahr S, Hentze H, Englisch S, et al. DNA fragments in the blood plasma of cancer patients: quantitations and evidence for their origin from apoptotic and necrotic cells. Cancer Res 2001;61(4): 1659–65.

9. Bronkhorst AJ, Wentzel JF, Aucamp J, et al. Characterization of the cell-free DNA released by cultured cancer cells. Biochim Biophys Acta 2016;1863(1): 157–65.

10. Thiery JP, Lim CT. Tumor dissemination: an EMT affair. Cancer Cell 2013;23(3):272–3.

11. McDonald DM, Baluk P. Significance of blood vessel leakiness in cancer. Cancer Res 2002;62(18): 5381–5.

12. Cristofanilli M, Budd GT, Ellis MJ, et al. Circulating tumor cells, disease progression, and survival in metastatic breast cancer. N Engl J Med 2004; 351(8):781–91.

13. Stroun M, Lyautey J, Lederrey C, et al. About the possible origin and mechanism of circulating DNA apoptosis and active DNA release. Clin Chim Acta 2001;313(1–2):139–42.

14. Joosse SA, Gorges TM, Pantel K. Biology, detection, and clinical implications of circulating tumor cells. EMBO Mol Med 2015;7(1):1–11.

15. Scholer LV, Reinert T, Orntoft MW, et al. Clinical Implications of Monitoring Circulating Tumor DNA in Patients with Colorectal Cancer. Clin Cancer Res 2017;23(18):5437–45.

16. Diehl F, Schmidt K, Choti MA, et al. Circulating mutant DNA to assess tumor dynamics. Nat Med 2008;14(9):985–90.

17. Aceto N, Bardia A, Miyamoto DT, et al. Circulating tumor cell clusters are oligoclonal precursors of breast cancer metastasis. Cell 2014;158(5):1110–22.

18. Alix-Panabieres C, Pantel K. Technologies for detection of circulating tumor cells: facts and vision. Lab Chip 2014;14(1):57–62.

19. Allard WJ, Matera J, Miller MC, et al. Tumor cells circulate in the peripheral blood of all major carcinomas but not in healthy subjects or patients with nonmalignant diseases. Clin Cancer Res 2004; 10(20):6897–904.

20. Saucedo-Zeni N, Mewes S, Niestroj R, et al. A novel method for the in vivo isolation of circulating tumor cells from peripheral blood of cancer patients using a functionalized and structured medical wire. Int J Oncol 2012;41(4):1241–50.

21. Ozkumur E, Shah AM, Ciciliano JC, et al. Inertial focusing for tumor antigen-dependent and -independent sorting of rare circulating tumor cells. Sci Transl Med 2013;5(179):179ra47.

22. Xu L, Mao X, Imrali A, et al. Optimization and evaluation of a novel size based circulating tumor cell isolation system. PLoS One 2015;10(9):e0138032.

23. Siravegna G, Marsoni S, Siena S, et al. Integrating liquid biopsies into the management of cancer. Nat Rev Clin Oncol 2017;14(9):531–48.

24. Postel M, Roosen A, Laurent-Puig P, et al. Droplet-based digital PCR and next generation sequencing for monitoring circulating tumor DNA: a cancer diagnostic perspective. Expert Rev Mol Diagn 2018; 18(1):7–17.

25. Shen SY, Singhania R, Fehringer G, et al. Sensitive tumour detection and classification using plasma cell-free DNA methylomes. Nat Nov 2018; 563(7732):579–83.

26. Siegel RL, Miller KD, Fuchs HE, et al. Cancer statistics. CA Cancer J Clin 2022;72(1):7–33.

27. Hennigan ST, Trostel SY, Terrigino NT, et al. Low Abundance of Circulating Tumor DNA in Localized Prostate Cancer. JCO Precis Oncol 2019. https://doi.org/10.1200/PO.19.00176.

28. de Bono JS, Scher HI, Montgomery RB, et al. Circulating tumor cells predict survival benefit from treatment in metastatic castration-resistant prostate cancer. Clin Cancer Res 2008;14(19):6302–9.

29. Nagaya N, Nagata M, Lu Y, et al. Prostate-specific membrane antigen in circulating tumor cells is a new poor prognostic marker for castration-resistant prostate cancer. PLoS One 2020;15(1):e0226219.

30. Miyamoto DT, Lee RJ, Stott SL, et al. Androgen receptor signaling in circulating tumor cells as a marker of hormonally responsive prostate cancer. Cancer Discovery 2012;2(11):995–1003.

31. Armstrong AJ, Halabi S, Luo J, et al. Prospective Multicenter Validation of Androgen Receptor Splice Variant 7 and Hormone Therapy Resistance in High-Risk Castration-Resistant Prostate Cancer: The PROPHECY Study. J Clin Oncol 2019;37(13): 1120–9.

32. Scher HI, Heller G, Molina A, et al. Circulating tumor cell biomarker panel as an individual-level surrogate for survival in metastatic castration-resistant prostate cancer. J Clin Oncol 2015;33(12):1348–55.

33. Heller G, McCormack R, Kheoh T, et al. Circulating Tumor Cell Number as a Response Measure of Prolonged Survival for Metastatic Castration-Resistant Prostate Cancer: A Comparison With Prostate-Specific Antigen Across Five Randomized Phase III Clinical Trials. J Clin Oncol 20 2018;36(6): 572–80.

34. Wyatt AW, Azad AA, Volik SV, et al. Genomic Alterations in Cell-Free DNA and Enzalutamide Resistance in Castration-Resistant Prostate Cancer. JAMA Oncol 2016;2(12):1598–606.

35. Goodall J, Mateo J, Yuan W, et al. Circulating cell-free DNA to guide prostate cancer treatment with PARP inhibition. Cancer Discovery 2017;7(9): 1006–17.

36. Morris MJ, Molina A, Small EJ, et al. Radiographic progression-free survival as a response biomarker in metastatic castration-resistant prostate cancer: COU-AA-302 results. J Clin Oncol 2015;33(12): 1356–63.

37. Mateo J, Porta N, Bianchini D, et al. Olaparib in patients with metastatic castration-resistant prostate cancer with DNA repair gene aberrations (TOPARP-B): a multicentre, open-label, randomised, phase 2 trial. Lancet Oncol 2020;21(1):162–74.

38. Lorente D, Olmos D, Mateo J, et al. Decline in Circulating Tumor Cell Count and Treatment Outcome in Advanced Prostate Cancer. Eur Urol 2016;70(6): 985–92.

39. Herberts C, Annala M, Sipola J, et al. Deep whole-genome ctDNA chronology of treatment-resistant prostate cancer. Nature 2022;608(7921):199–208.

40. Jordan B, Meeks JJ. T1 bladder cancer: current considerations for diagnosis and management. Nat Rev Urol 2019;16(1):23–34.

41. Chang SS, Bochner BH, Chou R, et al. Treatment of Non-Metastatic Muscle-Invasive Bladder Cancer: AUA/ASCO/ASTRO/SUO Guideline. J Urol Sep 2017;198(3):552–9.

42. Busetto GM, Ferro M, Del Giudice F, et al. The Prognostic Role of Circulating Tumor Cells (CTC) in High-risk Non-muscle-invasive Bladder Cancer. Clin Genitourin Cancer 2017;15(4):e661–6.

43. Gradilone A, Petracca A, Nicolazzo C, et al. Prognostic significance of survivin-expressing circulating tumour cells in T1G3 bladder cancer. BJU Int 2010; 106(5):710–5.

44. Rink M, Chun FK, Minner S, et al. Detection of circulating tumour cells in peripheral blood of patients with advanced non-metastatic bladder cancer. BJU Int 2011;107(10):1668–75.

45. Flaig TW, Wilson S, van Bokhoven A, et al. Detection of circulating tumor cells in metastatic and clinically localized urothelial carcinoma. Urology 2011;78(4): 863–7.

46. Naoe M, Ogawa Y, Morita J, et al. Detection of circulating urothelial cancer cells in the blood using the CellSearch System. Cancer 2007;109(7):1439–45.

47. Birkenkamp-Demtroder K, Nordentoft I, Christensen E, et al. Genomic Alterations in Liquid Biopsies from Patients with Bladder Cancer. Eur Urol 2016;70(1):75–82.

48. Christensen E, Birkenkamp-Demtroder K, Nordentoft I, et al. Liquid Biopsy Analysis of FGFR3 and PIK3CA Hotspot Mutations for Disease Surveillance in Bladder Cancer. Eur Urol 2017; 71(6):961–9.

49. Christensen E, Birkenkamp-Demtroder K, Sethi H, et al. Early detection of metastatic relapse and monitoring of therapeutic efficacy by ultra-deep sequencing of plasma cell-free DNA in patients with urothelial bladder carcinoma. J Clin Oncol 2019;37(18):1547–57.

50. Agarwal N, Pal SK, Hahn AW, et al. Characterization of metastatic urothelial carcinoma via comprehensive genomic profiling of circulating tumor DNA. Cancer 2018;124(10):2115–24.

51. Motzer RJ, Jonasch E, Agarwal N, et al. Kidney Cancer, Version 3.2022, NCCN Clinical Practice Guidelines in Oncology. J Natl Compr Canc Netw 2022; 20(1):71–90.

52. Janzen NK, Kim HL, Figlin RA, et al. Surveillance after radical or partial nephrectomy for localized renal cell carcinoma and management of recurrent disease. Urol Clin North Am 2003;30(4):843–52.

53. Bluemke K, Bilkenroth U, Meye A, et al. Detection of circulating tumor cells in peripheral blood of patients with renal cell carcinoma correlates with prognosis. Cancer Epidemiol Biomarkers Prev 2009;18(8): 2190–4.

54. Nel I, Gauler TC, Bublitz K, et al. Circulating Tumor Cell Composition in Renal Cell Carcinoma. PLoS One 2016;11(4):e0153018.

55. Wan J, Zhu L, Jiang Z, et al. Monitoring of plasma cell-free DNA in predicting postoperative recurrence of clear cell renal cell carcinoma. Urol Int 2013;91(3): 273–8.

56. Skrypkina I, Tsyba L, Onyshchenko K, et al. Concentration and Methylation of Cell-Free DNA from Blood Plasma as Diagnostic Markers of Renal Cancer. Dis Markers 2016;2016:3693096.

57. Yamamoto Y, Uemura M, Fujita M, et al. Clinical significance of the mutational landscape and fragmentation of circulating tumor DNA in renal cell carcinoma. Cancer Sci 2019;110(2):617–28.

58. Zill OA, Banks KC, Fairclough SR, et al. The Landscape of Actionable Genomic Alterations in Cell-Free Circulating Tumor DNA from 21,807 Advanced Cancer Patients. Clin Cancer Res 2018;24(15): 3528–38.

59. Hahn AW, Gill DM, Maughan B, et al. Correlation of genomic alterations assessed by next-generation sequencing (NGS) of tumor tissue DNA and circulating tumor DNA (ctDNA) in metastatic renal cell carcinoma (mRCC): potential clinical implications. Oncotarget 2017;8(20):33614–20.

60. Pal SK, Sonpavde G, Agarwal N, et al. Evolution of Circulating Tumor DNA Profile from First-line to Subsequent Therapy in Metastatic Renal Cell Carcinoma. Eur Urol 2017;72(4):557–64.

Targeted Molecular Imaging as a Biomarker in Urologic Oncology

Arvin Haj-Mirzaian, MD[a,b], Umar Mahmood, MD, PhD[a,b],*,
Pedram Heidari, MD[a,b]

KEYWORDS

- Molecular imaging • Radiopharmaceuticals • Urologic malignancies • Imaging biomarker • PET
- SPECT • Hyperpolarized MR

KEY POINTS

- Molecular imaging of urologic malignancies enables the accurate and early detection of malignant lesions and has markedly changed the management of these cancers, especially prostate cancer.
- Molecular imaging is superior to conventional imaging for detecting nodal and distant metastases.
- The choice of the molecular probe is dependent on cancer and the biological process studied.
- A vast array of processes could be targeted for the assessment of urologic malignancies, including cancer cell metabolism, cell surface, and intracellular receptors, angiogenesis, proliferation, extracellular matrix composition, and enzymatic activity.

INTRODUCTION

Urologic cancers account for a large proportion of all cancers worldwide.[1] Their rising incidence and mortality significantly burden health care systems globally.[1] In 2019, the prevalence and incidence rate of urologic malignancies increased by 1.5- to 2-fold since 1990[2]; this is likely due to the increasing population age and earlier diagnosis using new diagnostic tools.

In recent years, molecular imaging has gained widespread acceptance as a precision medicine tool, due to its better diagnostic performance than conventional imaging.[2] Molecular imaging approaches, such as positron emission tomography (PET), single-photon emission computerized tomography (SPECT), magnetic resonance imaging (MRI), ultrasound, and optical imaging, require the use of molecular probes, which specifically target a dysregulated biological process or pathway. In this regard, there are continued efforts to develop new biomarkers to improve diagnostic accuracy, prognostication, tumor characterization, and assessment of treatment response. This review discusses the current clinical applications of molecular imaging methods in urologic malignancies (**Fig. 1**).

PROSTATE CANCER

Prostate cancer (PCa) is the second most frequently diagnosed malignancy in men in developed countries and is a leading cause of cancer death worldwide.[3] Compared with conventional PCa detection methods, molecular imaging methods have shown better sensitivity and specificity in detecting PCa lesions.[4,5] Molecular imaging can localize the locoregional and distant metastatic sites at the presentation and provide valuable information for planning salvage treatments in patients with a rising PSA.[4] Here we highlight some recent clinical advances in molecular imaging of PCa (**Table 1**).

[a] Department of Radiology, Nuclear Medicine and Molecular Imaging, Massachusetts General Hospital, 55 Fruit St, Wht 427, Boston, MA 02114, USA; [b] Center for Precision Imaging, Athinoula A Martinos Center for Biomedical Imaging, Massachusetts General Hospital, 55 Fruit St, Wht 427, Boston, MA 02114, USA
* Corresponding author.
E-mail address: Umahmood@mgh.harvard.edu

Urol Clin N Am 50 (2023) 115–131
https://doi.org/10.1016/j.ucl.2022.09.011
0094-0143/23/© 2022 Published by Elsevier Inc.

Abbreviations	
ASCT	alanine-Serine-Cysteine transport
ASCT2	alanine, serine, cysteine transporter 2
BCa	Bladder cancer
BCR	Biochemical recurrence
CAIX	Carbonic anhydrase IX
ccRCA	clear cell Renal Cell Carcinoma
DHR	dihydrotestosterone
FCH	Fluorocholine
FDG	Fluorodeoxyglucose
FLT	fluorothymidine
GRPR	Gastrin-releasing peptide receptor
LAT1	L-type amino acid transporter 1
mCRPC	metastatic castration-resistant prostate cancer
MCT	Monocarboxylic acid transporter
MRI	Magnetic resonance imaging
MRSI	magnetic resonance spectroscopic imaging
PCa	Prostate cancer
PET	Positron emission tomography
PSA	Prostate-specific antigen
PSMA	Prostate specific membrane antigen
SPECT	Single photon emission computed tomography
SUV	Standardized uptake value
uPA	urokinase plasminogen activator
VEGFA	Vascular endothelial growth factor A
VPAC	vasoactive intestinal polypeptide receptor

Prostate-specific Membrane Antigen

Prostate-specific membrane antigen (PSMA) is a transmembrane protein localized to the cytoplasmic and apical side of the prostate epithelium. PSMA may play a role in cellular homeostasis, cell migration, angiogenesis, and endothelial repair.[6] PSMA expression in PCa is 1000-folds higher than the normal prostate tissue.[6] Targeting this transmembrane protein has shown promising results for detecting PCa. Various radiopharmaceuticals have been developed, most of which target a specific region of PSMA.

^{68}Ga-Gozetotide (aka ^{68}Ga-PSMA-11, ^{68}Ga-HBED-CC, or ^{68}Ga-HBED-PSMA) and ^{18}F-Piflufolastat (aka ^{18}F-DCFPyL) are the 2 FDA-approved PSMA-targeted radiopharmaceuticals for PET imaging of PCa. Both ^{18}F-Piflufolastat and ^{68}Ga-Gozetotide have a high affinity for the extracellular domain of PSMA, which explains their efficacy as imaging agents for PCa.[7] The critical difference is that ^{18}F-Piflufolastat has a longer half-life (110 minutes) than ^{68}Ga-Gozetotide (68 minutes), which benefits the supply and distribution.[6,7] Many other PSMA ligands combined with different

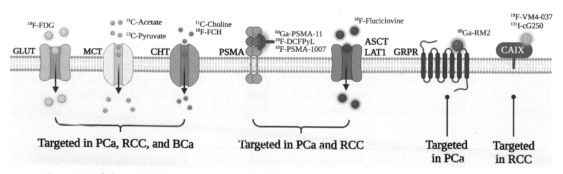

Fig. 1. Schematic of the most commonly used targeted biological pathways for molecular imaging in urologic malignancies, including PCa, RCC, and BCa (created with BioRender.com). GLUT, Glucose transporter; MCT, Monocarboxylic acid transporter; CHT, Choline transporter; ^{18}F-FDG, ^{18}F-Fluorodeoxyglucose; ^{18}F-FCH, ^{18}F-Fluorocholine; ASCT, Alanine-Serine-Cysteine transporter; LAT1, L-type amino acid transporter 1; GRPR, Gastrin-releasing peptide receptor; CAIX, Carbonic anhydrase IX.

Table 1
Summary of targeted biological agents and radiotracers used in molecular imaging for detecting urologic cancers and their diagnostic features

Cancer	Biological target	Imaging agent	Imaging modality	Features
PCa	*PSMA*	^{68}Ga-Gozetotide ^{68}Ga-PSMA I&T ^{68}Ga-PSMA-617	PET/MRI PET/CT	This imaging method detected primary PCa and provided accurate T-staging of PCa. The sensitivity of 70%–97% and specificity of 66%–84% were observed for detecting of primary lesions.
		^{18}F-Piflufolastat ^{18}F-DCFBC ^{18}F-PSMA-1007 ^{18}F-rhPSMA-7	PET/MRI PET/CT	^{18}F-PSMA-1007 has high labeling yield, excellent tumor uptake, and rapid with non-urinary excretion. The sensitivity of ^{18}F-labeled PSMA imaging was 95%–100% for T-staging of PCa.
		^{99m}Tc-MIP-1404 ^{99cm}Tc-PSMA I&S	SPECT	Although, the sensitivity of 94%–100% was observed for detecting the primary lesions using ^{99m}Tc-MIP-1404, this imaging method is suggested to be used for guided biopsy for patients with high suspicion and negative biopsies.
		^{111}In-capromab pendetide	SPECT	The sensitivity of 62% and specificity of 72% were reported. This modality has no priority to other imaging methods such as ^{18}F-FACBC in the detection of recurrent PCa.
	GRPR	^{68}Ga-RM2	PET/CT	This modality showed a sensitivity of 81%–88% and specificity of 81% for the evaluation of primary lesions

(continued on next page)

Table 1
(continued)

Cancer	Biological target	Imaging agent	Imaging modality	Features
				and sensitivity of 70% for LN metastasis.
	Amino acid metabolism	^{18}F-fluciclovine or FACBC	PET/CT	Very limited role in the primary staging of PCa. Sensitivity of 86% and specificity of 75% for PCa detection.
		^{11}C-methionine	PET/CT	PET using ^{11}C-methionine had a sensitivity of 72.1% to 100% in suspicious individuals. Controversial difference between of ^{11}C-methionine and ^{18}F-FDG.
	Androgen receptor	^{18}F-FDHT	PET/CT	The sensitivity detection rates of 63% and specificity of 86%; and results correlated with higher PSA levels. It has been reported to be inferior to ^{18}F-FDG.
	Fatty acid metabolism	^{18}F-FCH [1]C-choline ^{18}F-fluorinated choline	PET/CT PET/MRI	Targeting lipid metabolism is more prominent in the evaluation of biochemical recurrence and metastasis of PCa and has limited diagnostic accuracy depiction of the primary tumor. Sensitivity of 62% and specificity of 76% for PCa detection.
		^{11}C-acetate or ^{18}F-Flouroacetate ^{18}F/^{11}C-acetate	PET PET/CT	Limited value observed in the detection of primary PCa. High sensitivity observed in distant metastasis. Sensitivity of 75% to 93% and

(continued on next page)

Table 1
(continued)

Cancer	Biological target	Imaging agent	Imaging modality	Features
				specificity of 73% for PCa detection.
	Glucose metabolism	^{18}F-FDG	PET/CT	Sensitivity of 37%–67% and specificity of 72% for PCa detection. It provides prognostic information regarding tumor aggressiveness and patients' outcome.
	Pyruvate-to-lactate metabolism	^{13}C-pyruvate ^{13}C-lactate	^{13}C MRI ^{13}C MRSI	High uptake observed in high-grade PCa and correlated with the high-grade PCa. This imaging method can be infused safely multiple times to evaluate the response to treatment of PCa.
	Bone calcification activity	^{18}F-NaF		This imaging method has the highest diagnostic accuracy for detecting bone metastasis of PCa.
	uPA	^{64}Cu-DOTA-AE105 ^{64}Cu-CB-TE2A-AE105 ^{68}Ga-NOTA-AE105	PET/MRI	PET/MRI targeting uPA receptors has shown promising result in the evaluation of tumor aggressiveness and primary prostate lesions.
	αvβ3 integrin	^{68}Ga-NOTA-RGD ^{68}Ga-DOTA-NT-20.3	PET	Probing αvβ3 integrin has shown promising results in the detection of invasion, metastasis formation and angiogenesis of PCa.
RCC	*CAIX*	^{18}F-VM4-037	PET	This is a well-tolerated PET agent that allows same day imaging of CAIX; It demonstrated moderate signal

(continued on next page)

Table 1
(continued)

Cancer	Biological target	Imaging agent	Imaging modality	Features
				uptake in primary tumors and excellent visualization of CAIX positive metastases.
		^{131}I-cG250	PET	^{18}F-FDG is superior to this imaging modality in detecting metastases in patients with metastatic RCC.
		^{124}I-girentuximab ^{124}I-cG250	PET	This modality can accurately and noninvasively identify ccRCC, with potential utility for approaching in patients with renal masses.
		^{89}Zr-girentuximab	PET/CT	This imaging method increases lesion detection compared to CT alone in newly diagnosed good and intermediate prognosis mccRCC patients.
	Fatty acid metabolism	^{11}C-choline	^{13}C MRI	The sensitivity and specificity of this imaging method were 88.0% and 66.7%, respectively. In comparison to ^{18}F-FDG PET/CT, this imaging method is significantly more useful for staging and restaging of RCC.
		^{11}C-acetate	PET	This method has sensitivity of 77% and specificity of 100% for diagnosing RCC. Also, this imaging method might be useful for assessing the early therapeutic

(continued on next page)

Table 1
(continued)

Cancer	Biological target	Imaging agent	Imaging modality	Features
				response in metastatic RCC.
	Amino acid metabolism	^{18}F-fluciclovine or FACBC	PET	This imaging method had very limited ability to detect clear cell carcinoma, but not in papillary cell carcinoma
	Pyruvate-to-lactate metabolism	^{13}C-pyruvate ^{13}C-lactate	^{13}C MRI ^{13}C MRSI	This imaging modality provided a functional assessment of response to treatment in ccRCC. Higher uptake of this imaging correlated with high-grade ccRCCs.
	GLUTs	^{18}F-FDG	PET	The sensitivity and specificity of FDG for renal lesions were 62% and 88%, respectively. For detecting extra-renal lesions, the sensitivity and specificity were 79% and 90%, respectively.
	Cell proliferation	^{18}F-FLT	PET	This modality can be used for evaluating response to treatment in RCC.
	PSMA	^{18}F-Piflufolastat	PET	RCC metastasis sites showed high uptake of this imaging agent. Unlike ccRCC, this modality is not suitable for detecting of renal cancer.
		^{68}Ga-PSMA	PET	This modality is a promising method for detecting RCC metastases. However, no additional diagnostic value in assessing the primary tumor was found.

(continued on next page)

Table 1
(continued)

Cancer	Biological target	Imaging agent	Imaging modality	Features
	$\alpha v\beta 3$ and $\alpha v\beta 5$ integrins	^{18}F-fluciclatide	PET	This imaging is well tolerated and demonstrated favorable characteristics for imaging $\alpha v\beta 3$ and $\alpha v\beta 5$ expression in RCC. Higher uptake was observed in chromophobe than in nonchromophobe RCC.
	VEGFA	^{89}Zr-bevacizumab	PET	This modality is favorable for detecting RCC metastasis and capturing response to treatment.
BCa	Glucose metabolism	^{18}F-FDG	PET/CT	The sensitivity and specificity of ^{18}F-FDG PET for detecting BCa lymph node metastasis were 56%–57% and 92%–95%, respectively.
	Fatty acid metabolism	^{11}C-choline ^{11}C-acetate	PET/CT	^{11}C-choline and ^{11}C-acetate for detecting lymph node staging of BCa with the pooled sensitivity and specificity of 66% and 89%.
	VPAC	^{64}Cu-TP3805	PET	This imaging technique revealed the sensitivity of 79% and specificity of 92% for detecting urothelial bladder cancer.
Pelvic cancer	Glucose metabolism	^{18}F-FDG	PET/CT	^{18}F-FDG PET/CT was 83% for upper urinary tract urothelial cancers; however, no relation was observed between the uptake and tumor stage/grade.

(continued on next page)

Table 1
(*continued*)

Cancer	Biological target	Imaging agent	Imaging modality	Features
Testicular Cancer	*Glucose metabolism*	^{18}F-FDG	PET/CT	The sensitivity of 78%, specificity of 86%, PPV of 58%, NPV of 94%, and accuracy of 84% for detecting seminoma.

Abbreviations: BCa, Bladder Cancer; CAIX, Carbonic Anhydrase IX; ccRCC, clear cell renal cell carcinoma; DHT, dihydrotestosterone; FACBC, fluorocyclobutanecarboxylic-acid; FDG, fluorodeoxyglucose; FDG, fluorodeoxyglucose; FLT, fluorothymidine; GRPR, gastrin releasing peptide receptor; LN, lymph node; mccRCC, metastatic clear cell renal cell carcinoma; MRI, magnetic resonance imaging; MRSI, magnetic resonance spectroscopic imaging; PCa, Prostate cancer; PET, positron emission tomography; PSA, Prostate-specific antigen; PSMA, Prostate-specific membrane antigen; RCC, renal cell carcinoma; uPA, urokinase plasminogen activator; VEGFA, Vascular endothelial growth factor A; VPAC, vasoactive intestinal polypeptide receptor.

radionuclides are in various stages of clinical development (see **Table 1**). Below we briefly discuss the diagnostic accuracy of the most used PSMA-targeted radiopharmaceuticals.

[68]Ga-Gozetotide was first used in 2012 and rapidly gained popularity due to its robust performance. For primary PCa, von Eyben and colleagues demonstrated that the lesion-based sensitivity and specificity for detecting primary PCa were 70%, and 84%, respectively.[8] The patient-based sensitivity was 91%.[9] There were strong correlations between a higher uptake value, and higher PSA level, tumor grade, and the likelihood of distant metastases.[8,9] For N-staging a recent meta-analysis showed that ^{68}Ga-Gozetotide has a pooled sensitivity of 84% and specificity of 95% in intermediate- and high-risk PCa.[10] For bone metastases, ^{68}Ga-Gozetotide is superior to bone scintigraphy in sensitivity (97% vs 86%, respectively) and specificity (100% vs 87%, respectively).[11]

Multiple ^{18}F labeled PSMA-binding radiopharmaceuticals have been developed to address the logistical limitations of ^{68}Ga-Gozetotide distribution. Additionally, the smaller [18]Fluorine positron range and structural modification of the ligands resulting in desirable pharmacokinetic changes allow for higher spatial resolution and detection of smaller lesions in the pelvis.

[18]F-Piflufolastat, ^{18}F-PSMA-1007, and ^{18}F-rhPSMA-7.3 are the most investigated ^{18}F-labeled PSMA-targeted radiopharmaceuticals. Despite their distinctive attributes, these imaging agents seem equally effective for diagnosing PCa.[12] Only ^{18}F-Piflufolastat is approved by the FDA for staging and restaging PCa.[12] CONDOR trial showed that the detection rate of ^{18}F-Piflufolastat was 59% to 66%, and the positive predictive value (PPV) was 78% to 93%.[13] OSPREY trial reported

that the median sensitivity and specificity of ^{18}F-Piflufolastat for the detection of pelvic nodes in high-risk primary PCa were 40% and 98%, respectively; the sensitivity for the detection of extraprostatic lesions in recurrent/metastatic PCa was 96%.[14] A meta-analysis of the studies showed that in PCa biochemical recurrence, the pooled detection rate was 89% for PSA ≥ 0.5 ng/mL and 47% for PSA < 0.5 ng/mL.[15]

^{18}F-PSMA-1007 has high diagnostic accuracy in detecting the primary PCa lesions, with a strong correlation between SUV_{max} and Gleason Score, PSA level, and tumor grade.[16] Biliary excretion of ^{18}F-PSMA-1007 is beneficial for primary staging in individuals with a high-risk PCa.[12] For nodal disease, ^{18}F-PSMA-1007 has a sensitivity and specificity 95% and 100%, respectively.[17] Higher sensitivity of ^{18}F-PSMA-1007 compared to ^{18}F-Piflufolastat for N-staging is likely due to its low urinary elimination, allowing for better visualization of small lymph nodes in the pelvis.

Multiple other PSMA-targeting radiopharmaceuticals have been developed and tested. ^{111}In-capromab pendetide was the first PSMA-targeting radiopharmaceutical that received FDA approval; however, due to targeting the intracellular domain of PSMA, the diagnostic performance was relatively poor.[18] ^{68}Ga-PSMA-I&T, ^{68}Ga-PSMA-617, ^{68}Ga-PSMA-R2, [89]Zr-DFO-huJ591, [89]ZR-DF-IAB2M, ^{99m}Tc-MIP-1404 are among the other PSMA imaging agents studied.[12,19] Although these agents have shown promising results, the effectiveness of these imaging methods is yet to be investigated on a large scale (**Fig. 2**).

Gastrin-releasing Peptide Receptor

Gastrin-releasing peptide receptor (GRPR) is a bombesin-family transmembrane G-protein-

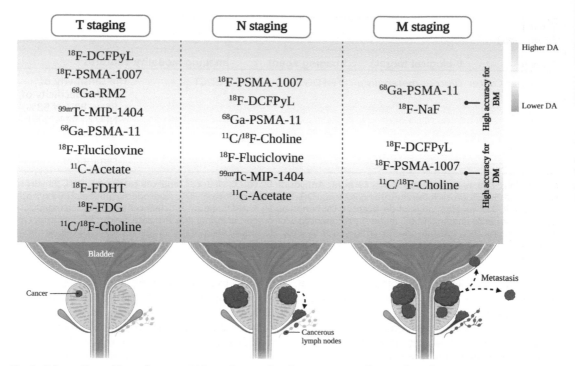

Fig. 2. Schematic ranking of targeted biomarkers and radiotracers according to their diagnostic accuracy in T-, N-, and M-staging of PCa (created with BioRender.com). DA, Diagnostic accuracy; DM, Distant metastasis; BM, Bone metastasis.

coupled receptor overexpressed in 63% to 100% of primary PCa.[20] High GPRR-mediated signaling enhances the proliferation of androgen-dependent and androgen-independent PCa cells. GRPR agonists and antagonists could be radiolabeled for PET and SPECT imaging. GRPR antagonists demonstrate superior imaging characteristics.[12] ^{68}Ga-RM2, a GRPR antagonist, had a sensitivity of 81% to 88% and specificity of 67% to 81% for primary PCa which is not significantly higher than mpMRI.[21–23] For lymph node metastases ^{68}Ga-RM2 had a sensitivity of 70%.[21] Compared with ^{18}F-Piflufolastat PET imaging, ^{68}Ga-RM2 showed significantly lower SUV$_{max}$.[24] Other promising antagonists, including ^{68}Ga-NeoBOM, ^{68}Ga-RM26, and ^{68}Ga-SB3, have also been reported to be safe and capable of detecting primary and metastatic PCa. However, a large-scale clinical trial has not tested these imaging methods.

Amino Acid Metabolism

[18]F-fluciclovine is a synthetically labeled amino acid (aka ^{18}F-FACBC, trans-1-amino-3-[18] F-fluorocyclobutanecarboxylic-acid or Axumin), is actively taken up by cancer cells through the up-regulated alanine, serine, cysteine transporter 2 (ASCT2) and large amino acid transporter 1

(LAT1). Unfortunately, ^{18}F-fluciclovine uptake is non-specific and there is overlap between uptake levels of benign and malignant lesions. This limits the ^{18}F-fluciclovine PET/CT ability to define the site of primary PCa.[25] In a meta-analysis, the pooled patient-based sensitivity, and specificity for PCa were 86.3% and 75.9%, respectively. In region-based analysis for detecting primary/recurrent disease, the sensitivity was significantly higher in the prostatic bed, than in extra-prostatic regions (90.4% vs 76.5%) while the specificity was higher for detecting extra-prostatic lesions than in the prostatic bed (89% vs 45%).[26] In addition, ^{18}F-fluciclovine PET/CT has a similar sensitivity to traditional imaging for detecting lymph nodes and bone metastases.[27] The FDA approved ^{18}F-fluciclovine PET/CT in 2016 for imaging of the BCR PCa. However, head-to-head comparison to PSMA PET imaging showed that for extraprostatic disease PSMA PET detects twice as many lesions as ^{18}F-fluciclovine PET.[28] Therefore, with the FDA approval of PSMA PET imaging agents, the use of ^{18}F-fluciclovine has become limited.

Glucose Metabolism

The Warburg effect in cancer cells shifts energy metabolism from oxidative phosphorylation to glycolysis. The rapid uptake and metabolism of glucose through GLUT allows for energy generation and proliferation. In this regard, ^{18}F-FDG, a glucose analog, is commonly used to detect cancer. ^{18}F-FDG converts to ^{18}F-FDG6P by hexokinase, accumulating in cancer cells.[29]

^{18}F-FDG PET/CT is of limited value for diagnosing the primary tumor and primary staging of lymph nodes or bone metastases. The sensitivity of ^{18}F-FDG PET/CT was reported at 37% to 67%, and specificity was 72% for the detection of primary PCa.[30,31] However, ^{18}F-FDG PET/CT imaging could provide prognostic information regarding tumor aggressiveness and patient outcomes. The higher intensity of ^{18}F-FDG uptake was correlated with higher pathologic grade, advanced stage, and lower cancer-related survival in PCa.[32]

Pyruvate-to-lactate Conversion

Rapid pyruvate-to-lactate conversion by lactate dehydrogenase isoform A (LDHA) is the signature of aggressive cancer.[33] The pyruvate-to-lactate conversion could provide information about the PCa grade.[34] This conversion can be imaged and quantified using hyperpolarized (HP) ^{13}C-pyruvate MRI.[34,35] HP ^{13}C-pyruvate MRI can provide real-time information about changes in cancer metabolism, which can be used for early response assessment.

Fatty Acid Metabolism

Fatty acid metabolism is prioritized in cells for synthesizing lipid membranes or signaling molecules rather than energy metabolism. As a component of the lipid membrane, choline is a biomarker for cell proliferation and division. Radiolabeled choline was used to image malignancies because the up-regulation of the choline kinase in tumors results in a high level of trapped labeled phosphatidylcholine in the membrane of cancer cells.[36] ^{11}C-choline and ^{18}F-fluorocholine (^{18}F-FCH) radiotracers are two of the most frequently used choline analogs in clinical practice. For primary staging of PCa they outperformed ^{18}F-FDG. In a meta-analysis by Evangelista and colleagues, the sensitivity and specificity of ^{11}C-choline/^{18}F-FCH PET/CT for the detection of primary lesions PCa were 62.6% and 76.3%, respectively; for the lymph node staging, the sensitivity and specificity were 49.2% and 95%, respectively.[37] For BCR PCa, the pooled detection rate of ^{18}F-FCH PET/CT was 66%, which is lower than 74% of ^{18}F-fluciclovine PET/CT. In addition, in PSA levels below 1 ng/dl, the lesion detection rate is approximately 40% and significantly below the detection rate of PSMA PET at all PSA levels.

Acetate is another molecule involved in fatty acid metabolism. Upregulation of acetyl-CoA synthase (ACeS), which converts acetate to acetyl-CoA, resulted in higher demand for acetate in PCa cells. Therefore, ^{11}C-acetate has been used as an imaging biomarker for PCa.[38] There is no relation between the ^{11}C-acetate uptake in the primary lesions and PSA levels or histologic findings. In a meta-analysis by Beheshti and colleagues, the sensitivity for the diagnosis of primary tumors was 75.1%, and specificity was 75.8%.[39] ^{11}C-acetate has nonspecific uptake in the prostate gland and typically misses a fraction of tumor foci, resulting in low accuracy in the detection of primary PCa. The sensitivity and specificity for metastatic PCa lesions were 68% and 78.1%, respectively.[40] ^{11}C-acetate PET/CT is superior to bone scintigraphy in detecting bone metastases in patients with untreated high-risk PCa.[41]

Other Targeted Biological Agents

Osteoid matrix deposition
[18]F-NaF PET/CT is highly effective in detecting PCa bone metastases.[42] A meta-analysis, revealed that the patient-based pooled sensitivity, and specificity, of ^{18}F-NaF PET/CT were 98%, and 90%, respectively.[43] ^{18}F-NaF PET/CT has superior sensitivity compared with bone scintigraphy; however, the higher cost of ^{18}F-NaF PET/CT, lack of outcomes benefit data, and approval of PSMA imaging with high accuracy for detecting bone and soft tissue lesions have limited its clinical use.

Androgen receptor
[18]F-16-fluoro-5-dihydrotestosterone (FDHT) PET/CT is used to measure androgen receptor (AR) expression. Eleven studies reported heterogeneous results of ^{18}F-FHDT PET in 323 patients.[44] Based on these reports, the patient-based and lesion-based positivity rates in detecting metastatic castration-resistant prostate cancer (mCRPC) ranged from 74% to 100% and 44% to 97%, respectively.[45,46] The scan positivity rate directly correlated with PSA levels.[47] Compared with 18F-FDG PET/CT, the sensitivity was inferior. Despite lower sensitivity, ^{18}F-FDHT PET/CT has a role in assessing AR heterogeneity in mCRPC in patients who are candidates for androgen deprivation therapy.[46]

Urokinase plasminogen activator surface receptor
The urokinase plasminogen activator surface receptor (uPA) is a cell membrane glycoprotein involved in the plasminogen activation. It is known as an aggressiveness marker.[48] uPA radioligands ^{64}Cu-DOTA-AE105 and ^{68}Ga-NOTA-AE105 have been used clinically in PCa.[48,49] Uptake level was

directly correlated to a higher Gleason score in primary PCa and lower survival in treated mCRPC.[49] Low uptake of in bone metastases is a limiting factor for broader adoption of these tracers.[49]

Integrin receptors

$\alpha v\beta 3$ integrin, a transmembrane cell adhesion receptor, involved in tumor angiogenesis, is overexpressed in PCa.[50] ^{18}F-Galacto-RGD targets the $\alpha v\beta 3$ integrin and showed a detection rate of 78.4% and 40% for bone and lymph node metastases, respectively.[51] These results are slightly inferior to the standard of care imaging.

RENAL CANCER

Renal malignancies are the sixth most frequently diagnosed cancer worldwide. Early detection of renal cancers can significantly impact the burden of this malignancy. Conventional imaging, such as CT and MRI, has long been the gold standard for RCC imaging. However, these methods are sometimes limited in differentiating RCC from other solid masses, such as lipid-poor angiomyolipoma (AML) or oncocytoma.[52] In this regard, molecular imaging methods for RCC diagnosis have made significant progress. PET imaging can target different biological molecules, such as carbonic anhydrase IX (CAIX), PSMA, glucose analogs, and thymidine kinase, to better detect RCCs. Later in discussion, we discuss the reported clinical approaches in molecular imaging of RCC (see **Table 1**).

Carbonic Anhydrase IX

CAIX, as a membrane-bound enzyme, catalyzes the conversion of carbon dioxide to bicarbonate, which has a crucial role in pH regulation in cancer cells, allowing these cells to adapt to the adverse conditions of the tumor microenvironment. Higher expression of CAIX in RCC has been correlated with decreased cell adhesion and enhanced migration, resulting in tumor invasion and metastasis.[53] In this regard, CAIX has been targeted with various radiotracers, including ^{18}F-VM4-037, ^{131}I-mG250, ^{131}I-cG250, and [124]I-cG250 ([124]I-girentuximab), and [89]Zr-girentuximab, to detect RCC.[52] These radiotracers showed promising results for the detection of RCC. For instance, [124]I-cG250 PET/CT had a sensitivity and specificity of 86% to 94% and 86% to 100%, respectively, for clear cell RCC (ccRCC).[54,55] Other radiotracers targeting CAIX, such as ^{18}F-VM4-037, [124]I-girentuximab, [89]Zr-girentuximab, ^{111}In-girentuximab, also showed high sensitivity and specificity, although the published clinical data about these tracers are relatively scarce.[56–58] Large-scale

clinical trials are still needed to establish this imaging method's performance.

Glucose Metabolism

There are data that targeting glucose metabolism using ^{18}F-FDG could help detect RCC lesions in specific situations. The sensitivity and specificity of ^{18}F-FDG PET/CT for primary intra-renal RCC lesions were 62% and 88%, respectively, and for extra-renal lesions and metastatic sites were 79% and 90%, respectively.[59,60] Metabolic tumor burden is prognostic for progression-free and overall survival in patients with metastatic RCC.[61] Although the ^{18}F-FDG PET/CT has a moderately high diagnostic accuracy for detecting metastatic RCC, other molecular imaging methods, such as CAIX imaging, have better performance.

Prostate-specific Membrane Antigen

PSMA expression is not limited to PCa and is demonstrated in the neovasculature of other cancers such as RCC. Limited clinical studies have evaluated the role of PSMA imaging in RCC. ^{18}F-Piflufolastat had higher sensitivity than CT or MRI. However, the diagnostic performance of ^{18}F-Piflufolastat for detecting the subtypes of RCC was inconsistent.[62,63] ^{68}Ga-Gozetotide PET/CT also has high uptake in the metastatic sites of RCC; however, due to high physiologic uptake in the normal renal parenchyma, no additional diagnostic value was observed in assessing the primary tumor using ^{68}Ga-Gozetotide PET/CT.[64] Overall, PSMA PET can be used as a biomarker for tumor neoangiogenesis in ccRCC metastases to stratify candidates for targeted anti-angiogenic therapies. Additionally, individuals with renal impairment or a contrast allergy can undergo the procedure without any risk of complications.

Other Pathways

Pyruvate-to-lactate metabolism
A few reports have evaluated the use of hyperpolarized ^{13}C-pyruvate MR imaging in RCC. Studies showed a trend toward a higher lactate-to-pyruvate ratio in high-grade ccRCCs compared with low-grade ccRCCs.[65] The kinetic rate constant for the conversion of pyruvate to lactate (kPL) was positively correlated to the WHO/ISUP tumor grade in the ccRCC.[66]

Lipid metabolism
In a clinical trial of 28 patients with RCC, the sensitivity and specificity of ^{11}C-choline PET/CT for the detection of RCC were 88.0% and 66.7%, respectively.[67] Compared with ^{18}F-FDG PET/CT, [11]C-

choline PET/CT was significantly more beneficial for staging and restaging RCC.[67]

Cell proliferation

^{18}F-FLT (3′-deoxy-3′-18F-fluoro-L-thymidine) is a thymidine analog used as a cellular proliferation biomarker. The uptake of ^{18}F-FLT indicates ongoing DNA replication, a proxy for cell division. Few clinical trials have evaluated ^{18}F-FLT PET/CT in RCC. It was shown that the uptake of ^{18}F-FLT decreases during treatment and returns to baseline with the treatment withdrawal.[68] However, ^{18}F-FLT imaging was not predictive of prognosis in metastatic RCC.[69] Overall, ^{18}F-FLT PET/CT imaging has shown promise for response assessment in RCC; but data are very scarce and needs further validation in a large-scale clinical trial.

Osteoid matrix

In a small population study with patients diagnosed with RCC bone metastases, Gerety and colleagues discovered that ^{18}F-NaF PET/CT could detect more RCC bone metastases than ^{99m}Tc-MDP bone scintigraphy/SPECT or CT alone.[70]

Vascular endothelial growth factors

RCC has a high rate of angiogenesis radiolabeled antivascular endothelial growth factor A (VEGF-A) antibodies such as [89]Zr-bevacizumab and ^{111}In-bevacizumab have been used to image RCC and its response to targeted therapies; both imaging agents showed a reduction in tumor uptake in response to targeted antitumor therapies, making them potential biomarkers for monitoring response to therapy.[71,72]

αvβ3 and αvβ5 integrins

αvβ3 and αvβ5 are highly expressed in tumor cells and activated endothelial cells. As a result, measuring integrins αvβ3 and αvβ5 expressions could help diagnose patients with RCC. Small clinical reports show that ^{18}F-Fluciclatide PET and ^{18}F-FPRGD2 PET/CT imaging have high uptake in RCC, but the uptake is dependent on the histologic subtype of the tumor.[73,74]

BLADDER CANCER

Bladder cancer (BCa) is the most frequent urinary tract cancer in the United States, with a higher incidence in men than women. The use of molecular imaging in BCa is often limited to detecting BCa metastases given the urinary elimination of most radiopharmaceuticals, which limits the detection of bladder wall lesions and reduces the diagnosis accuracy for locoregional metastases of BCa. Various biomarkers, including Vasoactive Intestinal Peptide Receptor (VPAC) and Fibroblast

Activation Protein (FAP), have been used to detect BCa by using ^{64}Cu-TP3805 and ^{68}Ga-FAPI, respectively. However, the following sections briefly discuss the diagnostic value of targeting glucose metabolism by ^{18}F-FDG and fatty acid metabolism by ^{11}C-choline and ^{11}C-acetate, which have been investigated in clinical trials (see **Table 1**).

Glucose Metabolism

In a series of meta-analyses, the pooled sensitivity and specificity of ^{18}F-FDG PET/CT for the detection of lymph node metastases of BCa were 56% to 57% and 92% to 95%, respectively.[75–77] In addition, ^{18}F-FDG PET/CT was shown to evaluate the response to treatment with a sensitivity of 75% and specificity of 90%.[78] Finally, compared with other conventional imaging methods, the diagnostic accuracy of ^{18}F-FDG PET/CT for detecting recurrent bladder cancer was significantly higher.[79]

Lipid Metabolism

A meta-analysis by Kim and colleagues evaluated the diagnostic accuracy of ^{11}C-choline and ^{11}C-acetate for lymph node staging of BCa, which showed a pooled sensitivity and specificity of 66% and 89%, respectively.[80] ^{11}C-choline and ^{11}C-acetate PET/CT showed low sensitivity and moderate specificity for detecting metastatic LNs in patients with BCa. A high rate of false-positive uptake due to inflammation or infection, limiting the staging utility of ^{11}C-acetate, especially after prior intravesical BCG therapy.[81]

OTHER UROLOGIC CANCERS

Molecular imaging has been used in other urologic malignancies, including testicular and ureteral cancers. However, most clinical studies have focused on ^{18}F-FDG PET/CT to evaluate these cancers. Later in discussion is a summary:

Testicular Cancer

A meta-analysis showed that ^{18}F-FDG PET/CT had a pooled sensitivity of 78%, specificity of 86%, PPV of 58%, NPV of 94%, and accuracy of 84% for detecting seminoma subtype of testicular cancer.[82] In addition, this study showed that ^{18}F-FDG PET/CT had better diagnostic accuracy in evaluating residual/recurrent lesions >3 cm compared with those <3 cm.

Pelvic and Ureteral Cancer

Previous studies have reported that the sensitivity of ^{18}F-FDG PET/CT for the detection of upper urinary tract urothelial cancers was 83%; however, no relation was observed between the uptake and tumor stage/grade.[83] In addition, it was suggested that ^{18}F-FDG PET/CT is more accurate than conventional imaging, including CECT for detecting local and distant recurrence of ureteral cancer after surgery, which can influence the patients' management.[84]

SUMMARY

In summary, nuclear medicine and molecular imaging are critical in diagnosing, staging, characterization, and prognosticating urologic malignancies. Overall, radiologists and urologists should choose the appropriate molecular imaging method based on the clinical findings of each patient. For detecting PCa, multiple tracers were developed, and each tracer has its features (see **Fig. 2**). Targeting PSMA using 18F-PSMA outperformed the other targeted biomarkers in T- and N-staging. In M-staging and detecting bone metastasis, ^{68}Ga-PSMA and ^{18}F-NaF have the highest accuracy compared with other tracers (see **Fig. 2**). Although targeting PSMA showed great diagnostic accuracy, it has a limited role in detecting primary lesions and T-staging of PCa. For diagnosis of RCC, targeting CAIX has higher diagnostic accuracy than other targeted biomarkers. In addition, although the role of molecular imaging in diagnosing BCa is evaluated in a limited number of studies, targeting glucose metabolism using ^{18}F-FDG revealed higher accuracy than conventional imaging methods. Targeting glucose metabolism performs better than other imaging methods for diagnosing other urologic cancers, including testicular and ureteral cancer.

CLINICS CARE POINTS

- Clinicians should choose the appropriate molecular imaging method based on the clinical findings of patients.
- For T-and N-staging in patients with PCa using molecular imaging, targeting PSMA by ^{18}F-Piflufolastat and ^{18}F-PSMA-1007 outperformed the other targeted biomarkers. For M-staging and evaluation of distant metastatic sites, targeting PSMA and bone calcification activity using ^{68}Ga-PSMA-11 and ^{18}F-NaF have shown higher accuracy than that of the other molecular imaging methods, respectively.
- In RCC, targeting CAIX has shown higher diagnostic accuracy in detecting primary lesions than that of the other targeted biomarkers. Diagnostic accuracy of targeting glucose metabolism using ^{18}F-FDG has been shown to be superior to CAIX in detecting metastatic sites of RCC.
- Although the role of molecular imaging in diagnosing other urologic malignancies, including BCa, testicular and ureteral cancers, has not been widely investigated, targeting the glucose metabolism using ^{18}F-FDG revealed higher accuracy than that of conventional imaging methods.

DISCLOSURES

Authors have no actual or potential conflict of interest concerning this article.

ACKNOWLEDGMENTS AND FUNDING SOURCE

P Heidari is supported by K08CA249047.

REFERENCES

1. Dy GW, Gore JL, Forouzanfar MH, et al. Global burden of urologic cancers, 1990–2013. Eur Urol 2017;71(3):437–46.
2. Savir-Baruch B, Werner RA, Rowe SP, et al. PET imaging for prostate cancer. Radiologic Clin 2021; 59(5):801–11.
3. Sharma S, Zapatero-Rodriguez J, O'Kennedy R. Prostate cancer diagnostics: Clinical challenges and the ongoing need for disruptive and effective diagnostic tools. Biotechnol Adv 2017;35(2):135–49.
4. Picchio M, Mapelli P, Panebianco V, et al. Imaging biomarkers in prostate cancer: role of PET/CT and MRI. Eur J Nucl Med Mol Imaging 2015;42(4): 644–55.
5. Wibmer AG, Burger IA, Sala E, et al. Molecular imaging of prostate cancer. Radiographics 2016; 36(1):142.
6. Mhawech-Fauceglia P, Zhang S, Terracciano L, et al. Prostate-specific membrane antigen (PSMA) protein expression in normal and neoplastic tissues and its sensitivity and specificity in prostate adenocarcinoma: an immunohistochemical study using multiple tumour tissue microarray technique. Histopathology 2007;50(4):472–83.
7. Ferreira G, Iravani A, Hofman MS, et al. Intra-individual comparison of 68 Ga-PSMA-11 and 18 F-DCFPyL normal-organ biodistribution. Cancer Imaging 2019;19(1):1–10.
8. von Eyben FE, Picchio M, von Eyben R, et al. 68Ga-labeled prostate-specific membrane antigen ligand positron emission tomography/computed tomography for prostate cancer: a

systematic review and meta-analysis. Eur Urol focus 2018;4(5):686–93.

9. Uprimny C, Kroiss AS, Decristoforo C, et al. 68Ga-PSMA-11 PET/CT in primary staging of prostate cancer: PSA and Gleason score predict the intensity of tracer accumulation in the primary tumour. Eur J Nucl Med Mol Imaging 2017;44(6):941–9.

10. Peng L, Li J, Meng C, et al. Can 68Ga-prostate specific membrane antigen positron emission tomography/computerized tomography provide an accurate lymph node staging for patients with medium/high risk prostate cancer? A diagnostic meta-analysis. Radiat Oncol 2020;15(1):1–10.

11. Zhao R, Li Y, Nie L, et al. The meta-analysis of the effect of 68Ga-PSMA-PET/CT diagnosis of prostatic cancer compared with bone scan. Medicine 2021;100(15).

12. Manafi-Farid R, Ranjbar S, Jamshidi Araghi Z, et al. Molecular Imaging in Primary Staging of Prostate Cancer Patients: Current Aspects and Future Trends. Cancers 2021;13(21):5360.

13. Morris MJ, Rowe SP, Gorin MA, et al. Diagnostic performance of 18F-DCFPyL-PET/CT in men with biochemically recurrent prostate cancer: Results from the CONDOR phase III, multicenter study. Clin Cancer Res 2021;27(13):3674–82.

14. Pienta KJ, Gorin MA, Rowe SP, et al. A phase 2/3 prospective multicenter study of the diagnostic accuracy of prostate specific membrane antigen PET/CT with 18F-DCFPyL in prostate cancer patients (OSPREY). J Urol 2021;206(1):52–61.

15. Sun J, Lin Y, Wei X, et al. Performance of 18F-DCFPyL PET/CT Imaging in Early Detection of Biochemically Recurrent Prostate Cancer: A Systematic Review and Meta-Analysis. Front Oncol 2021;11:649171.

16. Awenat S, Piccardo A, Carvoeiras P, et al. Diagnostic role of 18F-PSMA-1007 PET/CT in prostate cancer staging: a systematic review. Diagnostics 2021;11(3):552.

17. Giesel FL, Hadaschik B, Cardinale J, et al. F-18 labelled PSMA-1007: biodistribution, radiation dosimetry and histopathological validation of tumor lesions in prostate cancer patients. Eur J Nucl Med Mol Imaging 2017;44(4):678–88.

18. Manyak MJ, Hinkle GH, Olsen JO, et al. Immunoscintigraphy with indium-111-capromab pendetide: evaluation before definitive therapy in patients with prostate cancer. Urology 1999;54(6):1058–63.

19. Morris MJ, Pandit-Taskar N, Carrasquillo JA, et al. Phase I trial of zirconium 89 (Zr89) radiolabeled J591 in metastatic castration-resistant prostate cancer (mCRPC). Journal of Clinical Oncology 2013;31(6 suppl):31.

20. Bratanovic IJ, Zhang C, Zhang Z, et al. A Radiotracer for Molecular Imaging and Therapy of Gastrin-Releasing Peptide Receptor–Positive Prostate Cancer. J Nucl Med 2022;63(3):424–30.

21. Kähkönen E, Jambor I, Kemppainen J, et al. In vivo imaging of prostate cancer using [68Ga]-labeled bombesin analog BAY86-7548. Clin Cancer Res 2013;19(19):5434–43.

22. Touijer KA, Michaud L, Alvarez HAV, et al. Prospective study of the radiolabeled GRPR antagonist BAY86-7548 for positron emission tomography/computed tomography imaging of newly diagnosed prostate cancer. Eur Urol Oncol 2019;2(2):166–73.

23. Stephens A, Loidl WC, Beheshti M, et al. Detection of prostate cancer with the [68Ga]-labeled bombesin antagonist RM2 in patients undergoing radical prostatectomy. Journal of Clinical Oncology 2016;34(2 suppl):80.

24. Baratto L, Song H, Duan H, et al. A prospective study of 68Ga-RM2 PET/MRI in patients with biochemically recurrent prostate cancer and negative conventional imaging. Journal of Clinical Oncology 2020;38(15 suppl):e17536.

25. Parihar AS, Schmidt LR, Dehdashti F, et al. Detection of additional primary neoplasms on 18F-Fluciclovine PET/CT in patients with primary prostate cancer. J Nucl Med 2021;63(5):713–9.

26. Laudicella R, Albano D, Alongi P, et al. 18F-Facbc in prostate cancer: a systematic review and meta-analysis. Cancers 2019;11(9):1348.

27. Gusman M, Aminsharifi JA, Peacock JG, et al. Review of 18F-fluciclovine PET for detection of recurrent prostate cancer. Radiographics 2019;39(3):822–41.

28. Calais J, Ceci F, Eiber M, et al. 18F-fluciclovine PET-CT and 68Ga-PSMA-11 PET-CT in patients with early biochemical recurrence after prostatectomy: a prospective, single-centre, single-arm, comparative imaging trial. Lancet Oncol 2019;20(9):1286–94.

29. Wallitt KL, Khan SR, Dubash S, et al. Clinical PET imaging in prostate cancer. Radiographics 2017;37(5):1512–36.

30. Jadvar H. Is There Use for FDG-PET in Prostate Cancer? Semin Nucl Med 2016;46(6):502–6.

31. Bertagna F, Sadeghi R, Giovanella L, et al. Incidental uptake of 18F-fluorodeoxyglucose in the prostate gland. Nuklearmedizin-NuclearMedicine. 2014;53(06):249–58.

32. Shen K, Liu B, Zhou X, et al. The evolving role of 18F-FDG PET/CT in diagnosis and prognosis prediction in progressive prostate cancer. Front Oncol 2021;11:683793.

33. Woitek R, Gallagher FA. The use of hyperpolarised 13C-MRI in clinical body imaging to probe cancer metabolism. Br J Cancer 2021;124(7):1187–98.

34. Sushentsev N, McLean MA, Warren AY, et al. Hyperpolarised 13C-MRI identifies the emergence of a glycolytic cell population within intermediate-risk human prostate cancer. Nat Commun 2022;13(1):1–12.

35. Chen H-Y, Aggarwal R, Bok RA, et al. Hyperpolarized 13C-pyruvate MRI detects real-time metabolic

flux in prostate cancer metastases to bone and liver: a clinical feasibility study. Prostate Cancer prostatic Dis 2020;23(2):269–76.

36. Jadvar H. Prostate cancer: PET with 18F-FDG, 18F- or 11C-acetate, and 18F-or 11C-choline. J Nucl Med 2011;52(1):81–9.

37. Evangelista L, Cervino AR, Burei M, et al. Comparative studies of radiolabeled choline positron emission tomography, histology of primary tumor and other imaging modalities in prostate cancer: a systematic review and meta-analysis. Clin Translational Imaging 2013;1(2):99–109.

38. Kato T, Tsukamoto E, Kuge Y, et al. Accumulation of [11C] acetate in normal prostate and benign prostatic hyperplasia: comparison with prostate cancer. Eur J Nucl Med Mol Imaging 2002;29(11).1492–5.

39. Mohsen B, Giorgio T, Rasoul ZS, et al. Application of C-11-acetate positron-emission tomography (PET) imaging in prostate cancer: systematic review and meta-analysis of the literature. BJU Int 2013;112(8): 1062–72.

40. Haseebuddin M, Dehdashti F, Siegel BA, et al. 11C-acetate PET/CT before radical prostatectomy: nodal staging and treatment failure prediction. J Nucl Med 2013;54(5):699–706.

41. Strandberg S, Karlsson CT, Ogren M, et al. 11C-acetate-PET/CT compared to 99mTc-HDP bone Scintigraphy in primary staging of high-risk prostate cancer. Anticancer Res 2016;36(12):6475–9.

42. Beheshti M, Rezaee A, Geinitz H, et al. Evaluation of prostate cancer bone metastases with 18F-NaF and 18F-fluorocholine PET/CT. J Nucl Med 2016; 57(Supplement 3):55S–60S.

43. Sheikhbahaei S, Jones KM, Werner RA, et al. 18F-NaF-PET/CT for the detection of bone metastasis in prostate cancer: a meta-analysis of diagnostic accuracy studies. Ann Nucl Med 2019;33(5):351–61.

44. Gauthé M, Sargos P, Barret E, et al. Potential Targets Other Than PSMA for Prostate Cancer Theranostics: A Systematic Review. J Clin Med 2021;10(21):4909.

45. Vargas HA, Wassberg C, Fox JJ, et al. Bone metastases in castration-resistant prostate cancer: associations between morphologic CT patterns, glycolytic activity, and androgen receptor expression on PET and overall survival. Radiology 2014;271(1):220–9.

46. Larson SM, Morris M, Gunther I, et al. Tumor localization of 16β-18F-fluoro-5α-dihydrotestosterone versus 18F-FDG in patients with progressive, metastatic prostate cancer. J Nucl Med 2004;45(3): 366–73.

47. Dehdashti F, Picus J, Michalski JM, et al. Positron tomographic assessment of androgen receptors in prostatic carcinoma. Eur J Nucl Med Mol Imaging 2005;32(3):344–50.

48. Persson M, Skovgaard D, Brandt-Larsen M, et al. First-in-human uPAR PET: imaging of cancer aggressiveness. Theranostics 2015;5(12):1303.

49. Fosbøl MØ, Kurbegovic S, Johannesen HH, et al. Urokinase-type plasminogen activator receptor (uPAR) PET/MRI of prostate cancer for noninvasive evaluation of aggressiveness: comparison with Gleason score in a prospective phase 2 clinical trial. J Nucl Med 2021;62(3):354–9.

50. Zheng D-Q, Woodard AS, Fornaro M, et al. Prostatic carcinoma cell migration via αvβ3integrin is modulated by a focal adhesion kinase pathway. Cancer Res 1999;59(7):1655–64.

51. Beer AJ, Schwarzenböck SM, Zantl N, et al. Noninvasive assessment of inter-and intrapatient variability of integrin expression in metastasized prostate cancer by PET. Oncotarget 2016;7(19):28151.

52. Klinkhammer BM, Lammers T, Mottaghy FM, et al. Non-invasive molecular imaging of kidney diseases. Nat Rev Nephrol 2021;17(10):688–703.

53. Stillebroer AB, Mulders PF, Boerman OC, et al. Carbonic anhydrase IX in renal cell carcinoma: implications for prognosis, diagnosis, and therapy. Eur Urol 2010;58(1):75–83.

54. van Oostenbrugge T, Mulders P. Targeted PET/CT imaging for clear cell renal cell carcinoma with radiolabeled antibodies: recent developments using girentuximab. Curr Opin Urol 2021;31(3):249–54.

55. Divgi CR, Pandit-Taskar N, Jungbluth AA, et al. Preoperative characterisation of clear-cell renal carcinoma using iodine-124-labelled antibody chimeric G250 (124I-cG250) and PET in patients with renal masses: a phase I trial. Lancet Oncol 2007;8(4):304–10.

56. van Oostenbrugge TJ, Langenhuijsen JF, Oosterwijk E, et al. Follow-up imaging after cryoablation of clear cell renal cell carcinoma is feasible using single photon emission computed tomography with 111In-girentuximab. Eur J Nucl Med Mol Imaging 2020;47(8):1864–70.

57. Hekman MC, Rijpkema M, Aarntzen EH, et al. Positron emission tomography/computed tomography with 89Zr-girentuximab can aid in diagnostic dilemmas of clear cell renal cell carcinoma suspicion. Eur Urol 2018;74(3):257–60.

58. Turkbey B, Lindenberg ML, Adler S, et al. PET/CT imaging of renal cell carcinoma with 18F-VM4-037: a phase II pilot study. Abdom Radiol 2016;41(1): 109–18.

59. Tabei T, Nakaigawa N, Kaneta T, et al. Early assessment with 18 F-2-fluoro-2-deoxyglucose positron emission tomography/computed tomography to predict short-term outcome in clear cell renal carcinoma treated with nivolumab. BMC cancer 2019;19(1):1–9.

60. Wang H-Y, Ding H-J, Chen J-H, et al. Meta-analysis of the diagnostic performance of [18F] FDG-PET and PET/CT in renal cell carcinoma. Cancer Imaging 2012;12(3):464.

61. Hwang SH, Cho A, Yun M, et al. Prognostic value of pretreatment metabolic tumor volume and total lesion glycolysis using 18F-FDG PET/CT in patients

with metastatic renal cell carcinoma treated with anti–vascular endothelial growth factor–targeted agents. Clin Nucl Med 2017;42(5):e235–41.

62. Rowe SP, Gorin MA, Hammers HJ, et al. Imaging of metastatic clear cell renal cell carcinoma with PSMA-targeted 18F-DCFPyL PET/CT. Ann Nucl Med 2015;29(10):877–82.

63. Yin Y, Campbell SP, Markowski MC, et al. Inconsistent detection of sites of metastatic non-clear cell renal cell carcinoma with PSMA-targeted [18F] DCFPyL PET/CT. Mol Imaging Biol 2019;21(3):567–73.

64. Sawicki LM, Buchbender C, Boos J, et al. Diagnostic potential of PET/CT using a 68Ga-labelled prostate-specific membrane antigen ligand in whole-body staging of renal cell carcinoma: initial experience. Eur J Nucl Med Mol Imaging 2017;44(1):102–7.

65. Tang S, Meng MV, Slater JB, et al. Metabolic imaging with hyperpolarized 13C pyruvate magnetic resonance imaging in patients with renal tumors—Initial experience. Cancer 2021;127(15):2693–704.

66. Ursprung S, Woitek R, McLean MA, et al. Hyperpolarized 13C-Pyruvate Metabolism as a Surrogate for Tumor Grade and Poor Outcome in Renal Cell Carcinoma—A Proof of Principle Study. Cancers 2022; 14(2):335.

67. Nakanishi Y, Kitajima K, Yamada Y, et al. Diagnostic performance of 11C-choline PET/CT and FDG PET/CT for staging and restaging of renal cell cancer. Ann Nucl Med 2018;32(10):658–68.

68. Liu G, Jeraj R, Vanderhoek M, et al. Pharmacodynamic study using FLT PET/CT in patients with renal cell cancer and other solid malignancies treated with sunitinib malate. Clin Cancer Res 2011;17(24): 7634–44.

69. Horn KP, Yap JT, Agarwal N, et al. FDG and FLT-PET for early measurement of response to 37.5 mg daily sunitinib therapy in metastatic renal cell carcinoma. Cancer Imaging 2015;15(1):1–10.

70. Gerety E, Lawrence E, Wason J, et al. Prospective study evaluating the relative sensitivity of 18F-NaF PET/CT for detecting skeletal metastases from renal cell carcinoma in comparison to multidetector CT and 99mTc-MDP bone scintigraphy, using an adaptive trial design. Ann Oncol 2015;26(10):2113–8.

71. Desar IM, Stillebroer AB, Oosterwijk E, et al. 111In-bevacizumab imaging of renal cell cancer and evaluation of neoadjuvant treatment with the vascular endothelial growth factor receptor inhibitor sorafenib. J Nucl Med 2010;51(11):1707–15.

72. van Es SC, Brouwers AH, Mahesh SV, et al. 89Zr-bevacizumab PET: potential early indicator of everolimus efficacy in patients with metastatic renal cell carcinoma. J Nucl Med 2017;58(6):905–10.

73. Withofs N, Signolle N, Somja J, et al. 18F-FPRGD2 PET/CT imaging of integrin αvβ3 in renal carcinomas: correlation with histopathology. J Nucl Med 2015;56(3):361–4.

74. Mena E, Owenius R, Turkbey B, et al. [18F] Fluciclatide in the in vivo evaluation of human melanoma and renal tumors expressing αvβ3 and αvβ5 integrins. Eur J Nucl Med Mol Imaging 2014;41(10):1879–88.

75. Soubra A, Hayward D, Dahm P, et al. The diagnostic accuracy of 18F-fluorodeoxyglucose positron emission tomography and computed tomography in staging bladder cancer: a single-institution study and a systematic review with meta-analysis. World J Urol 2016;34(9):1229–37.

76. Crozier J, Papa N, Perera M, et al. Comparative sensitivity and specificity of imaging modalities in staging bladder cancer prior to radical cystectomy: a systematic review and meta-analysis. World J Urol 2019;37(4):667–90.

77. Ha HK, Koo PJ, Kim S-J. Diagnostic accuracy of F-18 FDG PET/CT for preoperative lymph node staging in newly diagnosed bladder cancer patients: a systematic review and meta-analysis. Oncology 2018;95(1):31–8.

78. Soubra A, Gencturk M, Froelich J, et al. FDG-PET/CT for assessing the response to neoadjuvant chemotherapy in bladder cancer patients. Clin Genitourinary Cancer 2018;16(5):360–4.

79. Zattoni F, Incerti E, Colicchia M, et al. Comparison between the diagnostic accuracies of 18F-fluorodeoxyglucose positron emission tomography/computed tomography and conventional imaging in recurrent urothelial carcinomas: a retrospective, multicenter study. Abdom Radiol 2018;43(9):2391–9.

80. Kim S-J, Koo PJ, Pak K, et al. Diagnostic accuracy of C-11 choline and C-11 acetate for lymph node staging in patients with bladder cancer: a systematic review and meta-analysis. World J Urol 2018; 36(3):331–40.

81. Schöder H, Ong SC, Reuter VE, et al. Initial results with 11C-acetate positron emission tomography/computed tomography (PET/CT) in the staging of urinary bladder cancer. Mol Imaging Biol 2012; 14(2):245–51.

82. Treglia G, Sadeghi R, Annunziata S, et al. Diagnostic performance of fluorine-18-fluorodeoxyglucose positron emission tomography in the postchemotherapy management of patients with seminoma: systematic review and meta-analysis. Biomed Res Int 2014;2014:852681.

83. Asai S, Fukumoto T, Tanji N, et al. Fluorodeoxyglucose positron emission tomography/computed tomography for diagnosis of upper urinary tract urothelial carcinoma. Int J Clin Oncol 2015;20(5): 1042–7.

84. Tanaka H, Yoshida S, Komai Y, et al. Clinical value of 18F-fluorodeoxyglucose positron emission tomography/computed tomography in upper tract urothelial carcinoma: impact on detection of metastases and patient management. Urologia Internationalis 2016; 96(1):65–72.

Biomarkers in Testicular Cancer
Classic Tumor Markers and Beyond

Jillian Egan, MD[a], Keyan Salari, MD, PhD[a,b,c],*

KEYWORDS

- Testicular cancer • Germ cell tumor • Serum tumor marker • microRNA • Biomarkers

KEY POINTS

- cSTM (AFP, bHCG, LDH) remain critically important in the diagnosis, prognostication and surveillance of patients with TGCT
- cSTM are limited by low sensitivity (40-60%) for initial diagnosis of TGCT and are often negative in low-stage disease, pure seminoma, and teratoma.
- miRNA are emerging serum biomarkers in TGCT, with miR-371a-3p in particular demonstrating the most favorable performance data compared to cSTM
- Current miRNA are unable to detect teratoma, which remains an elusive histology for biomarker discovery
- ctDNA and CTCs are two additional emerging biomarkers, but further study is needed to determine their future role in TGCT

INTRODUCTION

Testicular cancer represents approximately 0.5% of all adult neoplasms in the United States, with approximately 6 cases per 100,000 men per year.[1] The majority of cases are germ cell tumors (GCT), divided into seminoma and nonseminomatous germ cell tumors (NSGCT). Testicular cancer is most common in young adults, with more than 50% of new cases occurring in men aged 20 to 34 years. During the last several decades, the incidence of testicular cancer has been increasing, particularly among Hispanic, Asian, and Pacific Islander populations in the United States.[2,3] Despite the increase in incidence, death from testicular cancer is fortunately rare. Prognosis is largely based on stage, with 5-year cancer specific survival of 99% for clinical stage (CS) I disease. In the era of cisplatin-based chemotherapy, even

patients with advanced disease have a favorable prognosis, with overall cure rates greater than 80%.[4–8] Given the overall excellent prognosis associated with this disease, emphasis has shifted to minimizing harms associated with the treatment and decreasing overtreatment of these otherwise young, healthy patients.

Biomarkers play a key role in a variety of clinical contexts for patients with testicular germ cell tumors (TGCT) to guide management with the goal of minimizing both overtreatment and undertreatment of the disease. The classic serum tumor markers (cSTMs) for GCT—α-fetoprotein (AFP), beta subunit of human chorionic gonadotropin (βhCG), and lactate dehydrogenase (LDH)—have been used for diagnosis, risk stratification before treatment, monitoring disease response throughout the course of treatment, and as a crucial component of surveillance. Unfortunately,

Funding: None.
a Department of Urology, Massachusetts General Hospital, Harvard Medical School, Boston, MA, USA;
b Center for Genitourinary Cancers, Massachusetts General Hospital Cancer Center, Boston, MA, USA;
c Cancer Program, The Broad Institute of MIT and Harvard, Cambridge, MA USA
* Corresponding author: Keyan Salari, MD, PhD, Department of Urology, Massachusetts General Hospital, 55 Fruit St, GRB-1106H, Boston, MA, 02114.
E-mail address: ksalari@mgh.harvard.edu

Urol Clin N Am 50 (2023) 133–143
https://doi.org/10.1016/j.ucl.2022.09.002
0094-0143/23/© 2022 Elsevier Inc. All rights reserved.

urologic.theclinics.com

Table 1
Summary of classic serum tumor markers characteristics

Marker	Half-Life (Days)	Marker Elevation Pattern				
		Pure Seminoma	Yolk Sac Tumor	Choriocarcinoma	Embryonal Carcinoma	Teratoma
AFP	5–7	-	+++	-	+/−	+/−
βhCG	1–3	+/−[a]	+/−	+++	+/−	-
LDH	4–5	+/−	+/−	+/−	+/−	+/−

+++, Marker nearly always positive and in high amount proportional to volume.
+/−, Marker may be elevated but not always.
-, Marker never or seldom elevated.
[a] Typically low-level elevation, <500 IU/L.

the overall sensitivity of these tumor markers is low and cSTMs are often negative in patients presenting with low-stage disease or histologic subtypes that do not overproduce these markers, such as seminoma and teratoma (**Table 1**). As such, these markers are often insufficient to establish a diagnosis or reliably monitor disease status,[9] prompting further investigations aimed at identifying novel biomarkers with superior performance characteristics. Imaging modalities such as high-frequency ultrasound, computed tomography scans, and magnetic resonance imaging provide complementary information for diagnosis, staging, and surveillance of testicular cancer but these are beyond the scope of this review. Here, we will focus our discussion on classic and emerging serum-based biomarkers for TGCT, including cSTMs, microRNA (miR), circulating tumor DNA (ctDNA), and circulating tumor cells (CTCs).

Classic Serum Tumor Markers

cSTMs, consisting of AFP, βhCG, and LDH, are pivotal in the diagnosis and management of TGCT along with physical examination and ultrasonography.[10] cSTMs became essential tools in the late 1970s.[11,12] Historically, cSTMs are drawn at diagnosis and following radical orchiectomy, as well as at regular intervals to monitor response to treatment. In addition, they are an integral part of surveillance protocols for patients with TGCT following completion of therapy to monitor for relapse.[10] A summary of patterns of elevation of cSTMs in various histologic subtypes of TGCT can be found in **Table 1**. The European Association of Urology recommends obtaining cSTMs preoperatively, postorchiectomy, and before the initiation of systemic treatment of metastatic disease.[5] Similarly, the American Urologic Association guidelines advise cSTM measurement at the time of diagnosis before the treatment of any patient with a mass suspicious for testicular cancer.

They further recommend that cSTMs should be repeated postorchiectomy at appropriate half-life time intervals following radical orchiectomy for staging and risk stratification.[4]

AFP is synthesized in the fetal yolk sac, liver, and intestine and serves as a major serum-binding protein.[9,13] Peak levels are reached around 12 to 14 weeks gestation and should begin to decrease after birth, with levels reducing below 15 ng/mL at 1 year of life.[13] The half-life of AFP is 5 to 7 days (see **Table 1**). Therefore, postorchiectomy, levels should normalize for most patients in approximately 1 month, or 4 to 5 half-lives, in the absence of residual or metastatic disease.[10,13] AFP first emerged in the 1970s as a biomarker for TGCT, where in a cohort of testicular and ovarian GCT patients, serum levels of AFP were noted to be elevated in all patients with active disease and correlated with disease activity.[14] The authors also reported an association between the amount of endodermal sinus/yolk sac components in the tumor and AFP levels because AFP was noted to be elevated in patients with ovarian tumors containing endodermal sinus tumor admixed with teratoma or embryonal tumor.[14] Further study exclusively in patients with TGCT confirmed that AFP can be elevated in yolk sac tumor and embryonal carcinoma but never elevated in pure choriocarcinoma or pure seminoma.[13] Historically, AFP is elevated in 50% to 70% of low-stage NSGCT and 60% to 80% of advanced NSGCT.[10] Although traditional teaching is that teratoma does not produce cSTMs, AFP can be mildly elevated in up to 20% to 25% of teratoma (see **Table 1**), possibly due to mucinous gland components or hepatoid differentiation.[9,13] AFP levels can be normal in patients with low-stage disease and has a sensitivity of only 13.6% for detecting TGCT if used in isolation.[15]

In addition to being elevated in the first year of life, there are several other conditions aside from TGCT that can result in elevated serum AFP.

Table 2 American Joint Committee on Cancer S-staging for testicular cancer			
	Classic Serum Tumor Markers		
S Level	LDH (U/L)	βhCG (IU/L)	AFP (ng/mL)
S0	Normal (N)	Normal	Normal
S1	<1.5×N	<5000	<1000
S2	1.5–10×N	5000–50,000	1000–10,000
S3	>10×N	>50,000	>10,000
Sx	Not available	Not available	Not available

Values based on postorchiectomy measurement of cSTMs after appropriate number of half-lives.
Abbreviation: N, normal.

Hepatocellular carcinoma, lung cancer, pancreatic cancer, gastric adenocarcinoma, benign liver disease, postoperative states after gastrointestinal or hepatic surgery and systemic cytotoxic drug treatment can all elevate AFP,[9,10] and therefore, one must consider these diagnoses as possible causes of false positives. Further, stable mild elevations of AFP have been observed in patients without active GCT and thus should be interpreted with caution.[16]

hCG is produced by some GCT as either an intact molecule (composed of both alpha and beta subunits) or the beta subunit alone. It is normally secreted by placental syncytiotrophoblasts and has a half-life of 24 to 36 hours (see **Table 1**).[9,13] Thus, βhCG levels are typically expected to normalize in less than 1 week after orchiectomy for stage I patients in the absence of residual or metastatic disease. Unlike AFP, in 15% to 20% of pure seminomas mild elevation of βhCG can be observed[9] but this is rarely greater than 500 IU/L.[13] More pronounced elevations occur in NSGCT, where 10% to 40% of low-stage NSGCT and 40% to 60% of advanced NSGCT will have elevated βhCG,[10,17] corresponding to a sensitivity of 37.3%.[15] The most marked elevation is seen with pure choriocarcinoma but moderate elevations can be seen in embryonal carcinoma and mixed GCT (see **Table 1**).

βhCG is a glycoprotein in the same family as LH, FSH, and TSH. All are heterodimers with an alpha and beta subunit and can be found in healthy men at low levels. In fact, βhCG levels increase in both men and women with age. In men, this is related to decreased testicular function with aging.[18] This natural increase can make βhCG difficult to interpret, especially when borderline. False elevation can also be seen with hypogonadism for similar reasons. The radioimmunoassay that is often used to detect βhCG cross reacts with LH and FSH due to common subunits. Therefore, the increase in LH with hypogonadism can cross react with the βhCG assay and result in a false positive. This should correct within 48 to 72 hours after administration of testosterone, and therefore, a testosterone suppression test can be used to resolve such ambiguous cases.[10,19,20] Notable sources of false-positive elevations of βhCG can also be seen with hepatocellular carcinoma, cholangiocarcinoma, pancreatic and gastrointestinal cancers, breast cancer, kidney cancer, and bladder cancer.[9,10] Finally, historical data have indicated that marijuana use may falsely elevate βhCG,[21] presumably related to the effects of cannabinoids on the hypothalamus-pituitary axis.[22] However, this claim has been refuted because it has not been reproducible in other cohorts.[23]

LDH is notoriously the least specific cSTM for GCT. LDH has 5 unique isoforms, with LDH isoform 1 (LDH1) being the biomarker utilized in testicular cancer. LDH catalyzes the interconversion between lactate and pyruvate and is released during cell death.[13] Von Eyban and colleagues[24] demonstrated the utility of LDH1 as a biomarker in 1988 when they reported that the majority of patients with TGCT had elevated LDH, with the highest elevation seen in stage III disease. Since that time, the elevation in LDH has been interpreted as an indicator of cell turnover and burden of disease,[9] with levels greater than 2000 U/L often indicating bulky disease. LDH should also be monitored after the initial therapy because an increase after the treatment can be indicative of recurrence.[13]

In a study by Dieckmann and colleagues, the authors reported sensitivities of the cSTMs both individually and in combination. Across all patients with TGCT, sensitivity of AFP was 15%, βhCG 38%, LDH 47%, and approximately 50% for all 3 markers combined. For seminoma, the sensitivity of AFP, βhCG, LDH, and the panel of all 3 was 2%, 30%, 28%, and 48%, respectively. For nonseminoma, AFP had a sensitivity 42%, bHCG 39%, and all 3 markers together had a sensitivity of 60%.[17]

cSTMs are used in all aspects of GCT management. At the time of diagnosis, the degree of cSTM elevation has been shown to be prognostic,[13] warranting the unique inclusion of serum biomarkers in the AJCC staging system for TGCT (ie, TNMS staging; **Table 2**). Further, cSTMs play an integral role in the International Germ Cell Cancer Collaborative Group (IGCCCG) risk stratification system in conjunction with other clinical factors to determine prognosis and chemotherapy course.[6–8] First

Table 3
International germ cell cancer collaborative group risk classification

Risk Group	Definition		Original (1997)				Update (2021)[a]			
	Seminoma	Nonseminoma	Seminoma		Nonseminoma		Seminoma		Nonseminoma	
			5 y PFS (%)	5 y OS (%)	5 y PFS (%)	5 y OS (%)	5 y PFS (%)	5 y OS (%)	5 y PFS (%)	5 y OS (%)
Good[a]	Any primary site and No NPVM and Normal AFP, any βhCG, any LDH	Testis/RP primary and no NPVM and S0/S1	82	86	89	92	89	95	90	96
Intermediate	Any primary site and +NPVM and Normal AFP, any βhCG, any LDH	Testis/RP primary and no NPVM and S2	67	72	75	80	79	88	78	89
Poor	–	Mediastinal primary or +NPVM or S3	–	–	41	48	–	–	54	67

cSTMs drawn postorchiectomy.

Abbreviations: NPVM, nonpulmonary visceral metastasis; RP, retroperitoneum.

[a] 2021 IGCCCG update identified LDH as an additional, independent prognostic factor and utilized an updated cutoff for LDH in risk stratification system (ie, >2.5×N and <2.5×N in otherwise good-risk patients).

published in 1997,[6] and recently updated in 2021,[7,8] the IGCCCG risk groups describe the adverse factors associated with prognosis in advanced GCT. In the initial study of more than 5000 men with seminoma and NSGCT, the degree of cSTM elevation, mediastinal primary site, and presence of nonpulmonary visceral metastasis were all independently associated with overall survival (OS) and progression free survival (PFS) in patients with NSGCT. For patients with seminoma, only presence of nonpulmonary visceral metastasis was associated with prognosis. Using these risk factors, patients were categorized into good-risk, intermediate-risk, and poor-risk NSGCT and good-risk and intermediate-risk seminoma (Table 3). Of note, a poor-risk group does not exist for seminoma, reflecting its overall more favorable prognosis compared with NSGCT.[6] The IGCCCG risk groups were updated in 2021, including a change in the LDH cutoff to 2.5 times the upper limit of normal as well as updated estimates of PFS and OS, likely reflecting improvements in guideline-directed patient care over the past several decades (see Table 3).[7,8]

After diagnosis, serial measurements of cSTMs are followed during and after treatment to monitor response. In the absence of residual disease, cSTMs normalize according to half-life, and this expected decline may have prognostic implications. In a study from Memorial Sloan Kettering Cancer Center in 1990, the authors found that cSTMs decline in keeping with marker half-lives was associated with longer median OS as well as higher complete response rate (89% vs 29% with and without an appropriate decline, respectively).[25] In multivariable analysis, prolonged time of STM decline was the most significant independent predictor of OS. Based on this study, prolonged marker decline may indicate a higher risk for treatment failure. In addition, it is important to note that a longer delay between treatment and cSTMs decline can be seen with radiation or chemotherapy compared with surgery.[25]

There are several important caveats pertaining to cSTMs. First, although pure seminoma and teratoma classically do not produce elevated cSTMs, approximately 15% to 20% of pure seminoma will produce mildly elevated βhCG levels (rarely greater than 500 IU/L) and mild cSTM elevation can occasionally be observed in pure teratoma (see Table 1).[9,13] In addition, due to false positives and false negatives, interpretation of cSTM levels should incorporate the whole clinical context of the patient to ensure spurious cSTM results do not drive management decisions. For example, low levels of cSTMs have been found among patients on surveillance after testicular

cancer treatment that are not necessarily associated with residual or active disease.[9,16] In a multicenter study from 2017, 10 patients (out of 593 examined) had a mildly elevated AFP following treatment, defined as an AFP above normal but less than 30 ng/mL.[16] Among these patients, only 20% had documented disease recurrence over a median period of 42 months. These patients did receive additional chemotherapy in response to the elevation but had unchanged, mildly elevated AFP levels after treatment. An additional patient with mildly elevated AFP underwent retroperitoneal lymph node dissection (RPLND), and pathology demonstrated no active tumor. With further investigation, a definitive cause was never found in any of these patients for this subclinical elevation, which remained stable over the study duration period. The authors concluded that mildly elevated and stable AFP in the absence of any other clinical evidence of active disease can be safely monitored.[16] Ideally, these patients should be managed with surveillance to avoid the unnecessary harms of treatment. One occasional potential source of a mild stable elevation of cSTMs may be heterophile antibodies interfering with the laboratory immunoassay. This phenomenon has been described specifically with βhCG and is known to potentially occur with other immunoassays as well.[26,27]

Although cSTMs are essential for the management of testicular cancer, the aforementioned limitations of low sensitivity (particularly in seminoma and teratoma) and false-positive elevations represent an unmet clinical need in TGCT detection and surveillance driving ongoing biomarker discovery and development efforts.

MicroRNA

Starting in the 1990s, miR have been investigated as novel biomarkers in a variety of malignancies and first emerged as a promising biomarker for TGCT in 2011.[28] miR are noncoding, small, single-stranded RNA molecules consisting of approximately 20 base pairs.[9,15,17] They are responsible for regulating the expression of approximately one-third of human genes influencing cell cycle, development, proliferation, apoptosis, and differentiation. They have been found to be altered in many conditions, with differing patterns in benign versus malignant disease.[15] Although the human genome expresses more than 900 miR, only 31 are expressed by stem cells,[29] narrowing the search for miR relevant for TGCT.

miR were initially detected in tumor tissue specimens and subsequently found to be detectable in

Table 4
Performance characteristics of miR371a-3p for detection of testicular germ cell tumor

Primary Diagnosis

Study	Cohort	Sensitivity	Specificity	PPV	NPV	AUC
Syring et al,15 2015	All GCT	85	99	—	—	0.929
van Agthoven et al,35 2017	All GCT	90	91	94	79	0.962
Dieckmann et al,37 2019	All GCT	90	94	97	83	0.966
	Seminoma	90	96	—	—	—
	Nonseminoma	95	96	—	—	—
Pre-RPLND						
Lafin et al,31 2020	Chemotherapy Naïve	100	92	—	—	0.965
Leão et al,32 2018	Postchemotherapy	100	54	—	—	0.874

the serum and other extracellular fluids of TGCT patients.[15,17] In the first report of miR expression in testis tumor tissue, 2 miR, miR-372a-3p, and miR-373a-3p, were found to be abundantly expressed in GCT cell lines, and LATS2, a negative regulator of the cell cycle, was determined to be the most likely target of these miR.[30] Accordingly, these miR can promote the transition from G1 to S phase of the cell cycle, presumably leading to replication and tumor growth. After their discovery in GCT tissue samples, miR were detected in extracellular fluid and found to be stable in a variety of environments. Whereas serum messenger RNA is quickly degraded, miR are often protected by a protein complex that preserves RNA integrity and prevents degradation,[15,17] rendering them appealing as potential biomarkers in TGCT patients.

With further investigation, miR-367-3p, miR-371a-3p, and miR-373-3p were found to be increased in GCT compared with both healthy controls and men with nonmalignant testicular disorders. miR-371a-3p was found to have the highest sensitivity and specificity, 84.7% and 99%, respectively, with an area under the curve (AUC) of 0.929.[15] Across most (primarily retrospective) studies, miR-371a-3p has emerged as the most sensitive and specific miR for TGCT,[9,15,17,29,31–35] with equal or improved performance characteristics compared with a panel consisting of several miR. Findings have been consistent across studies, with sensitivities ranging 84% to 100% and specificity 91% to 100% (**Table 4**).[9,15,17,29,31–33,35,]36,37 In 2017, Dieckmann and colleagues17 published the first prospective study evaluating a panel of 4 miR and miR-371a-3p alone. The authors found equal performance characteristics between the miR panel and miR-371a-3p alone and in a subsequent prospective validation study confirmed miR-371a-3p to have a sensitivity and specificity of 90.1% and

94%, respectively37. Notably, the performance of the miR was higher than that of all 3 cSTMs combined.

Beyond distinguishing benign from malignant disease, differences in miR expression have been identified based on histologic subtype and disease stage. Levels of miR expression have been shown to be lower in seminoma compared with NSGCT, consistent with prior data demonstrating an inverse relationship between the degree of tumor differentiation and miR expression levels.[37] As a result, teratoma and seminoma have the lowest levels of miR expression, and embryonal carcinoma tends to have the highest.[17] A strong correlation between miR expression and both disease activity and tumor burden has also been reported. miR expression correlates with primary tumor size, is higher in metastatic versus localized disease, and decreases rapidly in response to therapy,[37] with a half-life of less than 24 hours.[9] In addition, patients with relapse demonstrate an increase in this biomarker, with a sensitivity and specificity of 82.6% and 96.1%, respectively.[37]

miR has now been studied in a variety of clinical contexts for TGCT patients. Due to the superior performance characteristics compared with cSTMs, miR could be potentially helpful in controversial clinical situations where treatment decisions are less certain. For example, miR might help predict the presence of microscopic metastatic disease in low-stage patients and guide decisions regarding adjuvant therapy versus surveillance. Another context in which the greater sensitivity of miR might prove useful is in patients with advanced disease with a residual mass after chemotherapy. Nappi and colleagues[29] investigated the role of miR-371a-3p in postorchiectomy patients with diagnosed seminoma or NSGCT. Patients were classified from low to high risk of relapse based on various clinical characteristics. The more challenging clinical scenarios mentioned above were captured primarily by their "moderate risk" group. This included patients with CS IB NSGCT with no suspicious imaging findings or elevation in cSTMs, CS I seminoma, or NSGCT with either suspicious imaging findings or indeterminate elevation in cSTMs and patients with a postchemotherapy residual mass with indeterminate cSTMs. Although this moderate risk group is heterogenous, miR-371a-3p performed favorably in this cohort, with a specificity of 100% and sensitivity of 92%, which was better than cSTMs in these challenging clinical contexts. In their low-risk group, specificity and sensitivity were both 100%. In the high-risk group, specificity and sensitivity were 100% and 97%, respectively.[29] Further study reporting performance characteristics of miR in each of these clinical contexts is warranted.

Lafin and colleagues[31] prospectively evaluated the performance characteristics of serum miR levels in predicting the presence of viable GCT among chemotherapy-naïve patients with CS I-II GCT undergoing primary RPLND. In addition to the conventional panel of 4 miR (including miR-371a-3p) for the detection of GCT, miR-375 was also evaluated in this study given a recent report indicating high expression in teratoma tissue.[38] Using RPLND pathologic condition as the reference, the authors found miR-371a-3p to be the most discriminatory miR for viable GCT compared with either benign or teratoma, with 100% sensitivity and 92% specificity corresponding to an AUC of 0.965 for detecting viable GCT in the retroperitoneum (see **Table 4**). However, none of the miR, including miR-375, was associated with the presence of pure teratoma.[31] Similarly, in a study of advanced NSGCT patients undergoing postchemotherapy RPLND, Leao and colleagues[32] found that postchemotherapy (pre-RPLND) miR-371a-3p levels predicted viable GCT but not teratoma in the retroperitoneum. Using a hypothetical cutoff of less than 3 cm for postchemotherapy residual masses to consider miR positivity to guide surgical intervention, miR-371a-3p demonstrated a sensitivity of 100% and specificity of 54% in detecting viable residual GCT (see **Table 4**). The authors concluded that serum miR-371a-3p is highly predictive of viable GCT in the retroperitoneum and proposed an algorithm in which postchemotherapy masses less than 3 cm are observed in the setting of a negative miR signature, whereas masses greater than 3 cm or rapidly growing are recommended to undergo RPLND regardless of miR signature due to the higher risk of teratoma.[32] These findings warrant prospective validation in future studies.

Mego and colleagues[33] retrospectively analyzed the utility of miR3-71a-3p in chemotherapy-naïve patients before the initiation of therapy. Of note, this included CS I patients undergoing adjuvant chemotherapy after orchiectomy. Pretreatment miR-371a-3p expression was found to be associated with IGCCCG risk group, number of metastatic sites, presence of retroperitoneal, mediastinal, and pulmonary lymphadenopathy, and S stage. This held true for miR as both a continuous and dichotomous variable. miR levels were correlated with improved PFS and OS on univariate analysis but using multivariable analysis, miR was not predictive of PFS or OS independent of IGCCCG risk category.[33]

Although promising as a sensitive and specific biomarker for nonteratomatous GCT, the current miR under study is limited by their inability to detect teratoma. Most miR (including miR-371a-3p) are not significantly differentially expressed in teratoma compared with healthy controls or patients with nonmalignant testicular disease.[9,17,31,35,39,40] This limits the utility of miR in the postchemotherapy residual mass setting, as up to 40% of these patients harbor teratoma.[32] Notably, miR-375 was recently reported to be highly expressed in teratoma and yolk sac tumor tissue (but poorly expressed in seminoma and embryonal carcinoma), leading to the hypothesis that miR-375 alone or in combination with miR-371a-3p might be useful for detecting patients with teratoma.[38] To address this question, Nappi and colleagues[41] recently conducted a prospective, multi-institutional study of 100 GCT patients divided in 2 cohorts of patients. The discovery cohort consisted of patients with pathologically confirmed teratoma before RPLND and patients with no/low risk of harboring teratoma (CSI GCT patients on surveillance after orchiectomy with no evidence of relapse and metastatic seminoma patients before chemotherapy). The validation cohort consisted of metastatic postchemotherapy patients with NSGCT with residual masses greater than 1 cm after chemotherapy or radiologic complete response. In the discovery cohort, the AUC for detecting teratoma for miR-375, miR-371, and combined miR-375 + 371 was 0.93, 0.59, and 0.95, respectively. In the validation cohort, the AUC significantly dropped to 0.55, 0.74, and 0.77 for miR-375, miR-371, and miR-375 + 371, respectively. Although the authors concluded that the combination of miR-371a-3p and miR-375 is a promising predictor of teratoma and may be particularly useful for identifying teratoma in the postchemotherapy setting, the lower performance in the validation cohort as well as other studies refuting an association between miR-375 and teratoma raises concerns about reproducibility of this finding across cohorts with differing patient characteristics and/or clinical settings.[31,42]

Finally, Lobo and colleagues[39] investigated the combination of miR-371 with hypermethylated RASSF1A. RASSF1A is frequently inactivated in other malignancies and was demonstrated to be inactive and hypermethylated in TGCT as well as Sertoli and Leydig cell tumors.[43] Blood samples collected from patients before radical orchiectomy were compared with healthy controls using a droplet digital PCR assay to detect hypermethylated RASSF1A. Levels of miR-371a-3p and hypermethylated RASSF1A were correlated with pathologic findings, and hypermethylated RASSF1A performed essentially equivalent to miR-371a-3p for seminoma and NSGCT but had superior detection of teratoma and GCNIS, detecting 88.9% and 100%, respectively. The combination of miR-371a-3p and hypermethylated RASSF1A exhibited improved detection of teratoma compared with cSTMs,[39] suggesting possible clinical utility that warrants further prospective validation.

miR represents promising biomarkers for TGCT in various clinical contexts. The majority of the existing data is retrospective and must be prospectively validated before adopting into clinical use. The primary limitation of the current miR under investigation is the detection of teratoma, which precludes their use in the postchemotherapy residual mass setting. Two clinical trials investigating the utility of miR in TGCT are underway. AGCT 1531 is investigating the role of active surveillance versus chemotherapy in patients with GCTs and incorporates a panel of 4 miR[44]; SWOG-S1823 aims to determine the positive predictive value of miR-371a-3p in determining the risk of relapse in early-stage seminoma and NSGCT.[45] Results of these trials may help to define the future role of miR in TGCT.

Circulating Tumor DNA

ctDNA has evolved into a useful biomarker for the detection and monitoring of a variety of malignancies but is currently in its early stages of investigation as a possible biomarker for TGCT. ctDNA are double-stranded segments of 150 to 200 nucleotides that are released into the bloodstream during apoptosis or necrosis.[9,46] Using PCR-based techniques, ctDNA can be isolated and quantified. In 2009, Ellinger and colleagues demonstrated that patients with both seminoma and NSGCT have higher absolute ctDNA content compared with healthy controls. ctDNA levels differentiated TGCT patients from controls with a sensitivity of 88% and specificity of 97%. Importantly, this cohort also included patients in whom cSTMs were negative. Levels of ctDNA were proportional to disease stage (stage III with increased ctDNA compared with stages I and II) and was associated with disease activity; ctDNA increased with progression and decreased in response to treatment. These data indicate that ctDNA may be a useful biomarker for GCT with the potential to improve clinical management of patients with testicular cancer.[46]

Circulating mitochondrial DNA (mDNA) has also been investigated as a possible biomarker because this too is elevated in patients with TGCT. In comparison with ctDNA, mDNA may be more useful given that there are hundreds of copies in each cell.[9,47] In one study of TGCT patients, mDNA levels were higher in TGCT patients compared with healthy individuals, with 94.3% and 59.5% specificity and sensitivity, respectively.[48]

Among emerging biomarkers in TGCT, ctDNA has the potential for clinical utility based on early studies. However, it currently remains an investigational biomarker and requires further study to determine whether it will prove useful for TGCT clinical management.

Circulating Tumor Cells

In addition to ctDNA, investigators are studying the role of CTCs as a biomarker for testicular GCT. CTCs are a subset of cells that can be found in serum of patients with solid tumors and have the potential to seed metastatic sites of disease.[49] Initial studies in GCT have used a variety of protein markers to identify CTCs—alkaline phosphatase, AFP, hCG, endodermal growth factor receptor, and combinations of these—but have demonstrated an overall low sensitivity (<60%) for detecting CTCs.[50–52] In addition, when detected, CTCs have not always been associated with tumor burden.[9] Another recent study detected CTCs in 11.5% to 17.5% of GCT patients.[53] However, when stratified by disease burden, a higher proportion of metastatic patients (41%) had detectable CTCs. In addition, all patients with cisplatin resistant or relapsed disease had detectable CTCs.[53] Notably, CTCs have been reported to be more commonly detected in NSGCT including teratoma, which could help to fill the current biomarker gap in the detection of this histologic subtype.[9] Currently, studies report many technical challenges, mainly with isolation and detection of CTCs, which has thus far limited clinical translation.[9]

Similar to ctDNA, CTCs represent an area in need of further investigation regarding their candidacy as a biomarker in TGCT. With improvements in our capability to identify and detect these cells, further research can be performed regarding their role in diagnosis and management of TGCT.

SUMMARY

For decades, cSTMs have been a cornerstone of the diagnosis, prognostication, and surveillance of patients with TGCT.[4,5,10] However, the sensitivity of AFP, βhCG, and LDH is limited, and these markers are often negative in seminoma, teratoma, as well as low-stage disease. Emerging biomarkers including miR, ctDNA, and CTCs may help us refine our management of patients with testicular cancer across the disease spectrum. miR371a-3p has thus far proven to be the most sensitive and specific of these novel biomarkers, with the caveat that it is insensitive to teratoma. miR-375 may be promising in this regard, as well as other emerging biomarkers such as ctDNA and CTCs. Prospective validation of these novel biomarkers is urgently needed before widespread clinical use can be adopted, but the existing data thus far suggests that new biomarkers—miR in particular—are likely to become an essential component in the management of patients with TGCT.

CLINICS CARE POINTS

- cSTMs (AFP, βhCG, LDH) remain critically important in the diagnosis, prognostication, and surveillance of patients with TGCT
- cSTMs are limited by low sensitivity (40%–60%) for the initial diagnosis of TGCT and are often negative in low-stage disease, pure seminoma, and teratoma
- miRNA are emerging serum biomarkers in TGCT, with miR-371a-3p in particular demonstrating the most favorable performance data compared with cSTMs
- Current miRNA are unable to detect teratoma, which remains an elusive histology for biomarker discovery
- ctDNA and CTCs are 2 additional emerging biomarkers but further study is needed to determine their future role in TGCT

DISCLOSURES

The authors have no relevant conflicts of interest to disclose.

REFERENCES

1. A Phase 3 Study of Active Surveillance for Low Risk and a Randomized Trial of Carboplatin vs. Cisplatin for Standard Risk Pediatric and Adult Patients With Germ Cell Tumors. Available at: https://clinicaltrials.gov/ct2/show/NCT03067181.
2. Nigam M, Aschebrook-Kilfoy B, Shikanov S, et al. Increasing incidence of testicular cancer in the United States and Europe between 1992 and 2009. World J Urol 2015;33(5):623–31.
3. Ghazarian AA, McGlynn KA. Increasing incidence of testicular germ cell tumors among racial/ethnic minorities in the United States. Cancer Epidemiol Biomarkers Prev 2020;29(6):1237–45.
4. Stephenson A, Eggener SE, Bass EB, et al. Diagnosis and treatment of early stage testicular cancer: AUA guideline. J Urol 2019;202(2):272–81.
5. Honecker F, Aparicio J, Berney D, et al. ESMO consensus conference on testicular germ cell cancer: Diagnosis, treatment and follow-up. Ann Oncol 2018;29(8):1658–86.
6. Mead GM. International germ cell consensus classification: a prognostic factor- based staging system for metastatic germ cell cancers. J Clin Oncol 1997;15(2):594–603.
7. Gillessen S, Sauvé N, Collette L, et al. Predicting outcomes in men with metastatic nonseminomatous germ cell tumors (NSGCT): Results from the IGCCCG update consortium. J Clin Oncol 2021;39(14):1563–74.
8. Beyer J, Collette L, Sauvé N, et al. Survival and new prognosticators in metastatic seminoma: Results from the IGCCCG-update consortium. J Clin Oncol 2021;39(14):1553–62.
9. Lobo J, Leão R, Jerónimo C, et al. Liquid biopsies in the clinical management of germ cell tumor patients: State-of-the-art and future directions. Int J Mol Sci 2021;22(5):1–22.
10. Wein Alan J, Kavoussi Louis R, Partin Alan W, et al. Campbell-walsh urology. 10th ed. Philadelphia, PA: Elsevier Saunders; 2016.
11. Javadpour N. The role of biologic tumor markers in testicular cancer. Cancer 1980;45(Suppl 7):1755–61.
12. Lange PH, Winfield HN. Biological markers in urologic cancer. Cancer 1987;60(3 Suppl):464–72.
13. Milose JC, Filson CP, Weizer AZ, et al. Role of biochemical markers in testicular cancer: diagnosis, staging, and surveillance. Open Access J Urol 2011;4:1–8.

14. Talerman A, Haije WG, Baggerman L. Alpha-1 anti-trypsin (AAT) and alphafoetoprotein (AFP) in sera of patients with germ-cell neoplasms: Value as tumour markers in patients with endodermal sinus tumour (yolk sac tumour). Int J Cancer 1977;19(6):741–6.

15. Syring I, Bartels J, Holdenrieder S, et al. Circulating Serum miRNA (miR-367-3p, miR-371a-3p, miR-372-3p and miR-373-3p) as Biomarkers in Patients with Testicular Germ Cell Cancer. J Urol 2015;193(1):331–7.

16. Wymer KM, Daneshmand S, Pierorazio PM, et al. Mildly elevated serum alpha-fetoprotein (AFP) among patients with testicular cancer may not be associated with residual cancer or need for treatment. Ann Oncol 2017;28(4):899–902.

17. Dieckmann KP, Radtke A, Spiekermann M, et al. Serum Levels of MicroRNA miR-371a-3p: a sensitive and specific new biomarker for germ cell tumours. Eur Urol 2017;71(2):213–20.

18. Stenman UH, Alfthan H, Hotakainen K. Human chorionic gonadotropin in cancer. Clin Biochem 2004;37(7):549–61.

19. Germa JR, Arcusa A, Casamitjana R. False elevations of human chorionic gonadotropin associated to Iatrogenic hypogonadism in gonadal germ cell tumors. Cancer 1987;60(10):2489–93.

20. Catalona WJ, Vaitukaitis JL, Fair WR. Falsely positive specific human chorionic gonadotropin assays in patients with testicular tumors: Conversion to negative with testosterone administration. J Urol 1979;122(1):126–8.

21. Garnick MB. Spurious rise in human chorionic gonadotropin induced by marihuana in patients with testicular cancer. N Engl J Med 1980;303(20):1177.

22. Harclerode J. Endocrine effects of marijuana in the male: preclinical studies. NIDA Res Monogr 1984;44:46–64.

23. Braunstein GD, Thompson R, Gross S, et al. Marijuana use does not spuriously elevate serum human chorionic gonadotropin levels. Urology 1985;25(6):605–6.

24. Von Eyben FE, Blaabjerg O, Petersen PH, et al. Serum lactate dehydrogenase isoenzyme 1 as a marker of testicular germ cell tumor. J Urol 1988;140(5 PART I):986–9.

25. Toner GC, Geller NL, Tan C, et al. Serum tumor marker half-life during chemotherapy allows early prediction of complete response and survival in non-seminomatous germ cell tumors. Cancer Res 1990;50(18):5904–10.

26. Soares DG, Millot F, Lacroix I, et al. Heterophile Antibody Interference led to Unneeded Chemotherapy in a Testicular Cancer Patient. Urol Case Reports 2016;9:1–3.

27. Bolstad N, Warren DJ, Nustad K. Heterophilic antibody interference in immunometric assays. Best Pract Res Clin Endocrinol Metab 2013;27(5):647–61.

28. Murray MJ, Halsall DJ, Hook CE, et al. Identification of microRNAs From the miR-371~373 and miR-302 clusters as potential serum biomarkers of malignant germ cell tumors. Am J Clin Pathol 2011;135(1):119–25.

29. Nappi L, Thi M, Lum A, et al. Developing a highly specific biomarker for germ cell malignancies: Plasma MiR371 expression across the germ cell malignancy spectrum. J Clin Oncol 2019;37(33):3090–8.

30. Voorhoeve PM, le Sage C, Schrier M, et al. A genetic screen implicates miRNA-372 and miRNA-373 as oncogenes in testicular germ cell tumors. Adv Exp Med Biol 2007;604:17–46.

31. Lafin JT, Singla N, Woldu SL, et al. Serum MicroRNA-371a-3p levels predict viable germ cell tumor in chemotherapy-naïve patients undergoing retroperitoneal lymph node dissection. Eur Urol 2020;77(2):290–2.

32. Leão R, van Agthoven T, Figueiredo A, et al. Serum miRNA predicts viable disease after chemotherapy in patients with testicular nonseminoma germ cell tumor. J Urol 2018;200(1):126–35.

33. Mego M, van Agthoven T, Gronesova P, et al. Clinical utility of plasma miR-371a-3p in germ cell tumors. J Cell Mol Med 2019;23(2):1128–36.

34. Abol-Enein H, Ghoneim MA. Functional results of orthotopic ileal neobladder with serous-lined extramural ureteral reimplantation: experience with 450 patients. J Urol 2001;165(5):1427–32.

35. van Agthoven T, Looijenga LHJ. Accurate primary germ cell cancer diagnosis using serum based microRNA detection (ampTSmiR test). Oncotarget 2017;8(35):58037–49.

36. Dieckmann KP, Spiekermann M, Balks T, et al. MicroRNAs miR-371-3 in serum as diagnostic tools in the management of testicular germ cell tumours. Br J Cancer 2012;107(10):1754–60.

37. Dieckmann KP, Radtke A, Geczi L, et al. Serum Levels of MicroRNA-371a-3p (M371 Test) as a new biomarker of testicular germ cell tumors: Results of a prospective multicentric study. J Clin Oncol 2019;37(16):1412–23.

38. Shen H, Shih J, Hollern DP, et al. Integrated molecular characterization of testicular germ cell tumors. Cell Rep 2018;23(11):3392–406.

39. Lobo J, van Zogchel LMJ, Nuru MG, et al. Combining hypermethylated rassf1a detection using ddpcr with mir-371a-3p testing: an improved panel of liquid biopsy biomarkers for testicular germ cell tumor patients. Cancers (Basel) 2021;13(20):1–15.

40. Chovanec M, Albany C, Mego M, et al. Emerging prognostic biomarkers in testicular germ cell tumors:

Looking beyond established practice. Front Oncol 2018;8(NOV):1–7.

41. Nappi L, Thi M, Adra N, et al. Integrated expression of circulating miR375 and miR371 to identify teratoma and active germ cell malignancy components in malignant germ cell tumors. Eur Urol 2021;79(1): 16–9.

42. Belge G, Grobelny F, Radtke A, et al. Serum levels of microRNA-371a-3p are not elevated in testicular tumours of non-germ cell origin. J Cancer Res Clin Oncol 2021;147(2):435–43.

43. Agathanggelou A, Cooper WN, Latif F. Role of the Ras-association domain family 1 tumor suppressor gene in human cancers. Cancer Res 2005;65(9): 3497–508.

44. A Phase 3 Study of Active Surveillance for Low Risk and a Randomized Trial of Carboplatin vs. Cisplatin for Standard Risk Pediatric and Adult Patients With Germ Cell Tumors. Available at: https://clinicaltrials.gov/ct2/show/NCT03067181.

45. NCT04435756. A Study of miRNA 371 in Patients With Germ Cell Tumors. Available at: https://clinicaltrials.gov/ct2/show/NCT04435756.

46. Ellinger J, Wittkamp V, Albers P, et al. Cell-Free Circulating DNA: diagnostic value in patients with testicular germ cell cancer. J Urol 2009;181(1): 363–71.

47. Afrifa J, Zhao T, Yu J. Circulating mitochondria DNA, a non-invasive cancer diagnostic biomarker candidate. Mitochondrion 2019;47:238–43.

48. Ellinger J, Albers P, Müller SC, et al. Circulating mitochondrial DNA in the serum of patients with testicular germ cell cancer as a novel noninvasive diagnostic biomarker. BJU Int 2009;104(1):48–52.

49. Yang C, Xia BR, Jin WL, et al. Circulating tumor cells in precision oncology: clinical applications in liquid biopsy and 3D organoid model. Cancer Cell Int 2019;19(1):1–13.

50. Hildebrandt M, Bläser F, Beyer J, et al. Detection of tumor cells in peripheral blood samples from patients with germ cell tumors using immunocytochemical and reverse transcriptase-polymerase chain reaction techniques. Bone Marrow Transpl 1998; 22(8):771–5.

51. Yuasa T, Yoshiki T, Tanaka T, et al. Detection of circulating testicular cancer cells in peripheral blood. Cancer Lett 1999;143(1):57–62.

52. Hautkappe AL, Lu M, Mueller H, et al. Detection of germ-cell tumor cells in the peripheral blood by nested reverse transcription-polymerase chain reaction for alpha-fetoprotein-messenger RNA and beta human chorionic gonadotropin-messenger RNA. Cancer Res 2000;60(12):3170–4.

53. Nastały P, Honecker F, Pantel K, et al. Detection of circulating tumor cells (CTCs) in patients with testicular germ cell tumors. Methods Mol Biol 2021;2195: 245–61.

The Evolving Landscape of Viral, Immune, and Molecular Biomarkers in Penile Cancer

Alice Yu, MD, MPH[a], Jad Chahoud, MD, MPH[a], Andrea Necchi, MD[b], Philippe E. Spiess, MD, MS, FRCS(C)[a],*

KEYWORDS

- Penile cancer • Biomarkers • Targeted therapy • Immunotherapy • HPV

KEY POINTS

- HPV is an important risk factor for penile cancer and HPV-specific targeted therapies is an area of active investigation.
- Several HPV-independent pathways have been identified, and some of these have investigational or approved targeted agents.
- Tumor mutational burden is a potential biomarker for improved response to immune checkpoint inhibitors.Scientific collaboration is essential to developing targeted therapies in patients with advanced penile cancer.

INTRODUCTION

Penile cancer is relatively rare in North America and Europe (<1% of all malignant neoplasms); however, it remains a significant health concern with a higher propensity of cases in many African, South American, and Asian countries.[1] It occurs primarily in older men with a peak incidence in the 6th decade of life.[2] The etiology of penile cancer is multifactorial and there are many risk factors including lack of neonatal circumcision, chronic inflammation, lichen sclerosis, tobacco use, obesity, poor hygiene, exposure to ultraviolet radiation, history of sexually transmitted diseases, and human papillomavirus (HPV) infection.[1,3] Pathogenesis of penile squamous cell carcinoma (PSCC) can be broadly dichotomized into HPV related and non–HPV-related pathways which will be discussed in detail in this review.

Penile cancer can be an aggressive disease and in advanced or metastatic cases, few options exist once patients progress after cisplatin-based treatments. The recent revolution in immunotherapy hold promises in expanding treatment options; however, further research in molecular biomarkers is needed to improve the personalization of care. In this review, we examined the current understanding of the pathogenesis of PSCC and reviewed novel biomarkers that can be explored in targeted therapy development.

HUMAN PAPILLOMAVIRUS-DEPENDENT PATHWAYS
Carcinogenesis

One of the most well-known risk factors for penile cancer is HPV infection which is linked to a variety of conditions such as cervical, penile, and oropharyngeal malignancies as well as benign diseases such as condyloma acuminata or genital warts. There are more than 100 different known HPV genotypes; however, only 20 have been shown to affect the genital tract.[4] HPV types 16, 18, 31, 33, 45, 56, and 65 are considered high risk due to their association with penile cancer, whereas

[a] Department of Genitourinary Oncology, H. Lee Moffitt Cancer Center & Research Institute, 12902 Magnolia Drive, Tampa, FL 33612, USA; [b] Department of Genitourinary Oncology, Vita-Salute San Raffaele University, Via Olgettina 60, 20132 Milan, Italy
* Corresponding author. Philippe E. Spiess. 12902 Magnolia Drive, Tampa, FL 33612.
E-mail address: philippe.spiess@moffitt.org

Urol Clin N Am 50 (2023) 145–150
https://doi.org/10.1016/j.ucl.2022.09.013

types 6 and 11 are known to be low risk for malignant transformation.[5]

HPV infection is prevalent in penile cancer, and the presence of HPV can be found in 20% to 70% of tumors.[6,7] This variation may be due to differences in sampling techniques, genital sites sampled, and populations studied.[8] Rates of infection also vary depending on histologic subtype. Basaloid and warty carcinomas are more consistently associated with HPV infection, suggesting that distinct pathogenic pathways may drive tumorigenesis.[7]

The pathogenetic mechanisms of HPV tumorigenesis is complex (**Fig. 1**). HPV encodes the E5, E6, and E7 oncogenes; however, only E6 and E7 are necessary for malignant transformation.[9] The activation of viral E5 oncogene may indirectly contribute to carcinogenesis by manipulating viral uptake in host target cells. The E5 gene product is a transmembrane protein that regulates the activation of epidermal growth factor receptor (EGFR) which subsequently leads to an increase in uncontrolled cell growth and cell migration.[10]

Viral oncogenes E6 and E7 are actively transcribed in HPV-infected cells and contribute to carcinogenesis by disrupting centrosome synthesis required for mitosis.[5] Specifically, viral E6 oncoprotein targets the p53 tumor suppressor protein which plays an important role in controlling cell proliferation and growth arrest. Thus, E6 binding and inactivation of p53 leads to the downstream effect of uncontrolled cellular growth.[11] Likewise, E7 oncoprotein activity on the tumor suppressor retinoblastoma-1 (RB1) gene blocks the feedback inhibition on p16(INK4a), resulting in an unregulated cell cycle and uncontrolled cell proliferation.[12]

It is important to note that some HPV-negative penile cancers have been linked to p53 and RB1 pathway disruptions as well (**Fig. 2**). Inactivation of p16(INK4a)[12] or p53[13] have been observed in HPV-negative cases, suggesting that carcinogenesis likely resulted from alternative genetic damage that disrupts similar targets.

Human Papillomavirus Prognosis

While HPV is an important risk factor for penile cancer, its role in disease prognosis is unclear. Some studies have linked HPV infection with positive clinical outcomes. In a cohort of 212 patients, the 5-year disease-free survival (DFS) in patients with HPV infection was 96% compared to 82% in the HPV negative group (P = 0.016).[14] Even after adjusting for pathological stage, tumor grade, lymphovascular invasion and age, HPV was an independent prognostic factor for DFS (HR 0.2, 95% CI 0.1–0.9, P = 0.03). Similarly, another cohort of 171 patients found improved 5-year survival in patients with HPV positive (92% vs 78%, P = 0.03).[15] Conversely, this effect was not seen in several other studies which have demonstrated no association between HPV and lymph node metastasis or 10-year survival rates.[16–18]

Targeted Therapies

HPV-specific targeted therapies are an area of active investigation. Due to the rarity of this disease,

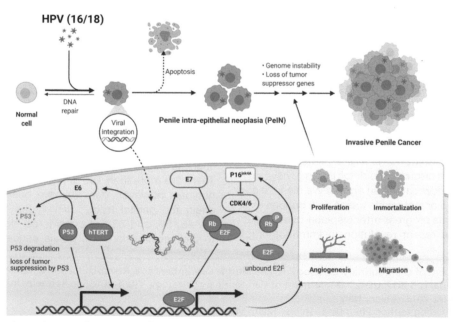

Fig. 1. HPV-dependent penile cancer pathogenesis. (*From* Vos G, et al. Chapter: Mechanism of Carcinogenesis and Progression. "Penile Carcinoma: Therapeutic Principles and Advances" (Springer, 2021).)

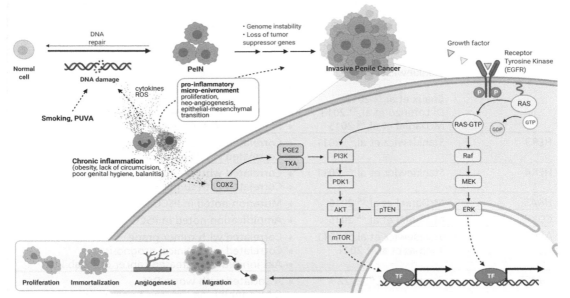

Fig. 2. HPV-independent penile cancer pathogenesis. (*From* Vos G, et al. Chapter: Mechanism of Carcinogenesis and Progression. "Penile Carcinoma: Therapeutic Principles and Advances" (Springer, 2021).)

research specifically in penile cancer is limited; however, some data can be extrapolated from other HPV-related malignancies. One phase II therapeutic vaccination study in women with HPV-16 or HPV-18-positive cervical cancer used a combination of synthetic plasmids to target E6 and E7 resulting in a 40% histopathological regression.[19]

Another promising advancement involves using HPV-targeted tumor-infiltrating lymphocytes (TILs) harvested from the primary tumor or sites of metastasis and transferred back to the donor patients to induce an antitumor immune response. In the metastatic cervical cancer setting, one study demonstrated a 33% (3/9) objective response including 2 long-term complete responses after infusion of HPV-16/18 E6 and E7 reactive TILs.[20]

Specific to PSCC, Aydin and colleagues were the first to demonstrate the feasibility of harvesting penile cancer TILS. Tumor samples from metastatic lymph nodes were propagated in high dose IL-2 and TILs were successfully expanded from 11 out of 12 samples. Five expanded samples secreted IFN- γ in response to autologous tumor.[21] These promising results suggest that adoptive T-cell therapy may play an important role in the treatment of HPV-related cancers in the future and that more research is needed in this space.

HUMAN PAPILLOMAVIRUS-INDEPENDENT PATHWAYS

Generally, non–HPV-related PSCC pathogenesis starts from DNA damage driven by chronic inflammatory states or smoking (see **Fig. 2**). There are

several biomarkers in HPV-independent penile cancer that have been identified (**Table 1**) and some of these have investigational or approved targeted agents.

Human Epidermal Growth Factor Receptor/ PTEN/Akt Pathway

The human epidermal growth factor receptor (HER) family is composed of EGFR, HER2, HER3, and HER4 transmembrane tyrosine kinase receptors.[22] High levels of EGFR are commonly found in penile carcinomas independent of histologic subtype, grade, and HPV status,[23,24] suggesting that this pathway has a significant role in HPV-negative penile carcinogenesis. Additionally, cytosolic presence of the phosphorylated form of EGFR is associated with increased risk of recurrence (OR 7.6, P = 0.009) and poor overall survival in N0-1 patients (HR = 9.0, P = 0.012).[25]

Studies have found that HPV-negative tumors expressed more activated EGFR than HPV-positive ones and this expression correlated with activated Akt, implicating EGFR as an upstream regulator of Akt signaling in penile cancer.[22] Therapeutic targeting of the HER/PTEN/Akt pathway has been studied in a single-arm phase II trial using dacomitinib, a second-generation, pan-HER tyrosine kinase inhibitor in 28 patients with locally advanced or metastatic PSCC, irrespective of their EGFR status.[26] The ORR for dacomitinib was 32.1%, with a median PFS of 4.1 months and OS of 13.7 months. This treatment was well tolerated and only 10% of patients developed grade 3 to 4 toxicity.[26]

Table 1
Biomarkers linked to HPV-negative penile squamous cell carcinoma

Biomarker	Authors	Findings
EGFR	Stankiewicz et al,[22] 2011	• Expressed more in HPV negative tumors • Correlated with pAkt
	Chaux et al,[23] 2013	• Expressed in penile tumor specimens
	Di Lorenzo et al,[25] 2013	• Predictive of recurrence
	McDaniel et al,[24] 2015	• Predictive of recurrence
HER3	Stankiewicz et al,[22] 2011	• Correlated with cytoplasmic Akt1 immunostaining • Correlated with tumor grade
HER4	Stankiewicz et al,[22] 2011	• Correlated with cytoplasmic Akt1 immunostaining • Correlated with tumor grade
HRAS	McDaniel et al,[24] 2015	• Mutation noted in PSCC
CDK4	McDaniel et al,[24] 2015	• Amplification noted in PSCC
Akt	Stankiewicz et al,[22] 2011 Thomas et al,[27] 2021	• Correlated with tumor grade • Correlated with clinical prognosis • Akt inhibition decreased cancer cell viability
C-MET	Thomas et al,[28] 2022	• Associated with worse DSS • C-MET inhibition reduced tumor viability
APOBEC-related mutation	Chahoud et al,[29] 2021	• Associated with higher TMB and worse overall survival
TIL	Vassallo et al,[31] 2015 Ottenhof et al,[30] 2018	• FOX-P3 associated with worse clinical prognosis • Low stomal CD8+ associated with LNM
TAM	Ottenhof et al,[30] 2018 Ahmed et al,[32] 2020	• CD163+ associated with LNM • CD68+ associated with improved survival
PDL-1	Udager et al,[34] 2016	• Increased expression associated with poor survival

Abbreviations: DSS, disease specific survival; LNM, lymph node metastasis; TAM, tumor-associated macrophage; TIL, tumor-infiltrating lymphocyte; TMB, tumor mutation burden.

c-MET

c-MET is one of the upstream modulators of the PI3K/mTOR/AKT pathway[27] and has recently been shown to impact penile cancer prognosis and elevated expression of c-MET was strongly associated with poor cancer-specific survival.[28] Moreover, the treatment of cell lines with c-MET inhibitors cabozantinib and tivantinib mediated an effective decrease in cell growth,[28] suggesting that these drugs deserve further investigation in their use in the treatment of metastatic disease.

Gene Mutation

Genomic whole-exome sequencing of penile cancer tissue uncovered actionable alterations in the Notch, DNA repair, kinase, and cell-cycle pathways. Penile squamous cell carcinoma samples showed an enrichment of 2 distinct mutational signatures that were associated with the oncogenic activity of AID/APOBEC and defective DNA mismatch repair and microsatellite instability.[29] These mutation signatures were comparable with head and neck squamous carcinomas. Additionally, among the mutant genes found in penile

cancer samples, 11 have been described in the DGIdb database as targetable by known drugs.

Immune Markers

As described earlier, the role of TILs in the host immune response to cancer has generated research interest and we know that immune infiltrating patterns may be an indicator of prognosis. Low stromal concentrations of CD8+ have been associated with higher rates of lymph node metastasis.[30] Additionally, high levels of tumor-infiltrating FOXP3+‴ Treg cells have been associated with worst DFS.[31]

Tumor-associated macrophages (TAMs) increase angiogenesis, enhance tumor cell mobility, and modulate immunotolerance. High densities of M1 (classic) subtypes such as CD68$^+$ TAMs have been shown to correlate with improved cancer-specific survival (CSS) ($p = 0.04$), overall survival (OS) ($p = 0.02$), and lower risk of regional recurrence ($p = 0.04$).[32] In contrast, M2 (alternative) macrophages such as CD163$^+$ may contribute to immune escape and has been shown to correspond with worse prognosis such as lymph node metastasis in penile cancer.[30]

The PD-1/PDL-1 axis has been demonstrated to play an important role in tumor immune escape, and in recent years, immune checkpoint inhibitors have emerged as a new therapy for many cancer types. 40–62% PSCC express $\geq$1% PD-L1 on tumor or infiltrating immune cells[33] and PD-L1 expression in penile cancer have been associated with poor cancer-specific survival.[34] Yet, there are scarce data on the use of PD-1/PDL-1 inhibitors in PSCC. Only case reports have described patients with metastatic PSCC who experienced durable response to Pembrolizumab.[35,36] There was a multicenter phase II trial that started in 2016 that ended prematurely due to poor accrual.

Tumor Mutational Burden (TMB) has been described in tumors with mismatch repair defect (MMR) or microsatellite instability defect (MSI) and is a potential biomarker for drug response. Increased expression of TMB may indicate increased expression of PDL-1, suggesting improved response of immune checkpoint inhibitors. The Food and Drug Administration (FDA) has approved the use of Pembrolizumab in patients with high TMB based on data from the KEYNOTE-158 trial which reported an objective response rate of 29% in patients with TMB $\geq$ 10 mutation/megabase.[37]

SUMMARY

Standard treatments in patients with recurrent or metastatic PSCC include cisplatin-based chemotherapy that often yields disappointing response rates. In the era of personalized medicine, targeted therapies have the potential to improve outcomes in patients with advanced PSCC, however, research in rare tumors can be challenging. Translational research in penile cancer is impeded by the scarcity of biobanks, cell lines, and xenograft models which lay the groundwork for testing novel therapies. Likewise, prospective clinical trials often face poor accrual and therefore early termination. Collaborative scientific effort is the key to the development of novel biomarkers and clinical trial design to improve outcomes for this rare disease.

CLINICS CARE POINTS

- Penile cancer pathogenesis is broadly dichotomized into HPV related and non-HPV-related pathways.
- This impacts identification of biomarkers and and development of targeted therapies.
- Increased expression of Tumor Mutation Burden (TMB) may indicate increased expression of PDL-1, suggesting improved response of immune checkpoint inhibitors.
- Pembrolizumab is FDA approved in patients with high TMB.

DISCLOSURES

Authors have no actual or potential conflict of interest concerning this article.

REFERENCES

1. Douglawi A, Masterson TA. Updates on the epidemiology and risk factors for penile cancer. Transl Androl Urol 2017;6(5):785–90.
2. Hernandez BY, Barnholtz-Sloan J, German RR, et al. Burden of invasive squamous cell carcinoma of the penis in the United States, 1998-2003. Cancer 2008;113(10 Suppl):2883–91.
3. Pow-Sang MR, Ferreira U, Pow-Sang JM, et al. Epidemiology and natural history of penile cancer. Urology 2010;76(2 Suppl 1):S2–6.
4. Leto M, Santos Junior GF, Porro AM, et al. Human papillomavirus infection: etiopathogenesis, molecular biology and clinical manifestations. An Bras Dermatol 2011;86(2):306–17.
5. Spiess PE, Dhillon J, Baumgarten AS, et al. Pathophysiological basis of human papillomavirus in penile cancer: Key to prevention and delivery of more effective therapies. CA Cancer J Clin 2016;66(6):481–95.
6. Stratton KL, Culkin DJ. A contemporary review of HPV and penile cancer. Oncology (Williston Park) 2016;30(3):245–9.
7. Olesen TB, Sand FL, Rasmussen CL, et al. Prevalence of human papillomavirus DNA and p16(INK4a) in penile cancer and penile intraepithelial neoplasia: a systematic review and meta-analysis. Lancet Oncol 2019;20(1):145–58.
8. Weaver BA, Feng Q, Holmes KK, et al. Evaluation of genital sites and sampling techniques for detection of human papillomavirus DNA in men. J Infect Dis 2004;189(4):677–85.
9. Chipollini J, Chaing S, Azizi M, et al. Advances in understanding of penile carcinogenesis: the search for actionable targets. Int J Mol Sci 2017;18(8).
10. Agarwal G, Gupta S, Spiess PE. Novel targeted therapies for the treatment of penile cancer. Expert Opin Drug Discov 2014;9(8):959–68.
11. Scheffner M, Werness BA, Huibregtse JM, et al. The E6 oncoprotein encoded by human papillomavirus types 16 and 18 promotes the degradation of p53. Cell 1990;63(6):1129–36.
12. Ferreux E, Lont AP, Horenblas S, et al. Evidence for at least three alternative mechanisms targeting the p16INK4A/cyclin D/Rb pathway in penile carcinoma,

one of which is mediated by high-risk human papillomavirus. J Pathol 2003;201(1):109–18.

13. Lopes A, Bezerra AL, Pinto CA, et al. p53 as a new prognostic factor for lymph node metastasis in penile carcinoma: analysis of 82 patients treated with amputation and bilateral lymphadenectomy. J Urol 2002;168(1):81–6.

14. Djajadiningrat RS, Jordanova ES, Kroon BK, et al. Human papillomavirus prevalence in invasive penile cancer and association with clinical outcome. J Urol 2015;193(2):526–31.

15. Lont AP, Kroon BK, Horenblas S, et al. Presence of high-risk human papillomavirus DNA in penile carcinoma predicts favorable outcome in survival. Int J Cancer 2006;119(5):1078–81.

16. Bezerra AL, Lopes A, Santiago GH, et al. Human papillomavirus as a prognostic factor in carcinoma of the penis: analysis of 82 patients treated with amputation and bilateral lymphadenectomy. Cancer 2001;91(12):2315–21.

17. Fonseca AG, Soares FA, Burbano RR, et al. Human papilloma virus: prevalence, distribution and predictive value to lymphatic metastasis in penile carcinoma. Int Braz J Urol 2013;39(4):542–50.

18. Steinestel J, Al Ghazal A, Arndt A, et al. The role of histologic subtype, p16(INK4a) expression, and presence of human papillomavirus DNA in penile squamous cell carcinoma. BMC Cancer 2015;15: 220.

19. Trimble CL, Morrow MP, Kraynyak KA, et al. Safety, efficacy, and immunogenicity of VGX-3100, a therapeutic synthetic DNA vaccine targeting human papillomavirus 16 and 18 E6 and E7 proteins for cervical intraepithelial neoplasia 2/3: a randomised, double-blind, placebo-controlled phase 2b trial. Lancet 2015;386(10008):2078–88.

20. Stevanovic S, Draper LM, Langhan MM, et al. Complete regression of metastatic cervical cancer after treatment with human papillomavirus-targeted tumor-infiltrating T cells. J Clin Oncol 2015;33(14):1543–50.

21. Aydin AM, Hall M, Bunch BL, et al. Expansion of tumor-infiltrating lymphocytes (TIL) from penile cancer patients. Int Immunopharmacol 2021;94:107481.

22. Stankiewicz E, Prowse DM, Ng M, et al. Alternative HER/PTEN/Akt pathway activation in HPV positive and negative penile carcinomas. PloS one 2011;6(3):e17517.

23. Chaux A, Munari E, Katz B, et al. The epidermal growth factor receptor is frequently overexpressed in penile squamous cell carcinomas: a tissue microarray and digital image analysis study of 112 cases. Hum Pathol 2013;44(12):2690–5.

24. McDaniel AS, Hovelson DH, Cani AK, et al. Genomic profiling of penile squamous cell carcinoma reveals new opportunities for targeted therapy. Cancer Res 2015;75(24):5219–27.

25. Di Lorenzo G, Perdona S, Buonerba C, et al. Cytosolic phosphorylated EGFR is predictive of recurrence in early stage penile cancer patients: a retropective study. J Transl Med 2013;11:161.

26. Necchi A, Lo Vullo S, Perrone F, et al. First-line therapy with dacomitinib, an orally available pan-HER tyrosine kinase inhibitor, for locally advanced or metastatic penile squamous cell carcinoma: results of an open-label, single-arm, single-centre, phase 2 study. BJU Int 2018;121(3):348–56.

27. Thomas A, Reetz S, Stenzel P, et al. Assessment of PI3K/mTOR/AKT pathway elements to serve as biomarkers and therapeutic targets in penile cancer. Cancers (Basel) 2021;13(10):2323.

28. Thomas A, Slade KS, Blaheta RA, et al. Value of c-MET and associated signaling elements for predicting outcomes and targeted therapy in penile cancer. Cancers (Basel) 2022;14(7):1683.

29. Chahoud J, Gleber-Netto FO, McCormick BZ, et al. Whole-exome sequencing in penile squamous cell carcinoma uncovers novel prognostic categorization and drug targets similar to head and neck squamous cell carcinoma. Clin Cancer Res 2021;27(9):2560–70.

30. Ottenhof SR, Djajadiningrat RS, Thygesen HH, et al. The prognostic value of immune factors in the tumor microenvironment of penile squamous cell carcinoma. Front Immunol 2018;9:1253.

31. Vassallo J, Rodrigues AF, Campos AH, et al. Pathologic and imunohistochemical characterization of tumoral inflammatory cell infiltrate in invasive penile squamous cell carcinomas: Fox-P3 expression is an independent predictor of recurrence. Tumour Biol 2015;36(4):2509–16.

32. Ahmed ME, Falasiri S, Hajiran A, et al. The immune microenvironment in penile cancer and rationale for immunotherapy. J Clin Med 2020;9(10):3334.

33. Azizi M, Aydin AM, Hajiran A, et al. Systematic review and meta-analysis-is there a benefit in using neoadjuvant systemic chemotherapy for locally advanced penile squamous cell carcinoma? J Urol 2020;203(6):1147–55.

34. Udager AM, Liu TY, Skala SL, et al. Frequent PD-L1 expression in primary and metastatic penile squamous cell carcinoma: potential opportunities for immunotherapeutic approaches. Ann Oncol 2016;27(9):1706–12.

35. Hahn AW, Chahoud J, Campbell MT, et al. Pembrolizumab for advanced penile cancer: a case series from a phase II basket trial. Invest New Drugs 2021;39(5):1405–10.

36. Chahoud J, Skelton WPt, Spiess PE, et al. Case report: two cases of chemotherapy refractory metastatic penile squamous cell carcinoma with extreme durable response to pembrolizumab. Front Oncol 2020;10:615298.

37. Marabelle A, Fakih M, Lopez J, et al. Association of tumour mutational burden with outcomes in patients with advanced solid tumours treated with pembrolizumab: prospective biomarker analysis of the multicohort, open-label, phase 2 KEYNOTE-158 study. Lancet Oncol 2020;21(10):1353–65.

Current and Future Biomarkers in the Management of Renal Cell Carcinoma

Stephen Reese, MD[a],*, Lina Calderon, MD[b], Sari Khaleel, MS, MD[a],
A. Ari Hakimi, MD[a]

KEYWORDS

- Renal cell carcinoma (RCC) • RCC biomarkers • Biomarkers

KEY POINTS

- Candidate biomarkers have been explored in several detection and disease settings.
- There remains an ongoing search for predictive biomarkers in the diagnosis and treatment of renal cell carcinoma, although many potential candidates have been explored.
- Current investigative efforts focus on tumor RNA expression as a biomarker, which is a potentially promising avenue of inquiry.

INTRODUCTION

Renal cell carcinoma (RCC) is a heterogeneous disease whose oncologic outcomes require an understanding of the underlying biology of disease, as more clinically indolent masses may be amenable to conservative management and more aggressive histology may require closer surveillance and benefit from multimodal therapy.[1,2] As recent advances in understanding the molecular pathophysiology of this disease have continued to evolve our management of advanced RCC, there has also been a rapid expansion in the research and development of biomarkers in the diagnostic, prognostic, and predictive domains for both localized and metastatic RCC (mRCC). Current approaches are directed toward serum, urine, liquid, and tissue biomarkers.

SERUM BIOMARKERS
"Classic" Biomarkers

Classic serum biomarkers remain an essential tool in the management of RCC patients independently or in conjunction with prognostic nomograms that incorporate clinical and laboratory data for prediction of patient survival. Two commonly used prognostic models in the mRCC setting include the International Metastatic RCC Database Consortium (IMDC) and The Memorial Sloan Kettering Cancer Center (MSKCC) models.[3,4] Both models were developed from retrospective studies of patients treated with systemic therapy (interferon alpha for MSKCC; vascular endothelial growth factor (VEGF)-inhibitors for IMDC) that identified predictors of overall survival and include patient performance status, time to diagnosis to systemic therapy, and classical serum markers calculated before initiation of systemic therapy, with slight differences in the used serum laboratory values, including hemoglobin, corrected serum calcium, neutrophil and platelet counts, and serum lactate dehydrogenase. The IMDC model[3] has been shown to outperform other prognostic models, including the Cleveland Clinic Foundation,[5] the International Kidney Cancer Working Group model[6] and the MSKCC model.[4,5] In addition, the IMDC

Funding: This was not funded.

[a] Department of Surgery, Urology Service, Memorial Sloan Kettering Cancer Center, 1275 York Avenue, New York, NY 10065, USA; [b] Department of Urology, Weill Cornell Medicine, 525 East 68th Street, Starr 9, New York, NY 10065, USA
* Corresponding author.
E-mail address: sreese479@gmail.com

Urol Clin N Am 50 (2023) 151–159
https://doi.org/10.1016/j.ucl.2022.09.003
0094-0143/23/© 2022 Published by Elsevier Inc.

model has been validated in several settings and patient cohorts, including patients previously treated with other systemic agents, immunotherapeutic agents, patients with de novo metastatic disease, those who have progressed from localized disease and in patients with non-clear cell carcinoma.[6–10] Although these classical models have been well validated, they lack specific biomarkers and genetic signatures that would help further risk-stratify patients and remain to be validated in the setting immune checkpoint combination therapies.

Vascular endothelial growth factor

VEGF is an important tyrosine kinase signaling molecule involved in vasculogenesis, angiogenesis, and endothelial cell growth. Five mammalian VEGF ligands exist as well as three primary VEGF receptor tyrosine kinases (VEGF 1/2/3).[10] VEGF is overexpressed in RCC, especially in tumors with inactivation of tumor suppressor gene VHL, a mutation noted in up to 90% of all clear cell RCC (ccRCC) tumors.[11] As a biomarker, circulating serum levels of VEGF have been evaluated as a predictor of response to targeted antiangiogenic therapies in ccRCC, particularly tyrosine kinase inhibitors. A retrospective analysis of a phase III trial of sunitinib versus interleukin (IL)-8 in ccRCC assessed the correlation of VEGF-A, VEGF-C, and sVEGFR-3 with survival outcomes, noting improved progression free survival (PFS) (21.7 vs 10.9 mo; hazard ratio [HR], 2.40; $P = 0.01$) and OS (Not reached (NR) vs 23.3 mo; HR, 1.68; $P = 0.07$) in sunitinib-treated patients with low baseline sVEGFR-3.[12] Similar results were found in analysis of the phase III TARGET trial, which randomized mRCC patients to sorafenib versus placebo, and found that lower levels of baseline plasma VEGF were associated with longer OS (18 vs 12.7 mo; HR 1.645, 95% CI: 1.19–2.28, $P = 0.003$), although higher baseline levels (>75th percentile) predicted improved response to systemic therapy in terms of PFS.[13] Other studies, however, have noted no significant association between pretreatment VEGF levels and response to sorafenib therapy[14] or sunitinib.[12] The utility of serum VEGF levels has not been assessed with more recently developed tyrosine kinase inhibitor (TKIs) or combination systemic therapy agents and may represent a source of future inquiry.

Cytokine and Angiogenic Factors

Cytokine and angiogenic factors (CAFs) are a group of cytokines and proteins that regulate pro-angiogenic, hypoxia-regulated factors, and inflammatory interleukin pathways. Although CAFs were initially studied to measure response to interferon-based therapy, they have been extrapolated to the novel systemic therapy space. One retrospective review of a phase II trial comparing sorafenib versus sorafenib + interferon described a six-marker CAF angiogenic signature (osteopontin, VEGF, carbonic anhydrase 9 [CAIX], collagen IV, VEGFR-2, and TRAIL) correlated with 5-fold increase in PFS with sorafenib compared with those negative for the signature (HR 2.25 vs 0.20; $P = 0.0002$).[1,5] Another study evaluating potential CAFs in patients with mRCC from phase II and III trials of pazopanib in the second-line therapy setting for mRCC demonstrated patients with high IL-8 ($P = 0.006$), osteopontin ($P = 0.004$) and TIMP-1 ($P = 0.006$) to have shorter PFS compared with those with low concentrations.[16] A separate analysis using the same phase III study proposed an "angiogenic signature" composed of seven CAFs [IL6, IL8, HGF, OPN, TIMP1, VEGF, and E-selectin],[17] finding patients with high scores on this angiogenic signature correlated with significantly shorter PFS in both the placebo (24 vs 11 weeks, $P = 0.001$) and pazopanib arms (25 vs 48 weeks, $P = 0.001$).

Shortcoming of many of the CAF studies include their reliance on retrospective analyses of small phase I–II studies of specific therapies, with limited or no external validation in other studies or the general population. For these reasons, CAFs have not been adopted in routine clinical practice and questions surround their ability to be generalized to a larger population of patients.

Circulating Tumor Nucleic Acids

Cell-free DNA (cfDNA) is small fragments ranging in length from 150 to 200 bp of DNA shed from tumor cells undergoing apoptosis and necrosis.[18] cfDNA offers a potential biomarker for monitoring treatment response, assessment of minimal residual disease after local treatment as well as in diagnosis of early-stage disease.[19]

Genomic alterations (GAs) in cfDNA, which include somatic mutations, copy number variations, gene fusions, and other mutations in cfDNA, may serve as a biomarker of treatment response in mRCC. An article by Pal and colleagues[20] examined 220 patients with mixed histology mRCC undergoing first- and then second-line systemic therapy and detected GAs in cfDNA in 78.6% of patients being studied. The most frequently altered GAs were TP53 (35%), VHL (23%), EGFR (17%), NF1(16%), and ARID1A (12%). A recent study demonstrated the challenges for using cfDNA as a biomarker.[21] In this study, the investigators sequenced primary tumor tissue as well as circulating tumor DNA (ctDNA) in 110 patients. They found a high number of GAs (554) in tumor tissue; however, only 24 GAs (or 6% of patients) were found in ctDNA suggesting a poor concordance with primary tumor as well as a low mutational detection of VHL (31.6%) in the small number of patients identified with GAs. Given the low yield in detection rates of mutational changes as well as poor concordance with the primary tumor, the current status of ctDNA as a biomarker remains unclear. Nevertheless, it remains an intriguing idea that patients can be monitored via a nucleic acid serum marker. However, challenges of poor detection and sampling error need to be overcome before its usefulness is demonstrated in clinical practice.

Early inquiries examining the absolute levels of cfDNA for differentiating healthy patients versus those with RCC remain mixed;[22,23] however, the use of cfDNA methylation patterns have demonstrated promise. In one study, examining methylation patterns of select tumor suppressor genes identified on cfDNA in patients with RCC ($n = 27$, including ccRCC and non-ccRCC) versus healthy controls ($n = 15$),[24] patients with RCC were noted have a higher frequency of hypermethylation of tumor suppressor genes identified on cfDNA, including APC (51.9%), FHIT (55.6%), and RASSF1 (62.9%). Although the sample size was small, using the methylation status of the three tumor suppressor genes, the study demonstrated an area under the curve (AUC) of almost 100% for differentiating RCC from healthy controls. Another study examined the methylation patterns of cfDNA in a larger cohort of 148 patients, identifying 300 differentially methylated regions between the patient groups.[19] The methylome signature was then validated in a randomly selected test set resulting in a mean AUC of 0.99 (95% CI, 0.985–0.995). Although these studies are limited by the small number of participants and their proposed signatures have yet to be validated in a large cohort, it remains a promising avenue for future investigations.

URINE BIOMARKERS

The excretion of urinary proteins to detect RCC has been an area of ongoing investigation. For example, Morissey and colleagues[25] investigated the urinary excretion of aquaporin-1 (AQP1) and perilipin-2 (PLIN2) in patients who underwent surgery for clear cell and papillary RCC and found a 35-fold and 9-fold increased urinary concentration of AQP1 and PLIN2 compared with sex- and aged-matched controls.

Similarly, urinary nucleic acids have been investigated to help differentiate patients with ccRCC

from healthy controls, presenting a potential noninvasive screening test to further characterize small renal masses on imaging. MicroRNA (miRNAs) are small (~22 nucleotide) noncoding single-stranded RNAs that play an important role in regulation of gene expression.[26] Studies have demonstrated miRNA signatures to be overexpressed in RCC and show stability in biologic fluids, including urine.[27–29] One group examined urinary miR-122-5p, miR-1271-5p, and miR-15b-5p levels in patients with ccRCC compared with controls and found higher expression levels in patients with RCC. When combined into a seven-parameter model, the sensitivity and specificity for differentiating between patients with RCC and controls were 96% and 65%, respectively.[30]

Another potential urinary biomarker is cfDNA methylomes. To examine the use of cfDNA methylomes, one group examined urinary cfDNA methylation patterns in patients with primarily localized RCC ($n = 30$) versus healthy controls ($n = 19$). Urinary cfDNA was able to discriminate between a cohort of localized disease and healthy controls with an AUC of 0.86 (95% CI 0.831–0.885).[19] This study demonstrates a proof of concept in a minimally invasive technique and promising technique but needs validation across a larger number of patients.

Use cases for urinary biomarkers seem to be in a screening program, noninvasive confirmatory tests to further characterize small renal masses on imaging and may have a role in other settings with nucleic acids are being shed systemically. Whether the current findings can be validated and extrapolated to a generalizable cohort and such tests find a use case, their utility in clinical practice remains to be seen.

TISSUE-BASED BIOMARKERS

Vascular Endothelial Growth Factor Tissue-based VEGF expression has also been studied as a potential biomarker for prognosis and treatment response. In one study of 40 patients who underwent cytoreductive nephrectomy for mRCC and subsequently treated with sunitinib,[31] expression levels of several markers were evaluated via immunohistochemical staining in the tumor specimen. The investigators found that strong VEGFR-2 expression (>10% of tumor cells) was shown to be significantly associated with favorable response to sunitinib as well as PFS [HR: 2.91 (1.15–7.41), $P = 0.003$). Another study looked at primary tumors from 23 metastatic ccRCC patients treated by sunitinib and examined Reverse transcription polymerase chain reaction (RT-PCR) expression levels of VEGF isoforms. They found that soluble isoforms of VEGF121 and VEGF165 were associated with response to sunitinib and that a low ratio of V121/V165 (<1.25) was associated with poor prognosis ($P = 0.02$).[32]

Tissue-based VEGF could be helpful in guiding adjuvant therapy after localized therapy or in a cytoreductive setting, although more studies and clinically proven adjuvant therapies would need to be validated for this to become clinically useful.

Programmed Death Ligand-1

Several trials examining immune checkpoint inhibitors have investigated the use of programmed death ligand-1 (PD-L1), a transmembrane protein important in suppressing the adaptive immune system and a target for novel immunotherapy agents, as a biomarker to predict treatment response in patients with advanced RCC (**Table 1**). Definitions of PD-L1 positivity on immunohistochemical staining varies, although it is generally defined as greater than 1% to 50% of tissue staining for the protein.[33]

Several immunotherapy clinical trials in the advanced RCC space have stratified patients based on PD-L1 positivity status, to examine if these patients are more likely to respond to therapy. In CheckMate 025, patients were randomized to receiving either nivolumab or everolimus and then further stratified based on PD-L1 expression ($\geq 1\%$). PD-L1 positivity predicted a worse overall survival; however, the trial noted an objective response irrespective of PD-L1 status.[34] CheckMate 214 randomized patients with mRCC to nivolumab and ipilimumab versus sunitinib.[35] An exploratory analysis was performed based on PD-L1 tumor expression and found that patients with $\geq 1\%$ PD-L1 expression treated with combination immunotherapy that the objective response rate was higher compared with the sunitinib arm (58% vs 22%, $P < 0.001$). In addition, PFS was greater in the nivolumab and ipilimumab group with PD-L1 expression $\geq 1\%$ versus <1% (22.8 months vs 11 months). In the Keynote-426 trial, in which patients with metastatic ccRCC were randomized to combination pembrolizumab plus axitinib or sunitinib patients demonstrated a clinical benefit with combination therapy across all arms regardless of PD-L1 status.[36]

In the Immotion151 trial, a randomized phase 3 trial, patients with mRCC were randomized to atezolizumab plus bevacizumab versus sunitinib.[37] Patients were further stratified based on PD-L1 expression. Patients with PD-L1 positive tumors demonstrated longer PFS (PFS: 11.2 vs 7.7 mo; HR, 0.74; 95% CI, 0.57–0.96, $P = 0.023$) and a higher complete response (43% vs 35%) in patients who received combination therapy versus sunitinib monotherapy; however, there was no difference in overall survival between the two groups.

Overall, PD-L1 positive status seems to confer an increased response to immunotherapy agents as well as signal improved PFS and possibly OS in treated patients. However, patients with both PD-L1 positive and negative tumors appear to demonstrate a clinically significant response to immunotherapy and PD-L1 status remains an unreliable marker of response, thus its use as a predictive biomarker remains limited.

NEXT-GENERATION BIOMARKERS

Next-generation sequencing technologies, including high-throughput RNA sequencing, are changing our understanding of genetic and molecular signatures. Although the incorporation of genomic mutations into prognostics models has improved performance,[39] transcriptional and epigenetic biomarkers may offer the opportunity to better classify ccRCC into clinically relevant molecular subtypes.[40,41]

One such approach has been to evaluate gene expression levels to classify clinical outcomes of patients. For example, monitoring cell cycle RNA expression levels using a measure of cell cycle proliferation (CCP score) in a cohort of patients who underwent surgery for localized disease was able to predict recurrence as well as cancer-specific mortality.[42] In another such approach Brannon and colleagues[43] identified two ccRCC subtypes with highly significant differences in gene expression, ccRCC type A and type B. In ccRCC type A (ccA), there was a higher expression of genes associated in pathways of angiogenesis, beta-oxidation, and pyruvate metabolism, whereas ccRCC type B (ccB) was enriched with expression of proteins that participate in cell differentiation, epithelial to mesenchymal transition, mitotic cell cycle, transforming growth factor beta, and Wnt targets. This classification was also shown to have a prognostic significance in high-risk patients, with ccA having a higher median overall survival of 8.6 years, versus 2 years in ccB ($P = 0.0002$), and a 5-year cancer-specific survival of 56% in ccA, and 29% in ccB patients.

Following this finding and its validation in a large cohort, Brooks and colleagues[40] applied next-generation RNA-sequencing (RNA-seq) to develop a 34-gene expression signature (GEC), named ClearCode34, to classify localized ccRCC tumors to tumor subtypes ccA and ccB. They showed patients with ccB recur earlier and more frequently than patient with ccA (HR 2.3, CI 1.6–3.3), and

Table 1
Summary of programmed death ligand-1 as a biomarker to predict outcomes and response to immunotherapy

Study	Outcome	PD-L1 Status
CheckMate 025[34]	Benefit observed in nivolumab arm irrespective of PD-L1 status *Overall survival (nivolumab vs everolimus):* ≥1% PD-L1: OS 21.8 vs 18.8 mo, HR 0.78; 95% CI 0.53–1.16 <1% PD-L1: OS 27.4 vs 21.2 mo, HR 0.76, 95% CI 0.60–0.97	Criteria for PD-L1 positive status: ≥1% vs <1% and ≥5% vs <5%[a]
CheckMate 214[35]	PD-L1 status associated with higher objective response and progression free survival *Objective response (ipilimumab/ nivolumab vs sunitinib):* ≥1% PD-L1: 58% vs 22% (*P* < 0.001) <1% PD-L1: 37% vs 28% (*P* = 0.03) *Progression free survival (ipilimumab/nivolumab vs sunitinib):* ≥1% PD-L1: 22.8 vs 5.9 mo, HR 0.46, 95% CI 0.31 to 0.67 <1% PD-L1: 11 vs 10.4 mo, HR 1, 95% CI 0.80 to 1.26	Criteria for PD-L1 positive status: ≥1% vs <1% and ≥5% vs <5%[b]
IMmotion 151[37]	PD-L1 status associated with progression free survival but not overall survival *Progression free survival (atezolizumab + bevacizumab vs sunitinib)* ≥1% PD-L1: HR 0.74, 95% CI 0.57–0.96 ITT: HR 0.83,95% CI 0.70–0.97 *Overall survival (atezolizumab + bevacizumab vs sunitinib)* ≥1% PD-L1: HR 0.84, 95% CI 0.62–1.15 ITT: HR 0.93, 95% CI 0.76–1.14	Criteria for PD-L1 positive status: ≥1% vs <1% Intention-to-treat (ITT arm) had up to 40% ≥ 1% PD-L1 expressivity.
JAVELIN Renal 101[38]	Patients in both overall population and PD-L1 positive group demonstrated increased progression free survival for experimental arm *Progression free survival (avelumab + axitinib vs sunitinib)* ≥1% PD-L1: HR 0.61, 95% CI, 0.47–0.79 Overall population: HR 0.69, 95% CI 0.56–0.84	Criteria for PD-L1 positive status: ≥1% vs <1% Overall population had 63.2% PD-L1 positive status
KEYNOTE 426[36]	Progression free and overall survival improved in experimental arm irrespective in overall population. Subgroup analysis demonstrated significant benefit in the ≥1% PD-L1 group	PD-L1 score of ≥1%. Positivity defined as a combined positive score of at least 1% (PD-L1-positive tumor cells/lymphocytes/ macrophages divided by the total number of cells.

(*continued on next page*)

Table 1
(continued)

Study	Outcome	PD-L1 Status
	Progression free survival (pembrolizumab + axitinib vs sunitinib) ≥1% PD-L1: HR 0.62, 95%CI 0.47–0.80 <1% PD-L1: HR 0.87 95%CI 0.62–1.23 *Overall survival (pembrolizumab + axitinib vs sunitinib)* ≥1% PD-L1: HR 0.54 (0.35–0.84) <1% PD-L1: HR 0.59 (0.34–1.03)	
KEYNOTE 564[2]	Improved disease-free survival and overall survival were associated with experimental arm. On subgroup analysis, ≥1% PD-L1 was significantly associated with a lower HR. *Disease-free survival (adjuvant pembrolizumab vs placebo)* ≥1% PD-L1: HR 0.67, 95% CI 0.51–0.88 <1% PD-L1: HR 0.83, 95%CI 0.45–1.51	PD-L1 score of ≥1%. Positivity defined as a combined positive score of at least 1% (PD-L1-positive tumor cells/lymphocytes/macrophages divided by the total number of cells. Overall population had 73.6% PD-L1 positive status in experimental arm

Abbreviations: HR, hazard ratio; PFS, progression free survival; OS, overall survival.
[a] Unable to measure outcomes in 5% PD-L1 cohort given small numbers.
[b] 5% PD-L1 expression was evaluated but not reported, but demonstrated similar trends compared with PD-L1 1% groups.

have three times more risk of dying from the disease (HR 2.9, CI 1.6–5.6).

The use of gene expression has also been evaluated to predict response to therapy. In the IMmotion 151 trial, a biomarker analysis of tumor gene expression was used to predict response to atezolizumab, bevacizumab, and sunitinib. Tumors with a higher expression of gene transcripts related to angiogenesis had a higher objective response rate and PFS in response to sunitinib, whereas patients with effector T-cell signatures had better objective response rate (ORR) and PFS in response to atezolizumab plus bevacizumab.[44] In a similar vein, the Javelin 101 trial proposed a 26 gene signature named the "Javelin Renal 101 Immuno Signature" which predicted greater PFS and overall survival in response to avelumab plus axitinib but not sunitinib.[38]

Another study examined tissue samples from patients in the Checkmate 009, 010, 025 trials and performed whole-exome sequencing, RNA-seq data, and measurements of CD8+ T-cell infiltrate via immunofluorescence.[45] The investigators did not find that tumor mutation burden, neoantigen load, human leukocyte antigen (HLA) zygosity, or CD8+ T cell infiltration were associated with a

response to PD-1 therapies, however, found that tumors with a high degree of immune cell infiltration was associated with an absence of PBRM1 mutation as well as chromosomal losses of 9p21.3. The full clinical significance of these findings is unclear; however, it underscores the complexity in predicting response to therapy in RCC tumors.

PBRM1 mutations, a protein involved in chromatin remodeling, have been examined as a potential biomarker in response to immunotherapy with conflicting results. Initial studies had suggested that the loss of function mutations in PBRM1 may serve as a marker of response to immunotherapy in patients with mRCC.[46,47] However, subsequent studies were unable to validate this finding and additional basic science work did not suggest that PBRM1 mutations enhanced immunogenicity; on the contrary, PBRM1 loss appeared to be associated with a less immunogenic tumor microenvironment (TME) that is typically associated with response to immunotherapy.[48,49] Currently, the data do not support a role for the use of PBRM1 as a biomarker to identify responders to immunotherapy.

Genomic mutations have also been used to enhance the predictive capabilities of traditional risk score models in the metastatic setting. Voss and colleagues[39] proposed the addition of BAP-1, PBRM1, and TP53 to the MSKCC risk-score model. In addition to the classic MSKCC model inputs (Karnofsky performance status score <80; elevated lactate dehydrogenase (LDGH), anemia, hypercalcemia, and time to first-line therapy), the proposed model included up to two additional points for various degrees of genetic mutations in BAP-1, PBRM1, and TP53. Patients were then stratified into four possible risk groups, ranging from favorable to poor risk. With the addition of genomic signatures, predictive model performance validated in a large patient cohort improved with the c-index increasing from $0 \cdot 60$ (95% CI $0 \cdot 56$–$0 \cdot 63$) to $0 \cdot 64$ ($0 \cdot 60$–$0 \cdot 69$). This model is a promising advance as insights into the oncogenic molecular landscape improve, no doubt, incorporation of genomic and transcriptomic signatures will improve the performance of predictive models in this setting.

The TME has been studied as a potential biomarker in ccRCC, as there has been increasing recognition that the TME plays an important role in tumorigenesis.[50] Although the TME has been identified as a critical determinant of tumorigenesis as well as therapeutic response, attempts at predicting TME activity, or therapeutic response in mRCC using genomic mutational signatures have been equivocal.[44,51] In contrast, molecular GESs that use transcriptomic RNA-seq to infer characteristics of the TME such as immune infiltration and angiogenesis or a myeloid inflammatory state have shown promising results in prognosis as well as predicting therapeutic response.[38,52–54] GESs of TME therefore may represent a promising line of future inquiry for understanding prognosis and therapeutic response.

Overall, these molecular signatures were based on retrospective analyses of treatment-naive patients undergoing trials for specific systematic therapies, which could limit their generalizability as therapeutic biomarkers. In the future, these biomarkers should be assessed prospectively in patients receiving different therapeutic and clinical setting to assess their generalizability.

SUMMARY

In summary, serum, urine, liquid, and tissue biomarkers have been proposed to evaluate RCC in several clinical settings. There is currently an ongoing search for predictive biomarkers in the detection, recurrence, and treatment response space. The most promising biomarkers are those currently being proposed in the transcriptomic and translational space. As better understanding of tumor biology emerges in the future and currently proposed signatures can be extrapolated to a larger and more generalizable patient population, the goal of predictive medicine may be realized in clinical practice.

DISCLOSURE

A. Ari Hakimi is on the Merck Advisory board and is funded in part by the MSK P30 grant.

REFERENCES

1. Ravaud A, Motzer RJ, Pandha HS, et al. Adjuvant sunitinib in high-risk renal-cell carcinoma after nephrectomy. N Engl J Med 2016;375(23):2246–54.
2. Choueiri TK, Tomczak P, Park SH, et al. Adjuvant pembrolizumab after nephrectomy in renal-cell carcinoma. N Engl J Med 2021;385(8):683–94.
3. Heng DYC, Xie W, Regan MM, et al. Prognostic factors for overall survival in patients with metastatic renal cell carcinoma treated with vascular endothelial growth factor-targeted agents: results from a large, multicenter study. J Clin Oncol 2009;27(34):5794–9.
4. Motzer RJ, Bacik J, Murphy BA, et al. Interferon-alfa as a comparative treatment for clinical trials of new therapies against advanced renal cell carcinoma. J Clin Oncol 2002;20(1):289–96.
5. Mekhail TM, Abou-Jawde RM, BouMerhi G, et al. Validation and extension of the Memorial Sloan-Kettering prognostic factors model for survival in patients with previously untreated metastatic renal cell carcinoma. J Clin Oncol 2005;23(4):832–41.
6. Manola J, Royston P, Elson P, et al. Prognostic model for survival in patients with metastatic renal cell carcinoma: Results from the international kidney cancer working group. Clin Cancer Res 2011;17(16):5443–50.
7. Heng DYC, Xie W, Regan MM, et al. External validation and comparison with other models of the International Metastatic Renal-Cell Carcinoma Database Consortium prognostic model: a population-based study. Lancet Oncol 2013;14(2):141–8.
8. Kroeger N, Xie W, Lee JL, et al. Metastatic non-clear cell renal cell carcinoma treated with targeted therapy agents: Characterization of survival outcome and application of the International mRCC Database Consortium criteria. Cancer 2013;119(16):2999–3006.
9. McKay RR, Kroeger N, Xie W, et al. Impact of bone and liver metastases on patients with renal cell carcinoma treated with targeted therapy. Eur Urol 2014;65(3):577–84.
10. Tugues S, Koch S, Gualandi L, et al. Vascular endothelial growth factors and receptors: anti-angiogenic

therapy in the treatment of cancer. Mol Aspects Med 2011;32(2):88–111.

11. Turajlic S, Xu H, Litchfield K, et al. Tracking cancer evolution reveals constrained routes to metastases: TRACERx renal. Cell 2018;173(3):581–94.e12.

12. Harmon CS, Deprimo SE, Figlin RA, et al. Circulating proteins as potential biomarkers of sunitinib and interferon-α efficacy in treatment-naïve patients with metastatic renal cell carcinoma. Cancer Chemother Pharmacol 2014;73(1):151–61.

13. Peña C, Lathia C, Shan M, et al. Biomarkers predicting outcome in patients with advanced renal cell carcinoma: Results from sorafenib phase III treatment approaches in renal cancer global evaluation trial. Clin Cancer Res 2010;16(19):4853–63.

14. Escudier B, Eisen T, Stadler WM, et al. Sorafenib for treatment of renal cell carcinoma: final efficacy and safety results of the phase III treatment approaches in renal cancer global evaluation trial. J Clin Oncol 2009;27(20):3312–8.

15. Zurita AJ, Jonasch E, Wang X, et al. A cytokine and angiogenic factor (CAF) analysis in plasma for selection of sorafenib therapy in patients with metastatic renal cell carcinoma. Ann Oncol 2012;23(1):46–52.

16. Tran HT, Liu Y, Zurita AJ, et al. Prognostic or predictive plasma cytokines and angiogenic factors for patients treated with pazopanib for metastatic renal-cell cancer: a retrospective analysis of phase 2 and phase 3 trials. Lancet Oncol 2012;13(8):827–37.

17. Liu Y, Tran HT, Lin Y, et al. Circulating baseline plasma cytokines and angiogenic factors (CAF) as markers of tumor burden and therapeutic response in a phase III study of pazopanib for metastatic renal cell carcinoma (mRCC). J Clin Oncol 2011;29(15_suppl):4553.

18. Hahn AW, Nussenzveig RH, Maughan BL, et al. Cell-free circulating tumor DNA (ctDNA) in metastatic renal cell carcinoma (mRCC): current knowledge and potential uses3 (1). Kidney Cancer; 2019. p. 7–13.

19. Nuzzo PV, Berchuck JE, Korthauer K, et al. Detection of renal cell carcinoma using plasma and urine cell-free DNA methylomes. Nat Med 2020;26(7):1041–3.

20. Pal SK, Sonpavde G, Agarwal N, et al. Evolution of circulating tumor DNA profile from first-line to subsequent therapy in metastatic renal cell carcinoma. Eur Urol 2017;72(4):557–64.

21. Kotecha RR, Gedvilaite E, Ptashkin R, et al. Matched molecular profiling of cell-free dna and tumor tissue in patients with advanced clear cell renal cell carcinoma. JCO Precis Oncol 2022;6:e2200012.

22. Yamamoto Y, Uemura M, Nakano K, et al. Increased level and fragmentation of plasma circulating cell-free DNA are diagnostic and prognostic markers for renal cell carcinoma. 2018.

23. Lu H, Busch J, Jung M, et al. Diagnostic and prognostic potential of circulating cell-free genomic and mitochondrial DNA fragments in clear cell renal cell carcinoma patients. Clinica Chim Acta 2016/1// 2016;452:109–19. https://doi.org/10.1016/j.cca.2015.11.009.

24. Skrypkina I, Tsyba L, Onyshchenko K, et al. Concentration and methylation of cell-free DNA from blood plasma as diagnostic markers of renal cancer. Dis Markers 2016;2016. https://doi.org/10.1155/2016/3693096.

25. Morrissey JJ, Mobley J, Song J, et al. Urinary concentrations of aquaporin-1 and perilipin-2 in patients with renal cell carcinoma correlate with tumor size and stage but not grade. Urology 2014;83(1). 256.e9-256.e14.

26. Treiber T, Treiber N, Meister G. Regulation of microRNA biogenesis and its crosstalk with other cellular pathways. Nat Rev Mol Cell Biol 2019;20(1):5–20.

27. Youssef YM, White NMA, Grigull J, et al. Accurate molecular classification of kidney cancer subtypes using microRNA signature. Eur Urol 2011;59(5):721–30.

28. White NMA, Bao TT, Grigull J, et al. miRNA profiling for clear cell renal cell carcinoma: biomarker discovery and identification of potential controls and consequences of miRNA dysregulation. J Urol 2011;186(3):1077–83.

29. Wotschofsky Z, Busch J, Jung M, et al. Diagnostic and prognostic potential of differentially expressed miRNAs between metastatic and non-metastatic renal cell carcinoma at the time of nephrectomy. Clinica Chim Acta 2013;416:5–10.

30. Cochetti G, Cari L, Maulà V, et al. Validation in an independent cohort of MiR-122, MiR-1271, and MiR-15b as urinary biomarkers for the potential early diagnosis of clear cell renal cell carcinoma. Cancers 2022;14(5):1112.

31. Terakawa T, Miyake H, Kusuda Y, et al. Expression level of vascular endothelial growth factor receptor-2 in radical nephrectomy specimens as a prognostic predictor in patients with metastatic renal cell carcinoma treated with sunitinib. Urol Oncol Semin Original Invest 2013;31(4):493–8.

32. Paule B, Bastien L, Deslandes E, et al. Soluble isoforms of vascular endothelial growth factor are predictors of response to sunitinib in metastatic renal cell carcinomas. PLoS One 2010;5(5). https://doi.org/10.1371/journal.pone.0010715.

33. Ribas A, Hu-Lieskovan S. What does PD-L1 positive or negative mean? J Exp Med 2016;213(13):2835–40.

34. Motzer RJ, Escudier B, McDermott DF, et al. Nivolumab versus everolimus in advanced renal-cell carcinoma. N Engl J Med 2015;373(19):1803–13.

35. Motzer RJ, Tannir NM, McDermott DF, et al. Nivolumab plus ipilimumab versus sunitinib in advanced renal-cell carcinoma. N Engl J Med 2018;378(14): 1277–90.

36. Rini BI, Plimack ER, Stus V, et al. Pembrolizumab plus axitinib versus sunitinib for advanced renal-cell carcinoma. N Engl J Med 2019;380(12): 1116–27.

37. Rini BI, Powles T, Atkins MB, et al. Atezolizumab plus bevacizumab versus sunitinib in patients with previously untreated metastatic renal cell carcinoma (IMmotion151): a multicentre, open-label, phase 3, randomised controlled trial. Lancet 2019; 393(10189):2404–15.

38. Motzer RJ, Robbins PB, Powles T, et al. Avelumab plus axitinib versus sunitinib in advanced renal cell carcinoma: biomarker analysis of the phase 3 JAVELIN Renal 101 trial. Nat Med 2020;26(11): 1733–41.

39. Voss MH, Reising A, Cheng Y, et al. Genomically annotated risk model for advanced renal-cell carcinoma: a retrospective cohort study. Lancet Oncol 2018;19(12):1688–98.

40. Brooks SA, Brannon AR, Parker JS, et al. ClearCode34: a prognostic risk predictor for localized clear cell renal cell carcinoma. Eur Urol 2014; 66(1):77–84.

41. Serie DJ, Joseph RW, Cheville JC, et al. Clear cell type A and B molecular subtypes in metastatic clear cell renal cell carcinoma: tumor heterogeneity and aggressiveness. Eur Urol 2017;71(6):979–85.

42. Morgan TM, Mehra R, Tiemeny P, et al. A multigene signature based on cell cycle proliferation improves prediction of mortality within 5 yr of radical nephrectomy for renal cell carcinoma. Eur Urol 2018;73(5): 763–9.

43. Brannon AR, Reddy A, Seiler M, et al. Molecular stratification of clear cell renal cell carcinoma by consensus clustering reveals distinct subtypes and survival patterns. Genes & Cancer 2010;1(2): 152–63.

44. Şenbabaoğlu Y, Gejman RS, Winer AG, et al. Tumor immune microenvironment characterization in clear cell renal cell carcinoma identifies prognostic and immunotherapeutically relevant messenger RNA signatures. Genome Biol 2016;17(1):231.

45. Braun DA, Hou Y, Bakouny Z, et al. Interplay of somatic alterations and immune infiltration modulates response to PD-1 blockade in advanced clear cell renal cell carcinoma. Nat Med 2020;26(6):909–18.

46. Miao D, Margolis CA, Gao W, et al. Genomic correlates of response to immune checkpoint therapies in clear cell renal cell carcinoma. Science 2018; 359(6377):801–6.

47. Braun DA, Ishii Y, Walsh AM, et al. Clinical validation of PBRM1 alterations as a marker of immune checkpoint inhibitor response in renal cell carcinoma. JAMA Oncol 2019;5(11):1631–3.

48. Liu XD, Kong W, Peterson CB, et al. PBRM1 loss defines a nonimmunogenic tumor phenotype associated with checkpoint inhibitor resistance in renal carcinoma. Nat Commun 2020;11(1):2135.

49. Hakimi AA, Attalla K, DiNatale RG, et al. A pan-cancer analysis of PBAF complex mutations and their association with immunotherapy response. Nat Commun 2020;11(1):4168.

50. Rappold PM, Silagy AW, Kotecha RR, et al. Immune checkpoint blockade in renal cell carcinoma. J Surg Oncol 2021;123(3):739–50.

51. McDermott DF, Huseni MA, Atkins MB, et al. Clinical activity and molecular correlates of response to atezolizumab alone or in combination with bevacizumab versus sunitinib in renal cell carcinoma. Nat Med 2018;24(6):749–57.

52. Braun DA, Bakouny Z, Hirsch L, et al. Beyond conventional immune-checkpoint inhibition — novel immunotherapies for renal cell carcinoma. Nat Rev Clin Oncol 2021;18(4):199–214.

53. Hakimi AA, Voss MH, Kuo F, et al. Transcriptomic profiling of the tumor microenvironment reveals distinct subgroups of clear cell renal cell cancer: data from a randomized phase III trial. Cancer Discov 2019;9(4):510–25.

54. Rappold PM, Vuong L, Leibold J, et al. A targetable myeloid inflammatory state governs disease recurrence in clear cell renal cell carcinoma. Cancer Discov 2022. https://doi.org/10.1158/2159-8290. CD-21-0925.

9780323940191